Geriatric Nursing
Growth of a Specialty

About the Authors

PRISCILLA EBERSOLE, PhD, RN, FAAN, has been involved in geriatric/gerontologic nursing for 35 years. She has conducted national and international workshops, seminars, and presentations on aging. She has written, with coauthors, nine textbooks on geriatric nursing. She is a professor emerita, retired from San Francisco State University School of Nursing in 1995. She earned a certificate in gerontology from the University of Southern California, Los Angeles, and has held appointments in the Applied Gerontology Certificate Program at San Francisco State University and at the Ethel Percy Andrus Gerontology Center, University of Southern California. From 1981 to 1984 she was on leave from San Francisco State University to act as field director of the geriatric nurse practitioner project funded by the W. K. Kellogg Foundation and administered by the Mountain States Health Corporation in Boise, Idaho. In 1987 she was named Educator of the Year by the American College of Health Care Administration. In 1988 Dr. Ebersole was a visiting professor at Frances Payne Bolton School of Nursing, Case Western Reserve University in Cleveland, Ohio, where she occupied the Florence Cellar endowed gerontologic nursing chair. In 1997 Dr. Ebersole was inducted into the Hall of Fame at San Francisco State University. From 1991 until January 2006 she was the editor of the *Geriatric Nursing Journal*.

THERIS A. TOUHY, ND, APRN, BC, is an Associate Professor in the Christine E. Lynn College of Nursing at Florida Atlantic University in Boca Raton, Florida. Dr. Touhy has been a Clinical Nurse Specialist in gerontological nursing for 25 years combining teaching and research with practice in the long-term care setting. She received her master's degree in Nursing Care of the Aged from Northern Illinois University in Dekalb, Illinois, and her doctorate from Case Western Reserve University. She was the recipient of the Geriatric Faculty Award from the Hartford Institute for Geriatric Nursing/AACN in 2003 and the Marie Haug Award for Excellence in Aging Research, Case Western Reserve University, in 1998. She is coauthor with Dr. Ebersole, Dr. Patricia Hess, and Dr. Kathleen Jett of the textbook *Gerontological Nursing and Healthy Aging* as well as the forthcoming 7th edition of *Toward Healthy Aging*. Dr. Touhy has several research interests, most of which are focused on care of elders in nursing homes, particularly those with dementia.

Geriatric Nursing
Growth of a Specialty

Priscilla Ebersole, PhD, RN, FAAN
Theris A. Touhy, ND, APRN, BC

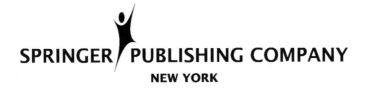

SPRINGER / PUBLISHING COMPANY
NEW YORK

Springer Publishing Company, Inc.
11 West 42nd Street
New York, NY 10036

Acquisitions Editors: Ruth Chasek and Sally J. Barhydt
Production Editor: Jeanne Libby
Cover design by Joanne Honigman
Typeset by Daily Information Processing, Churchville, PA

07 08 09 10 / 5 4 3 2

Library of Congress Cataloging-in-Publication Data

Ebersole, Priscilla.
    Geriatric nursing : growth of a specialty / Priscilla Ebersole,
Theris A. Touhy.
        p. ; cm.
    Includes bibliographical references and index.
    ISBN 0-8261-2649-9
    ISBN 978-0-8261-2649-8
    1. Geriatric nursing—United States—History. 2. Nurses—United
States—Biography. I. Touhy, Theris A. II. Title.
    [DNLM: 1. Geriatric Nursing. 2. Nurses.   WY 152 E16g 2006]
RC954.E2293 2006
618.97'0231—dc22

2005031308

Printed in the United States of America by Bang Printing.

Contents

Preface

This book describes the development of geriatric nursing as a specialty and the current state of geriatric nursing. It was written for both current and future generations of geriatric nurses—so they will know the work of those nurses who came before them, and so they can understand the full range of opportunity that exists at this time. The "pioneers" of geriatric nursing have given us a legacy that is fully defined and assembled for the first time in this book. This book also defines the scope of the specialty— how to become a geriatric nurse, what organizations and publications exist in the field, standards of practice, certification, and future directions.

This text has been developing for nearly 20 years. One is seldom on the scene when a whole new specialty begins to come to fruition. I was one of the lucky ones who met and interviewed many of the remarkable people who were in the forefront of geriatric nursing, laying the foundations for the flourishing profession as it is today. I began with little idea of what would or could be done with the information but just felt that their stories must be told. Between the years 1988 and 1993 I interviewed the geriatric nurse pioneers to whom I could gain access. Many of them are now gone and I am so pleased that they will be seen by readers as real people as well as highly accomplished leaders and nurses. The heart of this text is their stories, but the comprehensive nature of the work as it now has evolved is so much more.

With the guidance and confidence of Ursula Springer, the organizational abilities of Theris Touhy, and the editorial expertise of Ruth Chasek, we now feel that this text should be in the hands of every nursing student and practicing nurse. Geriatric care is the essence of nursing, and those who seek its origins, satisfactions, and possibilities will find this book exciting and useful. The primary goal of the text is inspirational, but it has sufficient scope to guide nurses to find resources, develop ideas, access research, and seek a future in geriatric care.

PRISCILLA EBERSOLE

Foreword

Few individuals have given so selflessly to the field of geriatric nursing as Priscilla Ebersole. In this text, *Geriatric Nursing: Growth of a Specialty,* Priscilla Ebersole traces the rudimentary first steps of our specialty through contemporary times. Dr. Ebersole (who would usually prefer the informal "Priscilla") traces our early history in gerontologic nursing care through the stories of remarkable leaders in our field. These stories include patient care vignettes as well as personal narratives related to grandparents and life events, which are especially effective.

In these pages, she provides the stories of people's lives and the way in which they shaped our field. Beginning with narratives of some of our most remarkable champions—Mary Opal Wolanin, Doris Schwartz, Irene Burnside, and Mary Harper to name a few—she takes us through their pioneering work that has provided the basis of our strength today. We should all be especially grateful to Dr. Ebersole for preserving this history.

To fully appreciate this book, one should understand the way Dr. Ebersole approaches any project. She is passionate, devoted, generous beyond compare, and fully immersed in her work. Dr Ebersole is also a central character in the story of gerontologic nursing. Far from an observer on the sidelines, I would argue that she has served as the linchpin between our history and our future. Ebersole understood early on the possibilities for improving gerontologic nursing care. Her textbook, *Toward Healthy Aging: Human Needs & Nursing Response,* with Patricia Hess, was one of the first comprehensive textbooks available to guide the education and practice of gerontologic nursing. She knew the importance of a conceptual framework to guide our practice, and her comprehensive text was organized using Maslow's hierarchy of needs with a holistic approach that distinguished our work from geriatric medicine. Now in its 6th edition, the Ebersole, Hess, and Luggen textbook is considered not only a classic but a text that is essential to any geriatric nursing library. Dr. Ebersole provided this text at a time when few people recognized this field as a unique specialty, and she was able to create a base for all of us from which to teach and conduct research. The book went beyond the traditional list of diseases and disorders, and provided a way to organize care that was holistic and humanistic. To this day, no one has articulated a better model for understanding the way in which we should care for older adults. Her compassionate stance, that love and belonging is a way to understand self-actualization of older people, is a commentary not only on her approach to care for older adults but on her approach to life.

As editor of *Geriatric Nursing* over the past 15 years, Dr. Ebersole has given selflessly in order to create a journal that speaks to the needs of practicing nurses in gerontologic settings. The journal, unique for its application to practice, has helped set standards for evidence-based practice in the care of older adults. Her passion for long-term care, and in particular nursing home care, is reflected in this journal, elevating the voice and status of long-term care nurses everywhere.

One understands others through a personal prism. I have come to love Priscilla through our friendship, our professional efforts, our mutual interests, and our commitment to family. How many of us have received one of her personal handwritten notes, bedecked with a photograph she has personally taken and selected for us? I have saved each one. Her generous spirit with letters of recommendation, nominations for awards, and introductions to others who can help and support us tells us legions about her as a human being. One need only ask the question, "how are your grandchildren?" to gain insight into this special person who has given so much.

We can thank leaders like Dr. Ebersole for the current status of geriatric nursing, which is robust and extremely promising. Her book makes a contribution by preserving our history and challenging current leaders to continue this work. I know Dr. Ebersole has much more she intends to accomplish, and she will.

TERRY FULMER, PhD, RN, FAAN
The Erline Perkins McGriff Professor and Dean
College of Nursing
New York University

Introduction

Many developed countries have provided numerous workable models of caring for their aged. Some we greatly admire. In the most notable of these, the Netherlands, the populations are relatively stable, the government is socialistic, health and social services are considered a right, and the aged are prepared in advance for their later years.

In the United States we have a unique, multicultural population; many émigrés from poorer countries come to the United States in their declining years, hoping for a better life for themselves and their descendants. This has made a uniquely complex, exciting, and challenging situation in geriatric care.

This text is designed to explore and present the growth and development of geriatric nursing from the 1940s until the present. Although it has been less than 70 years, much has transpired that has affected the status and opportunities for older persons within our borders. We have borrowed ideas and models from others, but no one approach to the aged can be sufficient given our diverse population.

The years after the institution of the Social Security Act of 1935 allowed many of the aged to emerge from destitution with at least a minimum level of protection against absolute deprivation. This is the genesis of aging in the United States as it is today. My own grandmother was a divorced lady who received no support from husband or state and died in 1934, before the advent of Social Security. She survived her later years on a small farm by selling berries, plants, and funeral pieces made from the flowers in her greenhouse.

World War II, the first conflict since the Civil War in which we were directly involved, moved us beyond our isolationist years and were watershed years for the aged. Arrangements with the Philippines and other allied countries gave some special immigration privileges to those who were our allies in the war. Veterans' benefits were vastly improved, and the work force shifted toward support of those who returned from the armed services; women and elders who had been the mainstay of the productive economy during the war years were no longer essential workers. Women reentered the home to produce the baby boom generation, and elders were retired from the working world. Concerns for the aged were not yet a high priority, as the percentage of those over age 65 was less than 10% and young families absorbed the nation's attention. Since that time the remarkable progress in medical technology, largely generated by the medical needs of injured veterans and inventions to support human life in space exploration, has been phenomenal, resulting in a vast increase in the number of elders who would not have survived in previous generations.

Those early years had widespread effects on nursing as many nurses returned from serving in the armed conflict with newfound awareness of their status. As ranking officers during the war they were respected and responsible for major life-and-death decisions. Many of the early geriatric nurse pioneers were among this group. Bernita Steffl graduated from nursing school just in time to enter the Army before the war was over. It was an exciting time for nurses, and she was anxious to be a part of it. Faye Abdellah, now retired, became a general and director of the U.S. Public Health Service. Her stint in the service greatly influenced her opportunities upon discharge. Mary Opal Wolanin met and married her husband while an army nurse and found that following him to his various assignments and working in diverse venues exposed her to a wide range of nursing situations that reaffirmed her interest in caring for the aged. Likewise, Irene Burnside met and married her husband while in the army nurse corps. She emerged from the experience with a new confidence in her influence that was later expressed in her leadership and mentorship of geriatric nurses. Doris Schwartz developed her leadership skills while in the service and worked in the rehabilitation of injured veterans upon discharge. Later she used this knowledge in rehabilitation of the aged. These and many others of that era are the mothers of modern geriatric nursing.

> "Do you realize that in the span of two lifetimes organized nursing was born, and within mine, geriatric nursing? Florence Nightingale was born in 1820 and I in 1910, the year she died." (personal reflections shared with me by Mary Opal Wolanin, who died in 1997)

It has been said before that wars and the status of women have been the impetus for significant progress in many spheres of modern life. This is true in the medical sphere and especially in geriatric nursing and the rehabilitation of elders.

The major geriatric organizations arose during and after World War II: The American Geriatrics Society was founded in 1942, the Gerontological Society of America in 1945, and the American Society on Aging (then the

Western Gerontological Society) in 1954. In just over 50 years, gerontologic care has emerged from a disregarded aspect of nursing and medicine
into the foremost concern of health care in the United States.

In this work, we have featured individuals who have made marked
contributions to the growth of the specialty of geriatric nursing. The im-
balance in space given to various individuals is in no way reflective of
their importance. We used the material available to us. Additionally, there
are many very important contributors who have not been included simply for lack of time, space, and contact information; thus, the history is
incomplete. We extend our regrets to those not mentioned. We are also
fully aware that the sociopolitical background, timing of events, and population shifts were the matrices essential to the emergence and flourishing of any individual's personal efforts to effect change in geriatric care.

It is worth noting that the silent majority, the unknown soldiers of
nursing who have carried on without kudos or special recognition, form
the substrate for testing the validity of research theories. They implement
daily compassionate care of the aged, incorporate best practices, use the
ideas brought forth by educators and researchers, and provide the milieu
that makes progress possible. These, the unsung, unrecognized, are collectively those who make things happen.

Numerous geriatric nurses have contributed their memories,
thoughts, and summaries of their accomplishments, which makes this
text interesting and challenging for future nurses. Throughout the text all
first-person comments not in quotes are those of Priscilla Ebersole, garnered from interaction with the geriatric nurse pioneers and other individuals. I found the interactions with them fascinating and their vision
profoundly affected me. I learned what could be accomplished by determination and persistence. All had an extraordinary concern for all individuals who were neglected and abandoned. We cannot thank them
enough for their input. Much of the dynamic specialty as it is today can
be attributed to their sustained efforts.

The inspirational debt owed to special elders in the lives of these remarkable people cannot be dismissed. Many chose to focus their efforts
on geriatric care because of particular interactions with elders during
their nursing practice, many because of involvement with grandparents.

Meeting Terri Touhy during a consultation was truly a serendipitous
event; there was an immediate connection. Throughout the work on this
text she has helped me organize, and has contributed ideas, chapters, and
her current knowledge and perspectives on the field. Her enthusiasm and
presence in the preparation of this book have been a gift. She writes:

> Dr. Ebersole has given me a privilege that I treasure by asking me to
> work with her on this book—a book that is truly a living legacy that
> she leaves to geriatric nursing.

In our early planning, I spent a weekend with her in her home discussing the focus and content of the text. For me, it was like being in a library of geriatric nursing history as we pored over her vast collection of memories and documents. I could hardly believe I was sitting in the kitchen of one of the geriatric pioneers I had so long admired. I recalled a workshop that she led on reminiscence therapy at a geriatric nursing conference in California in the very early '80s. It was the first conference I attended after earning my master's degree in 1979. She sparked my lifelong interest in reminiscence. Likewise, I used her textbooks in my teaching of geriatric nursing and in my own learning of the specialty. It has been an honor to have her as a mentor and friend whose contributions to my geriatric nursing knowledge have been immense. I treasure her friendship, wisdom, expert knowledge, passion, and commitment for care of older people.

My entrance into the specialty, like many other geriatric nurses, was via the back door. Studying for a master's in medical surgical nursing, I met Dr. Sarah Fuller, an early geriatric nurse researcher, who was developing a new master's program in nursing care of the aged at Northern Illinois University. As she showed me the syllabi of the new courses, I was struck by what I did not know about the care of old people. When she showed the video "Peege" in my first class, I was hooked forever.

I am grateful to her and to the other geriatric nurses who mentored me in my career, including May Wykle, Diana Morris, and Ruth Tappen. Those of us in geriatric nursing owe so much to those who laid the foundation and continue to inspire us daily.

It must be said: The terms gerontic nursing, geriatric nursing, and gerontologic nursing have been used rather indiscriminately throughout this text. "Gerontic" is an umbrella term coined by Laurie Gunther to cover the whole field; "geriatric" sometimes is thought to be too medical a term, but it is comparable in our use to "pediatric" care and concern with the whole person. "Gerontologic" was meant to encompass a broader perspective and includes research and theories about elders. Morley (2004) points out that the word gerontology is derived from the French *geronte,* meaning "man," and has nothing to do with aging. He suggests geratology as the appropriate term.

CHAPTER ONE

History and Development of Geriatric Nursing

We need to know not so much about where they are going as where they've come from, what they've had, what they've given up, how they feel about the past, for all that will color how they feel about the present. (Burnside, 1975, p. 1801)

Although Burnside, a geriatric nursing pioneer, was writing about older people, her words ring true as we look at the history of geriatric nursing and the significant work of the geriatric nursing pioneers. To understand the history of geriatric nursing today, we need to know where the pioneers have come from, what they've had available, what they've given up, and how they feel about the past, for all that colors and sets the course for the present and future.

In 1982, Barbara Davis, one of the geriatric nursing pioneers, saw the need for a historical inquiry of the history of the specialty of geriatric nursing and began a significant body of work documenting the historical evolution of the specialty and the impact of significant historical events and movements on nursing care of the elderly. Referring to a quote by Thelma Wells from England, Davis proposed to change the view that "early nursing history in the States, while characterized by outstanding leaders, fails to reveal any particular nurse leader primarily focused on work with the elderly. This . . . may reflect a lack of interest in gerontological nursing by American nursing researchers" (Wells, 1979, p. 187). The authors of this book are indebted to Barbara Davis for sharing with us her personal papers, deep insights, and scholarly research into the history of geriatric nursing to assist in the preparation of this chapter.

Historically, much of the development of nursing can be attributed to certain personal characteristics of the pioneering leaders. They were articulate; they did not take no for an answer; and they found a way around blocks. They had qualities of leadership such as energy, strength, dignity, and a sense of purpose. Some were ornery and autocratic (Achterberg, 1991). Reflecting on geriatric nurse pioneers as presented in chapters 2, 3 and 4, these qualities are apparent.

BACKGROUND AND SIGNIFICANCE

Nursing has always been about caring for the vulnerable. "The untrained nurse is as old as the human race; the trained nurse is a recent discovery" (Robinson, in Donahue, 1985). The geriatrically trained and educated nurse is most recent. Today there are still numerous nurses and physicians who believe that simply working with the old is sufficient and that special training is unnecessary.

History in nursing practice has experienced a revival of interest as nursing specialty organizations have emerged and flourished. It is edifying to trace the roots of their beginnings, because the strength of these specialty groups is nourished by their distinctive fundamental beliefs. Lambertson (1975, p. vii) provides a perspective on the value of historical nursing research and its meaning to professional specialty groups:

> Historical research contributes a valuable perspective to the analysis on current activities by providing a sense of continuity over time through analysis of persons, movements, events and concepts. Through the process of reconstructing events of the past and the analysis of why events occurred as they did, the historian has the capacity to assist professional groups in measuring, evaluating and predicting social change.

In examining the history of geriatric nursing, one must marvel at the advocacy and perseverance of nurses who have remained deeply committed to the care of older adults despite struggling against insurmountable odds over the years. For almost a century, nurses have been battling for reform, improvement of care, and professional nursing attention to the needs of older adults. The history of the specialty has been both helped and hindered by societal values and attitudes toward the elderly. The early history of nursing's concern for the elderly centered on institutional care, and although still of concern, nursing homes are now viewed as just one place on the continuum of care options. Schell noted "nurses' concern for the elderly poor of the almshouse foreshadowed the birth of gerontological nursing, a specialty conceived in the womb" (1993, p. 203).

THE BEGINNING SPECIALTY
OF GERIATRIC NURSING

Geriatric nursing emerged as a circumscribed area of practice only within the last five decades. Prior to 1950, geriatric nursing care was seen as the application of general principles of nursing to the aged client with little recognition of this area as a specialty similar to obstetric, pediatric, or surgical nursing. Content on geriatric nursing is not found in any early nursing text. Davis (1971) has related the similarities between the development of geriatric nursing and the development of two other nursing specialties, psychiatric/mental health nursing and pediatric nursing. From Davis's perspective, the formation of a body of knowledge in these two specialties was crucial to their recognition as specialties. When society became willing to use its resources to protect and care for children and individuals with mental illness, nursing emerged as a leader in the reform process. Reflecting on the similarities between pediatric nursing and geriatric nursing in development of their specialties, Davis (1980) said:

> An analogy is nursing care of the child in the early 1900s before there was full acceptance of the difference between the child and the adult. The oft-heard statement 'a child is a miniature adult' lost its credence when it was shown that the child, sick or well, had physiological and psychosocial needs which were different from those of the adult. As the child became treasured for his intrinsic value alone, rather than his ability to be productive and useful in the family and society, pediatrics as a medical specialty arose, followed by the specialization of pediatric nursing. Along with this came the anti-child-labor movement, school enforcement laws, and the development of services to protect the child. We can only speculate that a similar process might occur for the aged person. There is a variation, however, as nursing appears to be taking the lead instead of medicine, in developing its own specialty of nursing care of the aged. (p. 72)

Although most specialties in nursing practice developed from those identified in medicine, this was not the case with the specialty of geriatric nursing because health care of the elderly traditionally was considered to be within the domain of nursing. Nursing also has been credited for making a major contribution to the advance of gerontology as a profession over the past 25 years. In her farsighted thinking, Davis (1971) proposed that the specialty of geriatric nursing will have a strong enough base to develop into subspecialties similar to pediatric nursing with its subspecialty of neonatal nursing. Geropsychiatric nursing is already well accepted as a subspecialty and Davis's prediction is that there may be subspecialties by age such as one devoted to the young-old and the old-old. With the aging of the baby boomers, many geriatric nurses already see that we need to develop a new knowledge base related to the unique needs of this generation.

Considered nursing's newest and youngest specialty, geriatric nursing also has been referred to as nursing's forgotten or little understood specialty (Wells, 1979). In 1973, Sister Marilyn Schwab stated: "Care of the aged demands all the best skills known to nursing yet gerontological nursing is a relatively new specialty and many nurses still see it as the lowest rung on the professional ladder" (Schwab, 1973, p. 2049). Although interest in the specialty of geriatric nursing and numbers of nurses prepared academically are increasing, there is still a critical shortage of competent and compassionate professionals, especially in light of projections that 46% of all registered nurses will be providing direct care to elderly people by the beginning of the 21st century (Whall, 1996). Older adults account for 46% of all hospital days, 80% of home care visits, and 90% of long-term care residents. Newly licensed nurses report 62.5% of their patients are older adults and in most nursing specialties, the majority of patients are over the age of 65 (Berman & Thornlow, 2005; Wendt, 2003).Yet, the majority of nurses are still being educated without any specialized content in geriatric nursing. A statement by Wells in 1979 still rings true today in many settings:

> Because there is little awareness of the breadth and depth of gerontological nursing, many nurses believe it to be simply a kindly attention to the bedfast old. In their ignorance, they foster a passive acceptance of some of the most complex care problems in nursing such as mental disorientation, incontinence, and pressure sores. (Wells, 1979, p. 189)

ORIGIN OF GERIATRICS AND GERONTOLOGY

Hippocrates (Greek) and Celcus (Roman) studied the clinical aspects of aging under such names as Gerocomica and Geroncomia. Ignatiz Nascher, a Viennese physician who devoted himself to the study of old age, is credited with originating the word geriatrics in 1909 in an article in the *New York Medical Journal* (Nascher, 1909). Nascher lectured at medical society meetings and medical colleges to promote the practice of geriatric medicine as a specialty and published the first textbook on medical care of the aged in the United States in 1914 (Freeman, 1961; Nascher, 1914).

Although the term geriatrics originated in the United States with Ignatiz Nascher, we owe a great deal in the development of the principles of caring for the aged to the United Kingdom (UK). In 1935 Marjorie Warren, a physician at West Middlesex Hospital, established a practice

with the aged emphasizing enhanced environment, active rehabilitation, and motivational methods. Others of note who combined the best
of medicine and nursing concepts included Trevor Howell, Sir Ferguson
Anderson, Lawrence Sturdee, George Adams and Lionel Cosin, Robin
Kennedy, Doreen Norton, and Cicely Saunders (Morley, 2004). Two of
our pioneering nurses, Doris Schwartz and Thelma Wells, had their initial exposure to geriatric concepts in the UK.

Donahue (1985) notes that certain institutions of influence stand out
in nursing history as having a major impact on practice, as do certain
leaders. It seems hard to separate the influence of remarkable leaders and
conspicuous institutions in the march toward progress. The person cannot be disassociated from the institution when assessing the overall impact on the specialty. In geriatric nursing one might consider Duke
University School of Nursing and Virginia Stone as examples. Institutional
monoliths of substantial recognition invariably became so because of
money; major endowments with philosophic strings attached or particular beliefs to be expounded as can be seen so readily in the numerous outstanding Catholic and Jewish hospitals.

INFLUENCE OF MEDICINE

Medicine and nursing have been intertwined and interdependent even
though in the history of geriatrics there is a clear delineation in goals between nursing and medicine. In medicine the desire to cure, to extend life,
is rooted in the ancients' hope of and search for immortality. Medicine
strives to preserve life. Old people often have little life left and therefore
are unattractive subjects. The roots of nursing lie in succoring, relief of
suffering, and prevention of illness. Nursing strives to provide comfort
and a "good" death and intuitively understands that the most important
part of health care resides in the client or patient's perceptions. Thus, the
divergent goals have been influential in the development of the specialties.

John Morley (2004) has published an excellent history of geriatric
medicine that elucidates the growth of the specialty and the narrowing of
the boundaries between nursing and medicine. The parallel development
gradually has achieved a blend in which nurses and physicians have greater
appreciation for the particular skills and abilities each brings to health care.

Patricia Donahue has contributed a beautifully illustrated, artistic
work on nursing history. As she notes, "nursing is not merely a technique
but a process that incorporates the elements of soul, mind and imagination" (1985, p. ix). She traces the roots back to primitive animistic times
and the evolutionary process of nursing.

INFLUENCE OF SOCIAL, ECONOMIC, AND POLITICAL ERAS

There is a cyclic and ongoing relationship between nursing and the social and political trends of an era. Nursing is intertwined with political and institutional needs and priorities at local, state, and federal levels. Economics also are tied to the social and political factions and thus intimately bound to the prevailing priorities. In times of war there is an upsurge in physical and psychologic rehabilitation strategies that ultimately provide models for care of the aged. In times of affluence the aged are given deferential treatment, but in economic depressions tension builds between the generations and the notion of "greedy geezers" can be perceived from some of the middle generation as they wonder about their own retirement and whether any assistance will remain available. This chapter examines the history of geriatric nursing from 1800 to the present and discusses the social, political, and economic contexts and influences of significant events on the formation of geriatric nursing as a specialty.

1800–1930: POORHOUSES, ALMSHOUSES, AND THE CALL FOR REFORM

The origins of gerontological nursing began when Florence Nightingale, the founder of modern nursing, accepted a position as superintendent in an institution comparable to today's nursing home. The patients at the Institution for the Care of Sick Gentlewomen in Distressed Circumstances were primarily governesses and ladies' maids from wealthy English families. Because care of elders was provided by families during this time, the care Nightingale provided was unheard of (Wykle & McDonald, 1997). Nightingale's concern for the plight of frail and sick aged was continued by Agnes Jones, a wealthy Nightingale-trained nurse, who in 1864 was sent to work in the Liverpool Infirmary, a large Poor Law institution (Wells, 1979). During the time of the Industrial Revolution in England, social and economic pressures led to the development of the Poor Law. Workhouses (also called almshouses and poorhouses) were built as part of a system designed to discourage people who were able to work from seeking support from public funds. These institutions were designed to house the poor, who were divided into two groups: the deserving poor (those who were unable to work), and the undeserving poor (those who were perceived as morally corrupt because they were able, but unwilling, to work). Poor aged people housed in almshouses were not considered morally corrupt because of their age and inability to work (Hall & Buckwalter, 1990).

Although these institutions were not created to care for frail and sick aged, individuals without other resources had no choice but to become workhouse inhabitants. Care was provided by fellow inmates called pauper nurses.

> These "nurses" were uneducated, unsupervised, often ill, and sometimes alcoholics; the "care" was deplorable. In the first months of her duty, Miss Jones dismissed 35 pauper nurses for drunkeness and wrote that she found "men wore the same shirts for seven weeks. Bed clothes were sometimes not washed for months. The diet was hopeless[ly] meagre compared to a hospital standard. (Wells, 1979, p. 187)

With Miss Nightingale as her ally and mentor, Miss Jones and the 12 nurses under her direction not only improved standards of care at the institution, but also lowered the costs of maintaining the sick (Wells, 1979).

In the period of early colonization of the United States, very few people lived to an advanced (for that time in history) age. Consider that a child born in 1900 had a life expectancy of just 47 years (Stotts & Deitrich, 2004). If care was needed, it was provided by the family. There were some almshouses that were supported by funds or alms from the church members. Originally, there was no stigma attached to the almshouses. After the British took over the colonies, assistance to the needy began to take on the characteristics of English customs (Davis, 1971, p. 7). By the 1800s, almshouses, funded by the states, were considered a socially undesirable incentive to keep people working. Sick and well, prostitutes, children, the elderly, the insane, and vagrants were all housed together in this dreaded place of last resort. They were notorious for their poor care and crowded and unsanitary conditions and no attempts were made to provide care for the sick in these settings (Davis, 1971, p. 8).

Around 1867, some states began to differentiate welfare institutions and classify inmates. Children were the first to be removed from poorhouses and placed in orphanages or foster homes. The insane were transferred to insane asylums. Epileptics, the blind, and the deaf were taken to other custodial sites and jails and reformatories housed the criminals. This process of desegregation continued for many decades, continuing into the 1900s (Davis, 1971, p. 8). Davis noted that " a most outstanding contribution of the systematic classification of inmates was the impetus it gave to the rise and acceleration of medical and nursing care for large groups of people" (1971, p. 8). Nurses such as Lavinia Dock, and social activists such as Carolyn Crane, were among the first to address the needs of the elderly chronically ill in almshouses.

In 1906, Mrs. Carolyn Bartlett Crane, Chairman of the Charity Organization Department of the Women's Civic Improvement League of

Kalamazoo, Michigan, presented a paper to the Michigan State Nurses' Association entitled "A Neglected Field of Nursing: The County Almshouse." Mrs. Crane called for the immediate need for trained nurses to work in these institutions and for pupil nurse education in almshouses. She proposed an alliance between the Michigan State Nurses' Association and the Michigan State Federation of Women's Clubs to provide nursing care in almshouses. The nurses' association would provide the nurses and the women's clubs the salary.

A May 1906 editorial in the *American Journal of Nursing* provided comments on Crane's paper, endorsing the action of the nurses' association to confer with the women's clubs to raise funds to employ nurses in the almshouses, conduct a survey of almshouse conditions, and provide pupil nurse education.

In 1907, Mrs. Crane presented a passionate appeal to the Nurses' Associated Alumnae of the United States on behalf of the suffering and neglected sick poor in the county almshouses of the United States. In her paper, "Almshouse Nursing: The Human Need; The Professional Opportunity," she described deplorable conditions, neglect, preventable suffering, contagion, and death from lack of proper medical and nursing care. Mrs. Crane called the county almshouse a "hospital with the hospital part left out." Invoking the work of Dorothea Dix—who 50 years earlier had revolutionized the treatment of the indigent insane, blind, deaf, feeble-minded, and epileptic—she called upon nurses to provide scientific and humane care to the indigent aged. The following is an excerpt from that paper:

> Much of the bedside service must be left to feeble, stupid or vicious inmates . . . appetite disappears with the lack of any attention paid to the sick diet; bedsores come and stay, long nights drag on, with the keeper and matron and servants locked in their apartments a thousand miles away! It was but a few weeks ago that, in a poorhouse, an inmate arose in the night and murdered a sick man who disturbed his sleep with cries for water. There are many deaths in the night. . . . Of all the motley assemblage of human beings who were once carelessly assigned to oblivion in the county poorhouse, presently none will be left except the aged and infirm! The aged and infirm poor . . . homeless, friendless poor old men and women . . . these are—and will become more and more—the great body of our almshouse population . . . the thought of going to the poorhouse stirs in them a terror; that they go only as the last resort, often conducted by force, and literally "weeping" as "over the hills to the poorhouse they take their weary way. . . ." They go there to spend the remainder of their earthly days; feeble at first, to grow more feeble through advancing age, lack of employment and interesting events; sitting day by day, looking at blank cheerless walls, and blank cheerless

faces, and a blank cheerless future. Here is a fertile field of senile decay, of body, mind and spirit; the elect abode of cheerless, comfortless, hopeless, suffering old age. (Crane, 1907, p. 873)

In 1908, Lavinia Dock, in the *American Journal of Nursing,* published findings from a survey by Mrs. Crane and a group of Michigan taxpayers reporting scathing conditions in the Kalamazoo County Almshouse. Commenting on the findings, Dock called upon intelligent and able women to have not only positions in such institutions, but also a share of power "so that these evils, all of which lie strictly in the sphere of housekeeping and nursing,—two spheres which have always been lauded as women's own—might not occur" (Dock, 1908, pp. 520–523). In 1912, the ANA Board of Directors appointed an Almshouse Committee to continue to oversee nursing in these institutions (Davis, 1984).

During this time, another group of nurses and women's club members in Illinois also collected information on almshouses. They proposed a plan that included visiting nurses making rounds in almshouses and the addition of an almshouse rotation in the curriculum of nursing schools. In 1912, Dock wrote that there had been some accomplishments in the almshouse reform but noted, "even more than other institutions, however, almshouses are in the grasp of petty and venal politicians. Until women attain full citizenship, no thoroughgoing improvement can be made in them" (Dock, 1912, p. 228). Political pressures, low pay and status, job insecurity, and women's lack of political power hindered the progress of almshouse nursing.

Although early nursing attention was focused on the needs of ill older adults in almshouses, there were a few articles published in the *American Journal of Nursing* between 1903 and 1909 that described care of community-dwelling elders. Among these are one by Dock (1906) describing an 80-year-old man experiencing acute delirium, and another by Jessie Breeze (1909), a private duty nurse, describing the care of the aged. Burnside has described this last article as one of the most "incisive and instructive, beautifully written, and reading as though it were written today sensitively describing care of the aged (Burnside, 1988). Breeze wrote:

The care of old people requires just as much skill, tact, ingenuity, and patience as the care of children, and perhaps more, because one must keep in mind that old people cannot be treated like children even if childish and that feebleness of physical and mental powers is not accompanied by forgetfulness of early experiences. A genuine affection, gentleness, sympathy, and imagination sufficient to grasp the patient's point of view are necessary. (1909, p. 826)

During the period of 1910–1920 issues related to the war effort left little time or energy to devote to care of the elderly or conditions in almshouses. As the 1920s dawned, nursing staffs were disorganized and depleted (Kalisch & Kalisch, 1978). Still, in 1925, an editorial in the *American Journal of Nursing* called for nurses to consider a specialty in nursing care of the aged.

1930–1960: FROM ALMSHOUSE
TO NURSING HOME

By 1930, conditions in almshouses had changed little. Nurses continued their advocacy toward reform and appropriate care in these settings. Helen W. Munson, writing in the *American Journal of Nursing,* noted that with the development of social services such as mothers' pensions and workmen's compensation many almshouse residents were able to achieve independence and the population that remained was mostly elderly. She gave examples of neglect, indifference, lack of nursing care, and poor management in many facilities. Only three of the 27 almshouses visited had trained nurses on staff. Because almshouses were under local control, Munson commented that conditions reflected the extent of social enlightenment of the community. Despite yearly inspections there was no power to enforce recommendations, and conditions did not improve from year to year. Munson again challenged the profession of nursing to take action to improve almshouse care and consider the elderly as a special group needing nursing care.

> . . . The care of the chronically ill and especially of the chronically ill poor, is a nursing problem. Modern nursing, both in England and in this country, was started with the purpose of "cleaning up" just such conditions in hospitals as are still found in almshouses. Furthermore, there is just now a great deal more nursing service available than is being used. Doesn't it seem then that we should do something about it? (Munson, 1930, p. 1226)

By the 1930s, reformers had raised enough public support, particularly from the white middle class, for a comprehensive federal pension plan (The Social Security Act of 1935) to provide for old-age insurance and public assistance for needy aged who were not covered by insurance. To combat the fear of almshouse placement, Congress stipulated that federal monies could not be used to pay for care in almshouses or other public institutions. The names of these institutions changed. The insane asylum became the state hospital; a pauper was now known more respectfully as a poor person; the poorhouses and almshouses took on the names of county home and infirmary; and orphanages were known as children's homes. "However, much of this was window dressing—a change in name only" (Davis, 1971, p. 9).

During the next 10 years, many almshouses closed and some continued their function as public infirmaries for the aged and chronically ill. With the closing of almshouses, there was an increase in the number of private boarding homes providing care to elders. "Businessmen soon saw the opportunity for a profit making enterprise by buying large old private residences and renovating them into homes for the aged, or by constructing new buildings for the same purpose" (Davis, 1971, p. 9). Because retired and widowed nurses often converted their homes into such living quarters and gave care when their boarders became ill, they can be considered the first geriatric nurses and their homes the first nursing homes.

Some have reflected that although the Social Security Act of 1935 was designed to increase the independence of the aged, it contributed to the rise of commercial nursing homes and laid the foundation of this type of care for the rest of the century (Lacey, 1999). Elderly people needing the care provided by an institution were now able to buy care with their Social Security funds. A growing elderly population and increasing numbers of women employed outside the home contributed to an increase in nursing home use. With few exceptions, the problems found in almshouses were transferred to private nursing homes. Like almshouses, nursing homes during this period were unregulated; few employed professional nurses and most were providing poor care (Schell, 1993).

During the 1940s, nurses continued to express concern about the problems in these facilities and called for improvement and regulation. In several states, public health nurses carried out inspection of facilities, providing consultation, education, and supervision to nursing home operators. Deficiencies were found in many of the homes inspected, evaluations were made available to the public, and facilities were encouraged to adopt a rehabilitation focus in the care of the residents (Carson, 1947).

Beginning awareness of the specialty of gerontological nursing was developing during this time. In 1945, Sarah Gelbach, Assistant Superintendent of Nurses at Goldwater Memorial Hospital in New York, published an article describing nursing care for the aged. Recommending that nurses with special aptitude care for the aged, she also suggested geriatric education in medical and nursing schools to study "methods of deferring the onset of senility and retaining maximum efficiency for a substantial period beyond the fourth decade" (pp. 1113–1114).

Two nursing journal articles published in the 1940s also described model facilities in the United States. The Cuyahoga County Nursing Home in Ohio and a Jewish home for the Aged in New York were both described as centers of excellence for geriatric care (Gubersky & Burke,

1941; Marsh, 1941). Emphasizing rehabilitation, psychosocial care, professional nurse staffing, health promotion, and liaisons with collegiate nursing programs, these facilities were "forerunners of the best in modern institutional geriatric care" (Schell, 1993, p. 213). Both articles contain clinical information as relevant today as in the 1940s when they were published. Expansion of interest in the study of aging by other professional groups also occurred in the 1940s. In 1942, the American Geriatrics Society was founded, followed in 1945 by The Gerontological Society of America (Newton & Anderson, 1966) (Box 1.1).

Between 1900 and 1950, the number of elders in the United States had grown from 3 million to about 12 million, and the numbers of those 85 and older had grown by 25%. The nursing home industry began to flourish in the early 1950s. The Kerr-Mills Medical Assistance to the Aged Act provided direct payment to care providers. The American Nursing Homes Association lobbied for and won the right for nonprofit nursing homes to be built in conjunction with hospitals using Hill-Burton funds (Hall & Buckwalter, 1990). With new sources of income and funds made available for building, this was a period of rapid growth for both the hospital and nursing home industries. Still, there was a lack of facilities to care for the growing numbers of elders, as well as a lack of sufficient funds to pay for good care even when it did exist.

By the late 1950s, the gap between the need for long-term care and the available resources was critical. It was estimated that the need for nursing home beds was about 450,000, with only 221,000 beds available. About half of these beds were in facilities deemed fire hazards or medically inadequate. Perhaps more disconcerting was the dismal care provided to older adults with dementia, many of whom were cared for in state mental institutions. Several social workers who worked in mental institutions in the 1950s describe custodial care on back wards of the institution, treatment of agitation or aggressive behavior with Thorazine, and routine use of physical restraints. One author wrote of his 95-year-old demented great-grandmother being tied to the four corners of her bed where she remained until she died of pneumonia several weeks later (Lacey, 1999).

Positive changes during this period included an increased interest in research and study of aging. Beliefs about the universal, hopeless decline in aging were being challenged, and for the first time, focus was directed toward the possibility of healthy aging.

> Present-day aging is not normal because it is complicated by pathology and disease. Perhaps at a future date our society will contain individuals who have aged normally, when the most effective practices of medical science, nutrition, and sanitation have become known and adopted, and when cultural changes necessary to provide opportunity for continued personal development throughout life have been brought about. (Lacey, 1999, p. 110)

BOX 1.1 Description of the Cuyahoga County Nursing Home

The nursing home was opened in February 1939 with 140 beds; the capacity has since been increased to 179. The medical staff consists of a medical director, two resident doctors, and two medical students. A heart specialist and a neurologist visit and examine patients. The nursing staff consists of twelve graduate registered nurses besides the supervisor of nurses and the director. In addition, there are five graduate nurses and a group of male and female attendants. There is also a full-time physical therapist and a half-time occupational therapist and a full-time barber. With but two or three exceptions, our original staff remains intact. We anticipated that we might have trouble keeping our staff interested enough to remain in our employ for long, for we thought that caring for chronic cases might prove tiresome and would lack the excitement to be found in a general hospital. But we have had so many unusual cases and so much does happen that our nurses and attendants and doctors find ample interests. There is as much excitement when "Frankie" who was unable to walk for so long, took his first jaunt of a few steps, as there is anywhere in the city. And when "Reggie," who had such a bad heart that he was not expected to live the week out when transferred to the nursing home, got well enough to get around the ward and was finally allowed to dress, there was great rejoicing. We find that under carefully supervised medical and nursing care we have actually been able to return two hundred patients out of four hundred and eighty admitted in a year and a half to their homes, and some to their work.

Our nurses and attendants are kind and considerate of the old people. They jolly them when necessary, scold, if necessary, and do everything in their power to keep them comfortable and happy. We have a rule that each resident will have two baths a week. Many old people feel that one bath a week is plenty and we are encroaching on their rights to ask more. It has taken a great deal of patience to establish the routine of two baths a week. There are days when everyone seems to be on edge, which is to be expected. Rainy days when rheumatism seems worse, or breathing is more difficult, must be met with cheerfulness and tact. One must be most careful about going over clothes and dresser drawers for in this dresser rests all that is left of the patient's estate, and it is most precious.

Our doctors follow the treatment prescribed for the patients by the various hospitals and try everything possible to help the patients. Their concern is "What more can the Nursing Home do in addition to what the hospitals have done?" This spirit is reflected in the accomplishments of our medical and nursing staffs. One of our principal nursing problems is, of course, the danger of development of decubitus ulcers. These patients are given a special mixture of glycerin, witch hazel, grain alcohol, and water, which is followed by an oil rub. With patients admitted from the hospitals with very bad decubitus ulcers, it has taken a tremendous amount of painstaking care on the part of our staff to heal them. One of our patients who was incontinent was sent to a large hospital for treatment. She did not have a break in her skin when she left us, but when she returned she had a decubitus ulcer on her coccyx which went into the bone, and one on her hip which went almost to the bone. During this patient's stay in the hospital she had a retention catheter with constant drainage (which she did not have while in the nursing home), so there was not a wet bed to contend with, and such a dreadful condition should have been prevented. It has taken over a year to heal her ulcers but it has been done.

All patients have their temperature taken once daily. If any patient has a slight elevation or an increase in pulse and respiration, the doctor is notified at once. This might be the beginnings of pneumonia and must be checked at the onset. We feel that a poor cook is an expensive investment, so from the beginning we have had a most excellent chef. Our fresh vegetables and fruit are furnished by a farm project of the Cuyahoga County Relief Bureau.

Edith Marsh (1941). The care of the chronically ill. *American Journal of Nursing* (February 1941): 161–166.

Gerontological nursing also was coming of age in the 1950s. Newton and Anderson published the first book on nursing care of the aged in 1950. This classic text was reflective of the decade in which it originated, with emphasis on diseases of aging and the medical model of care. However, it has been hailed as a "landmark work that helped to dispel partially nursing's dependence on medicine for its literature" (Davis, 1984, p. 45). In 1952, the first published nursing research on chronic disease and the elderly appeared in the premier issue of *Nursing Research* (Mack, 1952). In the midst of growing concern over the quality of care in nursing homes, in 1958, ANA issued a Statement of Standards for Nursing Care in Nursing Homes (Davis, 1984). ANA was the first health professional group to support national health insurance for the elderly (Butler & Lewis, 1982). By the end of this period, growth of governmental involvement, increasing numbers of older people, and interest and research in gerontology provided the framework for the policy changes that occurred in the 1960s and 1970s.

1960–1985: MEDICARE, NURSING HOMES, AND THE BIRTH OF MODERN GERONTOLOGICAL NURSING

This era brought major changes and rapid growth in both health care and the nursing profession, including gerontological nursing. Gerontological nursing research increased both in quantity and quality, master's programs to prepare specialists were developed, and many strong gerontological nursing leaders emerged to guide the specialty. Virginia Stone provided an overview of the three distinct evolutionary stages that geriatric nursing had gone through since the turn of the century: (a) practice based on custodialism, (b) practice founded on imitation and intuition, and (c) practice supported by scientific theory (Stone, 1969). Schwartz (1969) identified the emerging needs in geriatric nursing: (a) identification of the core of knowledge specific to nursing assessment and care of the aged, (b) identification of those needs of the aged that require nursing attention or referral, and (c) the significance of the clinical nurse expert in gerontology (Davis, 1982). Pioneers such as Doris Schwartz, Barbara Davis, Delores Alford, Irene Burnside, Mary Opal Wolanin, Priscilla Ebersole, Laurie Gunter, Sister Marilyn Schwab, Bernita Steffl, Virginia Stone, and Sister Rose Therese Bahr led us into the birth of the specialty.

By 1961, 15 million Americans were older than 65 and life expectancy was approaching 70 and beyond. The first White House Conference on Aging, focused on health care, was held in 1961. Recommendations at the conference included nursing training in rehabilitation of nursing home residents and the importance of specialized training in geriatrics (Stotts & Dietrich, 2004).

In 1962, the ANA convened the first meeting of a conference group of 67 nurses from 27 states on gerontological nursing practice. Gerontological nursing was proposed as one of ANA's specialty divisions (Burnside, 1988). The year 1965 brought landmark legislation, the passage of nationalized health care for the aged in the form of Medicare and Medicaid. The Older Americans Act, providing grants to states for community services projects, was also passed that year. With the advent of Medicare and Medicaid, there were major changes in the way health care for the elderly was financed. People over 65, even poor Americans, were provided assurance of access to health care. Care for older adults shifted away from the family to the federal government (Stotts & Deitrich, 2004). Medicare provided payment for outpatient services, acute hospitalization, and some nursing home care. Although new sources of income were provided to nursing homes for post-hospital skilled care services, generally less than 5% of nursing home residents were eligible for this type of skilled care. However, Medicaid became a significant source of income for nursing homes with its coverage of custodial care for low-income elderly.

In the early years of Medicare and Medicaid, federal and state governments distributed large sums of taxpayer dollars to nursing homes but provided almost no oversight or regulation of the minimal federal standards that existed. Because of a persistent shortage of nursing home beds, the government was reluctant to enforce the standards or increase oversight. Quality of care in nursing homes continued to be of concern. Many entrepreneurial for-profit owners became wealthy by exploiting the new revenue sources, with reports of some pocketing funds instead of providing improved care for their residents. Six months after the Medicare legislation was enacted, only 25% of skilled nursing facilities met even the minimal standards of care (Lacey, 1999).

Interest in and support for the specialty of gerontological nursing continued to grow during this period. In 1966, the Division of Geriatric Nursing Practice was established within ANA, giving nursing care of the aged specialty status along with maternal-child, medical-surgical, psychiatric, and community health. Barbara Davis became the first full-time coordinator for the newly established Division. Davis noted

> a division was created if these criteria could be met: the presence of a unique body of knowledge and a large number of nurses employed in a field in which a health problem exists. Although the body of knowledge was skimpy, ANA's House of Delegates had the foresight to vote in a Division of Geriatric Nursing Practice. (Davis, 1980, p. 72)

Davis recorded the organization's role in developing this specialty in some of the first articles published on the historical evolution of geriatric nursing in the United States (Davis, 1968a, 1968b, 1982).

The Division developed a philosophy of care of the aged and definition of geriatric nursing. *Guidelines for the Preparation of Geriatric Nurse Practitioners and Nursing and Long-Term Care: Toward Quality Care of the Aged* were prepared by the division. The latter, considered a landmark report on long-term care in this country, was prepared at the request of the U.S. Senate Subcommittee on Aging. The newly formed division, with federal funding, conducted 42 continuing education conferences on geriatric nursing for about 3,000 nursing home nurses (Davis, 1980).

In 1968, there were 15,510 members in the geriatric practice division; by 1970, membership had grown to 37,811 (Moses, 1979). In 1973, the division was the first to publish standards of practice. These standards were revised in 1976 and the name of the division was changed to Gerontological Nursing Practice. An ANA committee staffed by Barbara Davis, and with Laurie Gunter as chairperson, developed certification criteria for geriatric nurses who wished to be credentialed. Priscilla Ebersole, editor of *Geriatric Nursing,* related that "to the committee's surprise, more than 100 nurses applied and kept the committee busy the entire Thanksgiving vacation reviewing applications" (1998, p. 49). In 1974, geriatric nursing was the first certification program offered by ANA, and 74 nurses were certified just 1 year later (Moses, 1979). Nursing was the first professional group to develop standards of care and certification in the field of gerontology (Davis, 1984). Table 1.1 presents a timeline for the development of gerontological nursing.

The study of aging accelerated during this period with more research and development of the scientific basis for much of the modern perspective on aging. Federal funding for nursing education encouraged growth in the numbers of nurses prepared at the master's and doctoral level and an increased interest in nursing science and theory building. Emphasis was placed on the profession's independent role and autonomous status (Davis, 1984). In the early 1960s, Doris Schwartz received some of the first funding from the Public Health Service for a study exploring a series of questions about the care of elderly chronically ill outpatients (Schwartz, 1960). The research was published in a book at a time when nursing research was seldom done, and if done, was not published in a book (Ebersole, 1997).

In 1966, Miller and colleagues published results of a 6-month study in a New York nursing home describing the differences in care requirements for older patients in nursing homes versus hospitals. Marked contrasts were noted in the areas of administrative relationships, psychosocial nursing, nursing clinical decision making, medication management, and comprehensive rehabilitation programs. The authors advocated for formal preparation for long-term care nursing and offered important suggestions for future research, many of which continue to be the focus of research today (Miller, Keller, Liebel, & Metrowitz, 1966) (Box 1.2).

The first master's program to prepare nurses as clinical nurse specialists in gerontological nursing was developed in 1966 by Virginia Stone at Duke University. This pioneer program was offered for 7 years and produced the first specialists in the field. The Duke program was based on the Reiter nurse specialist model (Davis, 1984). Reiter suggested that the long-term care setting afforded a greater degree of autonomy and initiative in nursing practice, more freedom to take professional responsibility and respond to nursing demands, and provided the opportunity to learn the "independent practice of the care of the patient before learning the dependent practice of the cure of patients" (Reiter, 1964, p. 66). According to Reiter, the involvement of nurses in the complexity of nonnursing tasks in acute care distracted nurses from improving practice. However, in long-term care the primary need of patients is not medicine's efforts to cure but rather "the rehabilitative, sustaining, nurturing

TABLE 1.1 Timeline of Professionalization of Gerontologic Nursing

1906	First article published in *American Journal of Nursing (AJN)* on care of the aged.
1925	*AJN* considers geriatric nursing as a possible specialty in nursing.
1950	Newton and Anderson publish first geriatric nursing textbook.
	Geriatrics becomes a specialization in nursing.
1962	American Nurses Association (ANA) forms a national geriatric nursing group.
1966	ANA creates the Division of Geriatric Nursing.
	First master's program for clinical nurse specialists in geriatric nursing developed by Virginia Stone at Duke University.
1970	ANA establishes Standards of Practice for Geriatric Nursing committee, chaired by Dorothy Moses; included Lois Knowles and Mary Shaunnessey.
1973	ANA defined Standards of Practice for Geriatric Nursing.
1974	Certification in geriatric nursing practice offered through ANA; process implemented by Laurie Gunter and Virginia Stone.
1975	*Journal of Gerontological Nursing* published by Slack; first editor, Edna Stilwell.
1976	ANA renames Geriatric Division "Gerontological" to reflect a health promotion emphasis.
	ANA publishes Standards for Gerontological Nursing Practice; Committee chaired by Barbara Allen Davis.
	ANA begins certifying geriatric nurse practitioners.
	Nursing and the Aged edited by Burnside and published by McGraw-Hill.
1977	First gerontological nursing track funded by Division of Nursing and established by Sr. Rose Therese Bahr at University of Kansas School of Nursing.
1979	*Education for Gerontic Nursing* written by Gunter and Estes; suggested curricula for all levels of nursing education.
	ANA Council of Long Term Care Nurses established; group first chaired by Ella Kick.
1980	*Geriatric Nursing* first published by *AJN;* Cynthia Kelly, editor.
1981	ANA Division of Gerontological Nursing issues statement regarding scope of practice.
1983	Florence Cellar Endowed Gerontological Nursing Chair established at Case Western Reserve University, first in the nation; Doreen Norton, first scholar to occupy chair.
	National Conference of Gerontological Nurse Practitioners established.
1984	National Gerontological Nurses Association established.
	Division of Gerontological Nursing Practice becomes Council on Gerontological Nursing (councils established for all practice specialties).
1986	ANA publishes survey of gerontological nurses in clinical practice.
1987	ANA revises and issues Scope and Standards of Gerontological Nursing Practice.
1989	ANA certifies gerontological clinical nurse specialists.
1990	ANA establishes a Division of Long-Term Care within the Council of Gerontological Nursing.
1992	ANA redefines long-term care to include life-span approach.
	John A. Hartford Foundation funds a major initiative to improve care of hospitalized older patients: Nurses Improving Care to Hospitalized Elderly (NICHE).
1993	National Institute of Nursing Research established as separate entity.
1994	ANA redefines Scope and Standards of Gerontological Nursing Practice.
1996	John A. Hartford Foundation establishes the Institute for Geriatric Nursing at New York University under the direction of Mathy Mezey.
2000	Recommended baccalaureate competencies and curricular guidelines for geriatric nursing care published by the American Association of Colleges of Nursing and the John A. Hartford Foundation Institute for Geriatric Nursing.
2001	ANA, in collaboration with the National Gerontological Nursing Association, National Association of Directors of Nursing Administration in Long-Term Care, and the National Conference of Gerontological Nurse Practitioners, publishes revised Scope and Standards of Gerontological Nursing Practice and reaffirms the need for competent gerontological nursing.
2003	Nurse Competence in Aging (funded by the Atlantic Philanthropies Inc.) initiative to improve the quality of health care to older adults by enhancing the geriatric competence of nurses who are members of specialty nursing associations (ANA, ANCC, John A. Hartford Foundation Institute for Geriatric Nursing).
2004	Nurse Practitioner and Clinical Nurse Specialist Competencies for Older Adult Care published by the American Association of Colleges of Nursing and the Hartford Geriatric Nursing Initiative.
	ANA Scope and Standards of Practice for all registered nurses referenced to include care of older adults.

measures that are recognized quite universally as independent nursing functions" (Reiter, 1964, p. 67). Gerontological nursing was seen by many of the early leaders as an area in which nursing had the potential to develop independently and demonstrate its unique contributions to the health and welfare of older adults.

BOX 1.2 Recommendations for Clinical Research

- The relationship of the physical environment to patient care and nursing techniques
- The relationship of patient disability to the type of bed required and other furniture needed
- The type of nursing education program best suited to prepare the nurse-administrator and the nurse-clinician
- The advantages and disadvantages of giving hypodermoclysis as compared with intravenous therapy
- Techniques of nursing care in psychosocial rehabilitation; feeding, bathing, and dressing the disabled patient
- Comparison of the effective use of bedpan, commode, and toilet in care of older people
- A meaningful study on patient restraints

Miller, M., Keller, D., Liebel, E., & Metrowitz, I. (1966). Nursing in a skilled nursing home. *American Journal of Nursing* 66(3): 321–325.

Funding from the Department of Health, Education and Welfare to develop curricula on aging in nursing schools began the growth of gerontological nurse practitioner and clinical nurse specialist programs in the mid 1970s. These programs were developed at both the certificate and master's level. Among them were the first PRIMEX program at Cornell under the direction of Doris Schwartz, and programs at the University of Colorado and State University of New York. An innovative program for the preparation of gerontological nurse practitioners was the Mountain States Gerontological Nurse Practitioner Program that prepared nurses from nursing homes for advanced practice roles (Buckwalter et al., 1997). In 1980 Kane and colleagues predicted a need for at least 12,000 gerontological nurse practitioners by the year 2010 and remarked that the growth of the nurse practitioner movement offered an attractive alternative to sole reliance on physicians, who demonstrated indifference to nursing home care. These authors also commented on nursing's tradition of care rather than cure and their ability to work more comfortably with nursing home staffs to upgrade their skills (Kane et al., 1980).

Issues related to gerontological nursing education at this time included the lack of faculty prepared in the specialty, negative attitudes of students and faculty toward gerontological nursing and older adults, and the dearth of content in schools of nursing on care of the aged. Controversy existed as to whether gerontological nursing should be integrated into nursing programs or taught as a specialty course similar to other specialties such as pediatrics, obstetrics, and psychiatric nursing (Gress, 1979).

Concerns over the quality of nursing home care continued in the 1970s and 1980s. In the early 1970s, Congressman David Pryor and consumer advocate Ralph Nader reported to Congress on their findings of poor care and abuses in some nursing homes (Lacey, 1999). Two books of the era describe the abysmal care and provide scathing critiques of the nursing home industry (Butler, 1975; Vladeck, 1980). The nursing profession continued its advocacy role in improvement of nursing home care. In 1975, The United States Senate Special Committee on Aging Subcommittee on Long-Term Care requested the ANA to prepare a paper on long-term care. Sister Marilyn Schwab chaired the committee that prepared the report "Nursing and Long-Term Care: Toward Quality Care for the Aging." The full text of the report was included in the Senate subcommittee series of reports on nursing home care in the United States: *Nurses in Nursing Homes: The Heavy Burden* (Gamroth, 1998; Schwab, 1973). Claire Townsend stated in that report: "Nurses have shown more responsibility than physicians and nursing home operators and for this the aged and the nation can be grateful" (Moses, 1979, p. 222).

Reports of widespread quality of care problems in nursing homes, proposed government regulation of the industry, and efforts of consumer advocacy groups led to the passage of the Omnibus Reconciliation Act of 1987 (OBRA). This was the most comprehensive nursing home reform law in history. Provisions of this law included physical and chemical restraint reduction, improved training of nursing home staff, a comprehensive assessment, Minimum Data Set (MDS) and the requirement that the facility must employ the services of at least one registered nurse 8 hours a day, 7 days a week. Despite recommendations for increased registered nurse staffing by both the Institute of Medicine and the American Nurses Association, OBRA 87 was passed with barely minimal staffing requirements. The nursing home industry protested even these minimum increases in staffing standards (Wunderlich et al., 1996).

The Teaching Nursing Home Program was an innovative demonstration project begun in 1982 to improve nursing home care and stimulate interest in gerontological nursing. Sponsored by the Robert Wood Johnson Foundation and the American Academy of Nursing, 11 collegiate nursing programs were funded to work in collaboration with skilled nursing facilities. The program was administered by the University of Pennsylvania School of Nursing under the direction of Mathy Mezey and Joan Lynaugh. The aims of the program were to "upgrade clinical care of patients in nursing homes by introducing a cadre of nurse specialists; to create an environment supportive of education of undergraduate and graduate nursing students, and students in other health professions; and to promote clinical research" (Mezey & Lynaugh, 1989). This innovative model has been called the most significant experiment to improve nursing home care in the last decade (Strumpf, 1994). Continuation of the programs beyond the funding stage was problematic for all sites. However, outcomes of the program indicated that the collaborative effort between schools of nursing and nursing homes has the potential to promote quality care, increase knowledge in care of the elderly, provide education and clinical experience for students, and assist in recruitment of nurses into long-term care (Dimond, Infield, Kethley, & Pfeiffer, 1997). The National Institute on Aging also launched its own teaching nursing home program in academic medical schools with the major focus on research.

With the increase in the number of nurses with master's and doctorates, gerontological nursing research increased in both quantity and quality. The literature in gerontological nursing increased substantially from 1955 to 1965 from 18 publications in 1955 to 71 in 1965 (Wells, 1979). Several overviews of the state of gerontological nursing research were published during this period and common trends noted were the lack of a nursing theoretic framework, minimal attention to the use of findings from biological, psychological, and sociologic sources, lack of clinical research, and a need for more longitudinal and replication studies (Burnside, 1988; Gunter & Miller, 1977). The bulk of research focused on nurses' attitudes toward care of the aged and psychosocial needs and interventions. Gunter and Miller remarked that there was "evidence of a developing nursing gerontology" (Gunter & Miller, 1977, p. 213).

Textbooks on gerontological nursing also increased during this time and by 1980 there were 13 (Burnside, 1988). Irene Burnside published the first reader in gerontological nursing issues in 1973, followed in 1976 by her publication of *Nursing and the Aged,* the first comprehensive text devoted entirely to geriatric nursing. This classic text, used in many of the early programs in the specialty, reflected the author's artistic and holistic approach to gerontological nursing. In 1975, the *Journal of Gerontological Nursing* was first published with Edna Stilwell as editor.

Other important events in the history of gerontological nursing during this time include the first presentation by a nurse (Laurie Gunter) to the International Congress on Gerontology in 1968, the first International Conference on Gerontological Nursing organized by Laurie Gunter and Barbara Davis in 1981, the establishment of the first Chair in gerontological nursing at an American university filled by Doreen Norton at Case Western Reserve in 1983, the formation of the National Conference of Gerontological Nurse Practitioners in 1983, and the National Gerontological Nurses Association in 1984 (Burnside, 1988). With a developing scientific base, advanced practice nursing education programs, and strong leaders, the specialty of geriatric nursing had come of age.

1985 TO PRESENT:
GERIATRIC NURSING COMES OF AGE

As we enter the 21st century, projections are that by 2030, 20% of the American population will be over the age of 65, with those over 85 showing the greatest increase in numbers. Today's older people are healthier, better educated, more affluent, and expect a much higher quality of life as they age than did their elders. Geriatric nurse educators, scholars, and clinicians continue their commitment to and advocacy for older people. Geriatric nurses have made substantial contributions to the body of knowledge guiding best practices in the care of older people. Nursing research has provided a solid knowledge base for important clinical issues such as restraint reduction, incontinence, care of people with Alzheimer's disease, informal caregiving, nutrition, health promotion, care environments, physical and emotional health, reminiscence therapy, and staffing issues in nursing homes (Fitzpatrick, Fulmer, Wallace, & Flaherty, 2000).

Geriatric nursing research has shown that better care is possible and should be expected. The task before us now is to communicate the knowledge to nurses who care for older adults in all settings. Geriatric nursing research has gained wide acceptance in the scientific community and geriatric nurses have taken their place as vital members of the interdisciplinary community of geriatric professionals. A testimony to the significant contribution of nurses to the study of gerontology is the current GSA presidency held by Dr. Terry Fulmer, the first nurse ever to hold that office. There remains an urgent need for increased funding for geriatric nursing research, particularly in the areas of new health care delivery models for older adults; clinical care concerns; and home, nursing home, assisted living, and community-based health care (Dimond et al., 1997; Wykle & McDonald, 1997).

Advanced practice nurses have demonstrated their skill as well as cost effectiveness across a variety of settings. "Advanced practice nurses will likely serve as a mainstay of care along with a cadre of other disciplines, in providing high quality interdisciplinary care to elders in ambulatory, long-term care and acute care settings" (Buckwalter et al., 1997, p. 11). The role of advanced practice gerontological nurses in nursing homes is well established and the positive outcomes of their care include patient satisfaction, decreased costs, less frequent hospitalizations, and improved quality of care (Dowling-Castronova, 2000).The geriatric nurse practitioner is and will continue to be a major influence on quality of care in nursing homes and other settings.

As our history progresses, some of the same issues confronting geriatric nurses at the beginning of the last century continue to be of concern today. The lack of professional nurses in nursing homes continues today and shockingly low nurse:patient ratios endanger resident care in many nursing homes (Harrington et al., 2000; Kovner, Mezey, & Harrington, 2000). Difficulty recruiting and retaining qualified personnel to provide direct care in nursing homes remains a critical problem.

Education for gerontological nursing, particularly at the undergraduate level, has not kept pace with demand and the problems that plagued us earlier continue. Despite gains, concern exists within the nursing profession about inadequate preparation and interest of students and faculty in geriatric nursing. The John A. Hartford Geriatric Nursing Institute, under the direction of Mathy Mezey and Terry Fulmer, is leading the way for advancement of geriatric nursing with funding for best practice care projects and development of geriatric nursing in undergraduate and graduate curricula. The John A. Hartford Foundation commitment is the largest of any foundation in nursing and has stimulated curricular reform, the development of academic centers of excellence, and predoctoral and postdoctoral scholarships, fostering the development of geriatric nursing research and practice.

A recent survey conducted by the John A. Hartford Foundation Institute for Geriatric Nursing (Hartford Institute), in collaboration with the American Association of Colleges of Nursing, compared gerontological content in baccalaureate nursing programs to baseline data collected by the Hartford Institute in 1997. Results suggest that there has been a "fundamental shift in baccalaureate curriculum toward incorporation of a greater amount of gerontological content, integration of content in a greater number of nursing courses, and more diversity of clinical sites used for gerontological nursing experiences" (Berman et al., 2005, p. 268). While these results are encouraging, there is a continued need to increase the numbers of faculty with preparation in gerontological nursing and to enhance the numbers of students and graduates choosing to work in the specialty.

Ensuring geriatric nursing competency in all students graduating from a nursing program is an imperative for improvement of health care to older adults. The Hartford Institute for Geriatric Nursing and the American Association of Colleges of Nursing (AACN) developed gerontological nursing competencies and curriculum materials for baccalaureate programs (http://www.aacn.nche.edu/Education/gerocomp.htm). Continued support for gerontological nursing education from the Foundation is provided through grants and awards for innovative curricula and models, faculty development, research, and leadership activities. Nationally recognized competencies in gerontological nursing also have been developed for graduate programs preparing advanced practice nurses in specialties other than gerontological nursing who will work with older adults (http://www.aacn.nche.edu/Education/Hartford/OlderAdultCare.htm).

Recognizing the critical need for a nursing workforce prepared to deliver quality care to the nation's aging population, and in light of the fact that few of the nation's 2.2 million practicing registered nurses have received any preparation in geriatric nursing, either in their educational programs or on the job, the ANA will be awarding grants in the Nurse Competence in Aging initiative. This 5-year program, funded by the Atlantic Philanthropies and representing a strategic alliance among ANA, ANCC, and the John A. Hartford Institute for Geriatric Nursing, is designed to improve the quality of health care to older adults by enhancing the geriatric competence—the attitudes, knowledge, and skills—of nurses who are members of specialty organizations. The Nurse Competence in Aging initiative will provide grant and technical assistance to national specialty nursing associations, conduct a national geriatric nursing certification outreach, and develop a web-based comprehensive geriatric nursing resource center. Additionally, the ANA has formed a partnership with the Gerontological Society of America to present *A New Look at the Old,* a new bimonthly series focusing on specific aspects of care for older adults (Stotts & Deitrich, 2004). Mezey and Fulmer (2002) suggested that efforts such as these will ensure that in the future, all older adults will be cared for by a nurse who has received special preparation in geriatrics.

Although the numbers of gerontological nurse practitioners and clinical nurse specialists have almost doubled in the last 9 years, the number prepared falls substantially short of national demands. By 2030, the projected need for full-time gerontological nurses in all settings is expected to reach 1.1 million (Klein, 1997). Approximately 14,000 gerontological nurse generalists (representing less than 1% of all RNs), 3,422 gerontological nurse practitioners (representing less than 6% of all APNs), and 710 gerontological clinical nurse specialists are certified (ANCC, 2003; Mezey, Harrington, & Kluger, 2005). Although graduates of all master's nursing programs have increased by 20%, only 3.1% of these graduates were prepared in geriatrics. There are currently 54 master's programs preparing advanced practice gerontological nurses, down from 80 in 1993, 65 in 1997, and 63 in 2000. The National Agenda for Geriatric Education White Papers has set forth a series of recommendations addressing actions needed to improve gerontological nursing education and practice in the present century (Buckwalter et al., 1997).

Historically, nurses have always been in the front lines caring for the aged. They have provided hands-on care, supervision, administration, program development, teaching, and research and to a great extent are responsible for the rapid advance of gerontology as a profession. Nurses have been, and continue to be, the mainstay of care of older adults (Mezey & Fulmer, 2002; Wykle & McDonald, 1997).

The solid foundation built by the geriatric nursing pioneers and the current leaders in the specialty, the commitment of geriatric nurses to "tackle difficult but exceptionally meaningful issues that impact profoundly on the health and quality of life for older adults" (Mezey & Fulmer, 2002, p. M440), the opportunities for decision making, independent action, and innovation (Davis, 1971, p. 10), and the significant contribution of geriatric nursing research to improved patient outcomes and health policy, position the specialty for continued growth, recognition, contribution, and value to society. Dare we say that geriatric nursing will be the most needed specialty in nursing as the number of older people in our society continues to increase and the need for our specialized knowledge becomes even more critical in every specialty and every health care setting?

In 1971, writing in *Imprint,* the student nursing organization's journal, Barbara Davis looked to the future of geriatric nursing and suggested that in the not-too-distant future, all nurses would be exposed to geriatric nursing in their basic nursing programs, graduate programs in geriatric nursing would become more numerous, geriatric nurses with doctorates would shape the future of the specialty, and there would be subspecialties in geriatric nursing branching out from a strong knowledge base. She closed her article as follows:

> The past, present, and future of nursing care of the aged is boundless. It is endless. It is the specialty which cares for the carriers of our culture, those who link us to our immediate past, and point to its consumers of the future—myself soon, and you, the Imprint readers who will be just a short distance behind me. (p. 73)

Those predictions have become a reality and more. The pioneers have charted the course for our future and we are continuing to create our legacy with pride, commitment, expertise, and unwavering devotion to the care of older people. Thirty-four years later, Berman and Thornlow, writing in that same journal, gave student nurses this advice:

> The opportunities for making a difference in geriatric nursing are endless. . . . There are no limits to what you can do in geriatric nursing. . . . As the number of older adults continues to rise, geriatric nursing opportunities will grow in leaps and bounds to meet the specialized health care needs of this population. . . . The time is right for you to become expert in geriatric nursing. (2005, pp. 25–26)

CHAPTER TWO

Geriatric Nurse Pioneers and Their Contributions

NURSES AT WAR

Nurses must often ferret out their origins and growth through thoughtful analyses of histories of wars and women. Both in reality and symbolically the gains in geriatric care have been as those of a war. We are privileged to have a wealth of data from the words and writings of geriatric nurses as they experienced the origins and growth of the specialty.

Most of the geriatric nurse pioneers in the United States began to appear in practice, academia, publishing, workshops, and conferences in the 1960s and early 1970s. We consider these the pioneers, although from the background in chapter 1 it is apparent that there were singular contributions and tentative efforts decades before. It is well known that we all build upon the work of those gone before us and "stand on their shoulders" as we progress. This chapter is designed to bring to the awareness of nurses, other professionals, and interested lay persons the foundations of geriatric nursing through some of the experience of its founders. We find them inspirational and hope our readers will as well.

To focus on the development of geriatric nurse pioneers in the health and illness arena one must look first at World War II. In that era the effects of war on the status of women was profound. Women took on civilian jobs to release men for war service. Youth, idealism, and their sense of adventure drew nurses to those in danger and need.

A very special group of particularly adventurous nurses emerged in the decades of the 1940s and 1950s. These nurses were quick to go to the battlegrounds to care for the ill and the casualties of the war. They preceded the MASH units and, in fact, preceded even the use of helicopter evacuation in most cases. The first jungle evacuation of the wounded occurred in Burma, toward the end of World War II, to transport the wounded when they were surrounded by enemy forces. Most of this was being done by L5 and L1 aircraft in the most difficult terrain and impossible airstrips (Zahorsky, 1989). Emerging from the devastation was a group of exceptionally strong-minded, capable, courageous, executive nurses. They could slog through mud, literally and figuratively, stand tall and stay on duty while under fire, and create hospitals where none existed. The humane concerns that drew them to care for these individuals, considered expendable, remained a driving force in the souls of many (Norman, 1999).

When the war was over many of those nurses did not return to the suburban housewife ideal of the 1950s but rather followed the call of their spirit: Some followed husbands who remained in the service, some sought positions in rehabilitation of returning veterans, some fought the wars of poverty and neglect, some went to public health service, most eventually entered academe and contributed to the knowledge and specificity of nursing education. Some had no biologic children but numerous ones in the profession. Their students became their progeny.

In the 1940s and 1950s the ill elderly were as abandoned as the wounded in Guadalcanal (Norman, 1999). They were expendable and of little interest to a nation embroiled in war and progress. The focus was on youth and the returning veterans. The old held no special position in the hearts of the nation. Some of the old and demented were housed in restored chicken coops; some existed in the back rooms of private homes, sometimes within isolated corners of institutions. Many were shuttled off to the back wards of psychiatric institutions.

All of the pioneers on whom we focus eventually directed their considerable energies to caring for the old. They came by many different routes. This select "band of angels" saw the neglected battlefield of the old and determined to care for their wounds and provide succor in the overgrown jungles of pain and chronic disability. Indeed, many advances in geriatric care are outgrowths of the technology of rehabilitation for injured veterans.

Bernita Steffl (see later in this chapter) says, "Some of the big changes in the professionalizing of nursing came about, or were greatly influenced, by the return of the World War II nurses to civilian life. Many of these strong minded women who had reached leadership positions in the military had visions of a more independent leadership role for nurses. Many went on for higher education using the benefits of the G.I. Bill of Education, and then into academia and took major roles in the development of collegiate status for nurses" (Steffl, 2004).

Mary Opal Wolanin

There are numerous outstanding individuals, but Mary Opal Wolanin provides the quintessential example: During her stint in the Army Air Force she married her husband, Tiger Wolanin, a career Army Air Force officer. She went with him from one base to another, working as a nurse wherever they were stationed. In the varied geographic and institutional situations she encountered, an awareness of the neglect of the old began to dominate her thoughts. She noted how the skill and dedication of the "pneumonia nurse" meant the difference between life and death for many elders. She also saw the total medical apathy demonstrated toward victims of stroke. They were simply ignored and forgotten. Those with dementia were stored in back wards of mental hospitals. Their civil rights were wantonly trampled.

Mary Opal Browne was born in Chrisney, Indiana, on November 1, 1910. Edwin Browne was homesteading a piece of land in the province of Saskatchewan, Canada. Florence Abbott Browne gave birth to Mary Opal at her parents' home in Indiana in order for her to be a United States citizen. There were two other girls before Florence divorced Edwin, moved back to Indiana, and later married a Kansas wheat farmer. Mary Opal began her "platform activities at the age of eight with roles in plays, programs and operettas as well as public speaking" (Wolanin, 1989, p. 1).

Mary Opal was studious and read every book available to her. While in a small rural high school in Westphalia, Kansas, she read about "trained nurses" and dreamed of becoming a romantic figure in a white uniform and cap and a red-lined navy blue cape just like the one in the World War I poster. After high school she was prepared, according to 1927 standards, to teach in a rural school and taught the first seven primary grades in a one-room school in Cottonwood, Kansas. She carefully saved money and entered Kansas City General Hospital School of Nursing in Kansas City, Missouri, in 1928. Unique for that era, courses were taught in a university. Upon graduation in 1931, Mary Opal was not yet old enough to take the RN Board examination, so she went to Cook County Hospital School of Nursing in Chicago and took a 6-month course in psychiatric nursing, then a very avant garde element of nursing curricula. Miss Fabin, her teacher, inspired her lifelong interest in psychiatric nursing.

When she finally was able to take her Boards the Great Depression made jobs scarce and she took one in a 10-bed hospital in Appleton City, Missouri. She dealt with everything, including typhoid fever and pneumonia epidemics. After 2 years she returned to school at Washington University in St. Louis to complete her college education. In the years that followed she worked as a "trail nurse" with a wilderness pack outfit, a tuberculosis nurse, and a surgical nurse until she was called up from the U.S. Reserves and in March of 1941 became a Second Lieutenant in the Army Nurse Corps (Fig. 2.1).

On October 29, 1942, she married HJ-Tiger Wolanin and left the Army Nurse Corps but followed Tiger in his assignments whenever possible. In 1944 she was in Mississippi teaching in a Cadet Nurse program

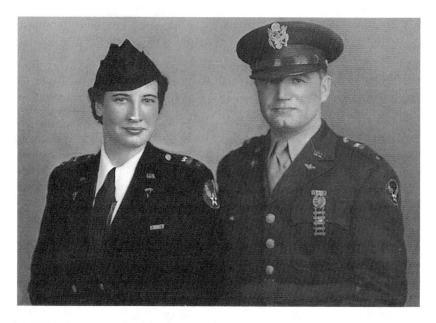

FIGURE 2.1 Mary Opal Wolanin and H. J. Tiger Wolanin after marriage in 1942.

and for the first time becoming fully aware of the discrimination of blacks. By 1947 she was in Arizona caring for Indians with tuberculosis. When Tiger returned from Okinawa and was assigned to an airforce base near Omaha, Mary Opal taught at the University of Nebraska school of Nursing. Back in Tucson with Tiger in 1951, she returned to school and obtained her bachelor's degree at the University of Arizona. There she learned about Hispanics and learned their language. Tiger was assigned to various places around the United States but Mary Opal remained in their home in Tucson for the next 36 years, except for a brief stint with Tiger in Florida where she worked with migrant families. In 1957 she began teaching at the University of Arizona, completed her master's degree in 1963, and remained there until she retired. During this time she continued to go to school part time working toward a doctorate until studies were interrupted by Tiger's stroke. She learned about stroke rehabilitation and developed a lasting interest in stroke care. It was then that her interest began to center on the care of the older person. Her appointment in 1968 to the Regional Medical Program resulted in a study of nursing homes and long-term care needs in Arizona. In 1973 she developed one of the first graduate programs in geriatric nursing at the University of Arizona while also beginning her research into confusion that resulted in publication of her classic text, *Confusion: Prevention and Care*, published by Mosby in 1981 (Fig. 2.2).

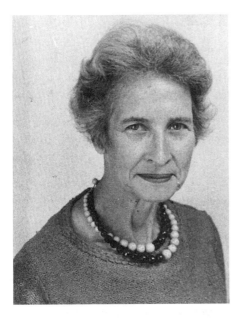

FIGURE 2.2 Mary Opal Wolanin at University of Arizona.

She provided consultation in gerontology and gerontological nursing in 37 states and seven countries. She funded monetary awards for Excellence in Gerontological Nursing Research at the University of Arizona and six other colleges in an effort to stimulate nurse scholars to study the problems of the aged. Her expertise was needed and was sought nationally and internationally until in 1985 her health problems and Tiger's frailty ended her speaking career. In 1987 they moved to the retirement center at Air Force Village II in San Antonio, Texas. Many of her devotees then went to her for counsel and encouragement and in addition she was the resident expert in the care of the aged. In 1988, a National Gerontological Nurses Association (NGNA) Scholarship was established and named in her honor. In 1990 she was awarded an Honorary Doctor of Science Degree by the University of Arizona based on her distinguished contributions in establishing gerontology and gerontological nursing as educational and research pursuits throughout this country. In 1996 she was inducted into the American Nursing Association's (ANA's) Hall of Fame (Fig. 2.3).

Gleanings From a Personal Interview With Mary Opal (1987, 1989)

"I didn't come into this field because as a child I loved old folks. I didn't know many old folks and I didn't have a chance to love them. Would I have loved them? I don't know. I wonder how many nurses came in by

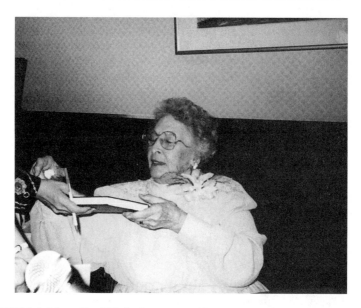

FIGURE 2.3 Mary Opal Wolanin autographing text, *Confusion: Prevention and Care*, 1982.

the back door as I did. If we were really truthful how many of us considered working with the elderly when we were thirty?

"When I was an 18-year-old student, I particularly remember one person with a fractured hip. She was put in a Thomas splint made of metal and covered with leather. She stayed on her back for a long time. I had a feeling of defeat as we knew so little about caring for older people. It never occurred to us that we were caring for an elderly woman with a fractured hip. Now we know that it isn't a 'fractured hip' but a *person* who has lived a long life, acquired certain idiosyncrasies and attitudes, certain feelings about right and wrong and definite feelings about themselves and their bodies.

"We have often missed the problems of the older person that come with illness, the depression, the loss of self-esteem, the loss of their feeling about their own body and the ability to trust that it will do as it always has. It was a very long time before I developed these insights. I still think hands on care, critically examined, is the only way we can really learn about older people. We must stop and look at what is happening to them and what's happening to ourselves and how we relate to them.

"I think the art of listening is the most important thing we nurses have. I call it an act of love when two people are on the same wave length, listening to the same thing intently. It's a new bond, it takes the two of them off somewhere if only for 3 minutes. It will never exist again. Just for that short time the two of you are really sharing and hearing what the other is saying and thinking. It's the most wonderful feeling to know that someone really understands you; it's really an act of love.

"How can we handle a world in which we are always playing Santa Claus and that's what we are doing, trying to make an unreal world. We like to see people get better but it is also a rule of life that people die. I think we have to be able to see that helping someone to die a good death is also a very satisfying experience and we are beginning to see a lot more of that. The hospice movement has helped a great deal.

"When I was a patient in Methodist hospital I had one particular LVN, a black nurse named Lois, who took care of me. I had a lot of quirky things happen to me and she could handle them. I felt like there wasn't anything so bad that Lois would be surprised by and that she couldn't take care of. It was a wonderful feeling to know that there was someone on my side like that. For awhile we heard a lot about advocates until it became a cliché but we should be advocates. I don't mean going around preaching about things but when the time comes, we should be on their side. Who stands up for this person who is having a hard time expressing themselves, who has just given up, who is too depressed to even try anymore. Who is their advocate? Even though you are a nurse, it is so different when it's your mother or father, or your own husband. When Tiger was in danger of a ruptured gall bladder and confused, I had to sign the consent form for surgery. As he went out the door on the stretcher, into surgery he said, 'Are we sure this is necessary?' I had awful forebodings. I thought he didn't want to go and I would have given anything to have someone to talk to me that minute and tell me I had done the only thing I could do as I could not let him die of a ruptured gall bladder.

"Neophytes are probably not the ones to begin geriatric care. I feel strongly that we need to attract the more mature nurses to caring for the elderly. If we set gerontological nursing aside as a highly skilled practice that only certain people could qualify for after considerable nursing experience it would add prestige to the field. It is the most skilled nursing one can do. I think it has to be an addition to the basic program. I would not go so far as to say we should have only master's prepared nurses but I do feel that in every course we give gerontological nursing content should be given. Child development should include both ends of the life cycle. I also think that every now and then we have to take a sabbatical from whatever we are doing, take time off and look at what's happening. I don't think we can do much without hands on experience but then need time to sit and contemplate and writing things down is one good way to contemplate. I found writing very gratifying" (Wolanin, 1990).

A reviewer of this manuscript commented that we need to consider these things in the present, just as in Wolanin's era.

In 1984, Cynthia Kelly wrote a piece for *Geriatric Nursing* about Mary Opal Wolanin, summarizing her many accomplishments and professional recognitions, ending with a lovely simile. "It is tempting to compare this nurse to a diamond, that many-faceted sparkling stone. Her favorite gem, however, is the opal. Her hobby is polishing the rare stones, making them into very special gifts. And like the luminous opal, this woman characteristically sheds a serene and steady glow. But just as a fine opal can display brilliant fire when held to the light, so Mary Opal can explode in fiery wrath, verbal and written, when she is lit up by any evidence of injustice or dishonesty. Long may she shine!" (Kelly, 1984, p. 340).

Memories of Mary Opal Wolanin

Mary Opal Wolanin died May 22, 1997. She was to geriatric nursing as Florence Nightingale was to organized nursing, and, indeed, Mrs. Wolanin sometimes noted that in only two lifetimes nursing has become what it is today. Florence Nightingale was born in 1820 and died in 1910; Mary Opal Wolanin was born in 1910 and died in 1997. She had thought she might complete her cycle in the year 2000 but that was not to be. Yet, she, like Florence, will remain with us always because of the strength and wisdom of their personalities.

Mary Opal's inherent dignity did not welcome first-name intimacy from strangers and passing acquaintances. She was proud of being Tiger's wife and Mrs. Wolanin. Those who attempted to intrude into her life too quickly were not welcomed. One story demonstrates this quite nicely. A young gerontologist who was learning about sex and aging asked, "Would you mind discussing your sexuality with me?" Mrs. Wolanin immediately replied, "I certainly would mind." She could be aloof but instantly compassionate when she sensed the need.

Mary Opal had little tolerance for carelessness or inefficiency. One anecdote illustrates this. Mary Opal often shared a hotel room with Cynthia Kelly when traveling. In one instance, she called the registration desk to let them know her husband would be calling. They did not have her name on the list of guests. She became rather irate and said, "What do you think my husband will say when he calls and finds I'm not here!" To the chagrin of the reservation agent and the amusement of Cynthia and Mary Opal the room charge was deleted (Ebersole, 1997). Mary Opal also kept a "Feudin' File" of situations she felt were unjust or needed pursuing. Some were rather tongue-in-cheek issues and amusing; some she took seriously.

Mrs. Wolanin not only advanced geriatric nursing in numerous ways but was the cardinal gerontine, having begun her career in geriatric nursing on retirement. She often said, "I made most of my major contributions after I was 70 years old." She had numerous students, proteges, and devoted friends and colleagues worldwide. She is sorely missed.

In retirement, Mary Opal Wolanin "took on the world full-time" (Phillips, 1997, p. 233). She established Awards of Excellence in several universities; gave speeches; and wrote books, journal articles, and essays intended to improve the care of frail and vulnerable elderly through research, education, and practice.

"Mary Opal and I shared many things. We wrote, traveled and gave presentations together. We talked and laughed a lot. She saw me through illnesses, personal upheaval, new jobs, setbacks and my father's death. She was always there for me and for others who shared her life. She was devoted to her husband and committed to her work. She taught me more about generosity and compassion than any person I have ever known. Once I asked how I could repay her. She said, 'Do it for someone else. Pass it on'" (Phillips, 1997, p. 233).

"Mary Opal left many legacies—her work, her determination, her generosity, and her love. Among her finest legacies, however, was her philosophy—'Pass it on.' I think if she wanted to be remembered for anything, it would be that" (Phillips, 1997, p. 233).

Mary Opal and Bea Steffl frequently worked together giving workshops in Arizona and enjoyed and learned from each other. Here are some memories from Bea Steffl:

"Some memories that stand out: in the 1970s, at one of the first meetings of the Arizona Nurses Geriatric Nursing Council, Mary Opal practically pounded the table when I suggested we change the name to *Gerontological* versus *Geriatric* because gerontological included the well older person as well as the 'geriatric' sick older person. She said, 'Let's call it what it is!!' We often laughed about that later and she, as well as the ANA, enlarged the concept to gerontological" (Steffl, 1997, pp. 233–234).

"One day in Seattle we were celebrating her birthday with a brunch in the hotel; we commented on, and later shopped for, the wonderful Washington apples. Mary Opal told us about those Spitzenbergs. I've never again been able to find them. We had numerous wonderful hour-long telephone visits when we cussed and discussed what was happening in gerontology and nursing education. Most of all, I always think about how she made each of us feel like a special, cherished friend, and, indeed, she had the capacity to make each of us special in some way. I will miss her" (Steffl, 1997, pp. 233–234).

"To Mary Opal, From Virginia Burggraf"

"The nursing world has lost one of its heroines, advocates, leaders and trailblazers. I have lost a dear friend, adopted mother, and mentor. I will miss our visits, which mapped out the future of gerontological nursing through research, education, and practice, as well as our vision for addressing confusion as an illness that can be prevented. . . . Your soft voice would empower me as I recall your words, 'Virginia, you need to . . . ,' while my vision would emerge as my eyes watered. . . . Although my faith has made it easy to imagine that the heavens are indeed blessed since you arrived, it will be difficult to grieve your earthly loss" (Burggraf, 1997, p. 234).

Doris Schwartz

Doris's career parallels the history of gerontology (*American Nurse*, 1989). She says, "When I was starting out in nursing 50 years ago there was no such thing as gerontological nursing." She first heard the terms after completing her duty in the Army Nurse Corps during World War II. "Older patients were generally thought of as adults who just happened to have lived a long time. The idea that caring for them required a special body of knowledge never crossed my mind" (*American Nurse*, 1989, p. 6). "I came into nursing at a time of its greatest development, its fastest development. Everything in nursing, in technology and in opportunity has changed in the 50 years that I have been a nurse" (Schwartz, 1990a).

Doris was born on May 30, 1915, and her earliest years were spent in Brooklyn. Her father emigrated from Vienna, Austria when he was 16 years old, expecting to join a great uncle as a candymaker. This did not work out and he spent his working life making wooden baskets until his death in 1926. Her parents were hard-working, thrifty people but her father had a charming tradition of saving "cherry money." During the weeks when cherries were ripe he would buy them in bulk, use the rejected wood and basket splints from the factory to construct unusual baskets, fill them with cherries, and sell them door-to-door. The "cherry money" was divided equally among her father, mother, brother Don, and herself. This could be used frivolously or in any way they chose. Doris kept that tradition throughout her life and when earning "cherry money" through writing, speaking, or consulting she would spend it to assist her "foster families" or other personal special projects (Schwartz, 1995).

"I grew up close to a colorful and strongly opinionated group of aunts and uncles—siblings of my mother. They lived long lives, and I shared in the care of the oldest of them, both in hospitals and at home, during the middle and later years of my own career. Six of them became recipients of geriatric care, and three of the six lived into their nineties. They provided a fine collection of personal preceptors, always quick to clarify for me what they thought 'a nurse ought to know,' either about how to give personal care or about becoming older" (Schwartz, 1990b).

Doris took her basic nursing education at Methodist Hospital in Brooklyn, 1939–1942, and bachelor's and master's degrees from New York University. While at Methodist Hospital she and the other fledgling nurses cared for Methodist missionaries from all over the world. They were great storytellers and deeply religious. The experiences with these missionaries and her mother's nine long-lived siblings made her very aware of the potential for independence of older people (Ebersole, 1997b).

Doris Schwartz was another nurse veteran of the war. Recruitment of military nurses was managed by the Red Cross Nursing Reserve and she was called up in 1943. She spent 1 year at Mitchell Field on Long Island, New York, and on V-J day in 1945 was assigned to the U.S Army Nurse Corps on the hospital ship *Marigold* in the Pacific Theater. The *Marigold* was the first American ship to enter Japanese waters and cared for hundreds of allied prisoners released from Japanese detention camps (Knollmueller, 1998, p. 68). From her journal dated September 2, 1945, Yokohama Harbor, "The morning peace was signed aboard the *Missouri* in the harbor of the bay. The eyes of the whole world were on this spot, and landing barges poured wave after wave of troops ashore in never ending lines" (Schwartz, 1995, p. 22).

The final months of her service were spent at the Percy Jones Army Rehabilitation Center at the General Hospital in Battle Creek, Michigan; Doris was discharged as a captain. Following that there was a period as a nurse in the Visiting Nurse Services of New York (VNSNY) at Red Hook on the Brooklyn waterfront. "The experience was rich with low-income, multiethnic individuals, immigrants who seldom spoke English. All had numerous health problems. There were also a group of aged merchant seamen too old or to sick to work who lived in 'flophouses' and a few grandparents that lived with their families on the crowded deck houses of narrow barges which plied the canals of New York State" (Ebersole, 1997b, p. 815).

Doris joined the faculty of Cornell-New York Hospital School of Nursing in 1951. Cornell had many innovative programs, one of which was the Cornell-Navajo Field Health Project initiated in 1955. Her love of public health nursing and concern for the neglected and underserved led her to a stint in Arizona with the U.S. Bureau of Indian Affairs. She kept a fascinating journal of that experience. In the early 1970s she co-directed the family nurse practitioner program at Cornell and then in 1976, the Primex program to prepare geriatric nurse practitioners. In 1975 she completed a Fogarty Fellowship for study of geriatric care at University of Glasgow, Scotland, under the direction of Sir Ferguson Anderson. Sir Ferguson Anderson occupied the first chair for geriatrics in the world, the Cargill Chair at Glasgow University, Scotland, established in 1965. The year with Sir Ferguson Anderson gave her many of the ideas she brought to the Primex program. Robin Kennedy, her preceptor at Glasgow, was an exchange physician in the United States in 1976; together they formulated and developed the course, held at Burk Rehabilitation Center, an arm of the Cornell Medical Center. In 1980 she received the Pearl McIver Public Health Nurse Award and after 29 years at Cornell planned to retire.

Shortly before that much-anticipated time she suffered a stroke and required a lengthy rehabilitation period. However, after recovery she spent 10 years as Senior Fellow at the School of Nursing, University of Pennsylvania, playing an advisory role to the Robert Wood Johnson Foundation Teaching Nursing Home Project. At the 100th anniversary of the VNSNY she was awarded the Lillian D. Wald Spirit of Nursing Award for her numerous contributions and dedication to public health nursing. Doris was a Charter Fellow of the American Academy of Nursing (AAN) and in 1997 was declared a Living Legend by the AAN (Fig. 2.4).

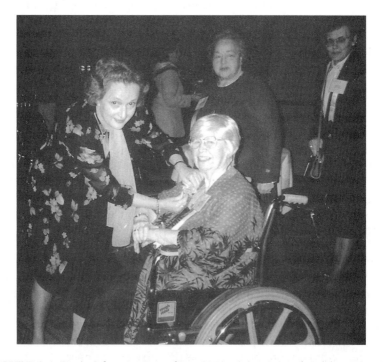

FIGURE 2.4 Doris Schwartz (seated) at ANA Living Legend Celebration with Neville Strumpf.

A Personal Interview With Doris Schwartz

Doris says she never decided to enter gerontic nursing. She simply saw more and more older people and recognized their nursing and social needs and was encouraged by George Reeder, a professor and director of the program at Cornell, to apply for the Fogarty Fellowship at the National Institutes of Health. It had been awarded previously only to physicians and senior scientists, but Doris was undaunted and applied.

"Thelma Wells and I worked together in Scotland with Sir Ferguson Anderson. . . . I had a wonderful time in Scotland with Sir Ferguson. . . . I worked there on the inpatient service with him. In Scottish hospitals there is a public health nurse assigned to every geriatric service, who follows patients in their homes and acts as a liaison between staff of the Queen's Visiting Nursing Service and the nurses and doctors on the inpatient units" (Schwartz, 1990a).

"Immediately upon my return I was appointed cochairman of the geriatric nursing practitioner program. Some of the people from the Kellogg GNP program were in our first class. There were no geriatric nurse practitioners at that time and no role models so we on the faculty were it. We, a doctor and nurse team, had to go with them. I worked with a Dr. Seligman and he taught other doctors how to work with them and Marge Miller and I taught the students how to work with doctors. Nurses had to be taught when to seek medical consultation and doctors need to know when to seek nursing consultation. . . . An interesting thing turned up repeatedly . . . and that was a great feeling of triumph in the young nurse whose patient told her or him something that the doctor had not known about the patient. There is a tendency, probably a normal human tendency, to want to rush over to the doctor and say, 'Yaa, yaa, look what I found out that you don't know!' Trying to help the student physician and the student nurse to understand their education teaches them to look for different things and the differences are valuable. . . . I would like to see every student nurse paired with an experienced physician and later with a medical student and given the opportunity to work with a couple of very difficult patients during the early part of their education and I *sure* would like to see that happen with *every* nurse practitioner."

At Cornell, the nurse practitioner programs were financed through a Primex Public Health service program. This arrangement included the provision that nurses from hospital schools, 2-year programs, and baccalaureate programs were all to be included. The government sent Peace Corps nurses, Mountain States Health Corporation sent nurses from nursing homes, and others came from various backgrounds. "This was 1972. The groups were small, 15 or 16 students. Mistakes were made, some were *sent* by their employers. We gathered in a most exciting group of people" (Schwartz, 1990a).

After retirement from Cornell and when working with the group at University of Pennsylvania, Doris visited numbers of nursing homes to assess their suitability for students and was "horrified at the amount of restraint that I saw being used. I couldn't believe that the increase in restraints was of the magnitude that it was since I had been teaching in the 1970s and 1980s. It was much worse. I talked about this with the Penn faculty. . . . In 1984 or 1985 I wrote to the editor of *Geriatric Nursing* spelling out how troubled I was at the tremendous overuse of restraints."

Doris's concern was published and she agreed to act as a "clearing house" for information from nurses who were doing something about this. She received a tremendous number of letters, mostly from staff nurses, equally as distressed as she. Neville Strumpf and Lois Evans took on the investigation and by 1990 some alternatives were being tested. Doris felt she had planted the seed for research into the problem that was now bearing fruit.

"My relationship and work with the people at the University of Pennsylvania has just been a pure, a golden streak in my life." Mathy Mezey had approached her saying, "Help me. You taught geriatric nurse practitioners. I never have. What do I need to do with this curriculum to make it possible for nurses to be concerned with all stages of the health care of older patients and really focus on their needs? . . . Mathy Mezey is a dream of a geriatric nurse, a dream of a person and she could teach anything to anybody. She built that course into what I think is the most superb course for geriatric, gerontic, gerontological nurses . . . whatever term . . . in the country.

"I resigned as of my 75th birthday which was the end of the term in June 1990."

Doris was given a 75th birthday party with students and faculty from many departments at Penn in addition to friends from Foulkeways. She was ostensibly retired and lived at Foulkeways, the Friend's life care community near Philadelphia. An announcement was made of a new chair in Gerontological Nursing to be named the Doris Schwartz chair. "I sat there with tears coming down my face and with a silly grin underneath the tears and I just couldn't believe it" (Schwartz, 1990a). An excerpt from a letter to Foulkeways residents, March 18, 1996, seems pertinent here, "and I sat where they sat and remained there astonished among them" (Ezekiel 3:15).

At the time of my interview, her newest concern was for elders who were caring for developmentally disabled adults and children. Those who previously died in childhood were now living much longer and their care was being provided by aged parents. "We have no place that can replace the care that they have given and, sad as its sounds, their prayer is really, 'If only he would die before I do'" (Schwartz, 1990b).

Her belief about student education is that their very first experience should be with healthy older people. "They would then learn to listen." She believed an early experience in acute care gives them a distorted view. "Then I'd like to see either an elective or a required course at the senior end of the experience in which those who became interested in older people would have an opportunity to do a more specialized and a more knowledgeable kind of nursing. . . . It is not our job to change older people but to help them be able to live as one wants to live and as one's personhood and basic experiences prepare one to live as long as one finds it possible, while moving from one plateau of life to another, one plateau of illness to another, gently, comfortable and to remain part of the world about them. This is what I think is terribly important" (Schwartz, 1990a).

Even now, more than a decade later, the lucidity and orderliness of Doris's thoughts, as expressed on tape and video, stun me.

Doris says, "The purpose of gerontological nursing is not to save lives, but to prevent untimely death and needless suffering. Both these goals include respect for human dignity—the preservation of personhood as long as life continues" (*American Nurse*, 1989, p. 6).

In Memory of Doris Schwartz

Doris Schwartz died at Foulkeways, August 22, 1999. Doris was featured as a Geriatric Nurse Leader in the January/February 1998 issue of *Geriatric Nursing* and in the July/August 1986 issue of *Geriatric Nursing*, then under the editorship of Cynthia Kelly. Her accomplishments, so varied and absorbing, were awesome, a geriatric nurse icon long before her death. Obituaries in *The New York Times* (8/28/99) and the *Philadelphia Inquirer* (8/28/99) featured some of the highlights of her life. The *Philadelphia Inquirer* noted that the diaries of her service in the Army Nurse Corps are stored in the Army's Military History Center in Washington, D.C.

I first heard of Doris when I was directing the Kellogg Foundation Geriatric Nurse Practitioner Project in 1981. But, Doris never retired. Until a month before her death she was busy participating in an Alzheimer's support group and a stroke support group at Foulkeways. In addition she was heavily involved in the work of the Friend's Meeting to provide assistance for elders taking care of adult children with developmental disabilities.

It is impossible to say what impressed me most about Doris but I believe it was her hardy and hearty outlook. Her last decade was exceedingly physically challenging but that did not keep her out of action. Frequently she would send short pieces to *Geriatric Nursing* about particular approaches to nursing care that she wished to share with our readers. The last time I saw Doris was at a GSA meeting in Philadelphia in 1998. She was as vital as always and there to attend the presentation to Cornelia Beck of the Doris Schwartz Research Award. Doris's legacy lives on in the Doris Schwartz Award given annually at the Gerontological Society of America convention. This award, perhaps the most prestigious in geriatric nursing, recognizes nurses of national and international prominence.

Doris wrote her memoirs in an autobiography published by Springer in 1995, "My fifty years in nursing," *Give Us to Go Blithely.*

Thanks to the marvelous curators of the Nursing History Library at University of Pennsylvania in Philadelphia, under the guidance of archivist Joan Lynaugh, the Doris Schwartz historic records are beautifully cataloged and preserved. In these archives I discovered that Doris, as a young woman, had routinely corresponded with Mary Beard, the wife of the famous historian James Beard. Doris was much more than a nurse, she was a humanitarian and even then aware of history and politics and sharing her ideas about the way things should be. In her honor, the Doris Schwartz Gerontological Nursing Research Award has been established by the John A. Hartford Foundation and the Gerontological Society of America (Fig. 2.5).

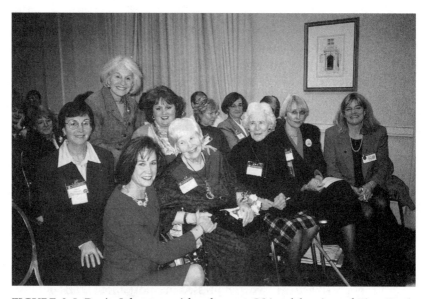

FIGURE 2.5 Doris Schwartz with others at GSA celebration of First Doris Schwartz Gerontological Nursing Research Award to Cornelia Beck. Left to right: Diane Mahoney, Mathy Mezey (standing), Cornelia Beck holding Doris Schwartz's hand, Cynthia Kelly, Terry Fulmer on the end.

Irene Burnside

Irene is probably best known for inspiring many of the next generation of nurses with her unstinting generosity, mentoring, and encouraging neophyte geriatric nurses, sharing opportunities to work with her, and sending us out to teach. Her focus on the psychosocial aspects of elder care was a new idea when she entered the field and began writing about it. She was particularly interested in elders with dementia and helped us understand there was meaning in whatever they were doing or saying. She led small groups of these elders and mentored us as we led similar groups.

"Irene Mortenson Burnside was born in Grove City, Minnesota, on October 4, 1923, the daughter of Walter Hollyer and Rebecca (Wortz) Mortenson. She lived with relatives in rural Minnesota after the age of 5 due to her mother's poor health and her parents' separation. Irene received elementary education in a one-room country school. It was Irene's aunt who nurtured both her astute awareness of environments and her passion for the fine arts, while her high school teacher Abigail Quigley McCarthy (former wife of Eugene McCarthy) instilled the importance of writing well, lessons she remembers fondly" (Bullough & Sentz, 2000, p. 39).

In 1941, Irene enrolled at age 17 in the diploma nurses training program at the Ancker Hospital School of Nursing in St. Paul, Minnesota, and joined the United States Cadet Nurse Corps as soon as it became available in 1943.

Women as young as 17 years old were eligible to join and were then provided tuition, books, a stipend, and a uniform with the provision that after completion they would serve for the duration of the war in a civilian or military hospital, the Indian Health Service, or other public health facility (Robinson & Perry, 2001).

The U.S. Cadet Nurse Corps comprised the largest and youngest group of uniformed women to serve their country during World War II. It existed during the years 1943–1948, under the auspices of the United States Public Health Service (USPHS). Lucile Petry (later Leone) was appointed director of the Corps. By October 15, 1945, 179,000 women had joined the Corps and 124,065 nurses were graduated from the 1,125 participating schools of nursing (U.S. Federal Security Agency, 1950).

During the last 3 months of nurses' training Irene had a rotation in psychiatric nursing care where she found the back wards filled with demented old people. She was made much more aware of the need for geropsychiatric care and this had a major impact on her future direction (Garand & Buckwalter, 1996). Irene graduated in 1944 but had to wait the few months until she was 21 to take the Minnesota State Board of Nursing Examination.

Irene was promptly called into action in the Army Nurse Corps and served in Okinawa and Osaka, Japan. She met her husband, Dean, while in the Corps and was married in 1946, after their discharges. She was a First Lieutenant when discharged. They had three children: Mark, Tonya, and Clark. Irene worked at various nursing jobs, but found shift work and child care expenses onerous. She decided to pursue her interest in the arts and enrolled in Denver University in Denver, Colorado, and was awarded a Fine Arts Degree in 1957. The family moved to Martinez, California, where she worked part time at the Contra Costa County Health Department and then at the Veterans Administration Hospital in Martinez. In 1966 she began graduate education and earned a Master of Science Degree in Nursing and a year later, a Post Master's Certificate in Adult Psychiatric Nursing, both from the University of California, San Francisco.

During her post master's education she conducted therapeutic group sessions for older persons. Irene led group therapy sessions in nursing homes from 1967 until 1969, resulting in publications with guidelines for group work with the elderly (Burnside, 1983, 1994; Burnside & Schmidt, 1994), and a life-long interest in reminiscence and its many benefits. In 2004, Haight and Gibson authored the 4th edition of *Working With Older Adults: Group Process and Techniques.* In 1995 Barbara Haight and Irene were the founding members and established the International Society for Reminiscence and Life Review. She continued to serve the Society on a continuing basis, organizing and giving presentations until her death.

Irene's pioneering work with the aged in groups attracted attention and she was invited to join the nursing faculty at University of California, San Francisco, in 1967. Her husband, Dean, died in 1970 and a new dimension was added to her sensitivity. From 1970 until 1972 she spent her summers at the Ethel Percy Andrus Gerontology Center, University of Southern California in Los Angeles, learning more about aging and gerontological research. From that grew a position as Coordinator of Nursing Education at the Ethel Percy Andrus Gerontology Center from 1976 until 1979, then under the direction of James Birren. In addition, she was writing, lecturing worldwide, conducting research, and encouraging others to enter the dynamically growing field. Her landmark text, *Nursing and the Aged,* was published in 1976 and was followed by two more editions (Fig. 2.6).

Her quest for more knowledge and research led her to the University of Texas School of Nursing doctoral program, in Austin, Texas. At the age of 66 Irene graduated with a PhD in Nursing. President George H. W. Bush was the commencement speaker and singled her and two others out to show that age is not a deterrent to educational achievement. In 1994 she was selected, as one of the most distinguished graduates, to give the commemorative address at the 50th anniversary of the Cadet Nurse

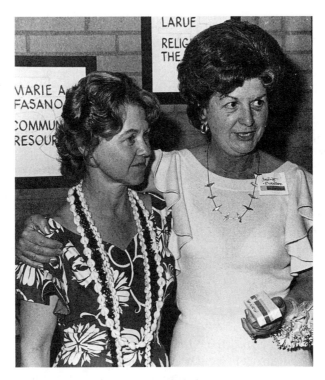

FIGURE 2.6 Priscilla Ebersole with Irene Burnside at USC party to celebrate publication of *Nursing and the Aged*.

Corps. Irene moved to Los Gatos, California, and taught at San Jose State University until her retirement.

Much of the evolution of geropsychiatric care and psychosocial nursing care during the past 50 years can be attributed to the extensive influence of Irene Burnside. In addition, her early upbringing by her grandfather had a lasting influence on her understanding of the aged. In personal correspondence with Linda Garand and Kathleen Buckwalter she shared some of her early years. Always adaptive and with an active imagination, she set up a schoolroom in a closet of her grandfather's house and taught piano lessons, using an accordion, to imaginary students. "I was a little kid in a closet, emulating a teacher. The nurse was on one side (of me) and the teacher on the other. I would make exams and grade papers. Relatives would let me have one shelf in the closet as my desk. It was a world I created for myself, a type of escape" (Garand & Buckwalter, 1996, p. 215). One of her aunts was a nurse, the first in the family to finish high school. They would often take long "nature" walks. Decades later, Irene took her students on nature walks to sharpen their observational skills and appreciation of the world around them. Her aunt's influence on Irene was profound and instilled in her determination not only to finish high school but to continue on to college. She credits her with laying the foundation of her career as a nurse and nurse educator.

Irene's awards, journal articles, and books are numerous and have been translated into many languages. Her influence has been felt throughout the world as she has presented speeches and provided consultation. Throughout her career, Irene focused on the psychosocial needs of elders, bringing and mentoring nurses into the field of geriatric nursing. Her contributions are far too numerous to list but it is clear that the writing lessons instilled by Ms. Abigail Quigley McCarthy bore productive fruit throughout her life.

The Premier Issue of *Geriatric Nursing* featured an article by Irene (Why Work With the Aged?) in which she mentions the educators, trailblazers, those who have led many into the work. Irene writes, "We just must communicate this sense of creative excitement and opportunity to students and to nurses, along with the sense of the great need for them and the rewards of the career" (Burnside, 1980, p. 33) (Fig. 2.7).

Memories of Irene Mortenson Burnside

From Priscilla Ebersole: Irene Renay Mortenson Burnside died on April 12, 2003, while living in San Diego. We first met in 1971, while as a student in the master's program at University of California, San Francisco, I

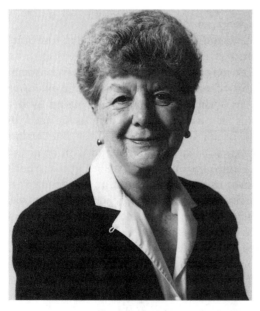

FIGURE 2.7 Irene Burnside.

enrolled in Irene's gerontological research class. There were few of us, which made it a double blessing. We read the gerontological research papers that had been published and presented our written critiques each week. There wasn't an abundance of them. I had never had such thoughtful comments on my written work: clear, astute, but always gentle. The disengagement theory (Cumming & Henry, 1961) was being ferociously argued at that time and I thought the theorists propounding continued active involvement were correct. (I was 43 years old!) Now, with age and more insight personally and professionally, I know there is no correct path for anyone. Each makes his or her own based upon health (yes, health comes first), energy level, wealth, personality bent, and opportunity. The class had great enthusiasm for our theory discussions. Bernice Neugarten's, *Middle Age and Aging* (1968) was our primary text.

I was simultaneously doing reminiscence groups at the Veterans Administration Hospital in Palo Alto, California, with Irene's guidance. When she suggested I take my group skills to a nursing home and do a reminiscence group workshop I was simply dumbfounded. Nancy McEuen was then a Surveyor for the State of California and thought she should bring something into the places that would enrich them rather than simply focus on their deficiencies. So, I went. This was the first baby step in my professional growth and Irene was the best support one could have. I was too naive to even know she was my mentor but she led me through writing, speaking, consulting and provided endless opportunities for me to polish my skills. I know that today I would not have had such an exciting and fruitful professional life had it not been for my infancy with Irene Mortenson Burnside.

From Bernita Steffl: "I first met Irene 60 years ago. My class were big sisters to her class at Ancker Hospital School for Nurses. We formed life-long bonds. During World War II, many of us joined the military and were scattered worldwide. Irene and I met again in 1970 while taking classes at the Andrus Gerontology Center. I had seen two of her publications and was impressed by them. This meeting led to 30 years of shared personal and professional adventures and teaching experiences, some with older adults of different ethnic groups in Canada and Hawaii. Her writing style and ability were unique and opened the door to looking at behavior and feelings in addition to the medical problems of the aged. There was a poetic quality to much of her work. . . . I will be forever grateful to Irene for two things: I learned that I could and should write, and I learned a philosophical approach to work with the aged that is now helpful in my own aging—always start by looking at what is left, not what is gone" (Steffl, in Ebersole, 2003, p. 233).

From Helen Monea (RN, MSN, retired faculty from University of California, San Francisco and San Francisco State University): "Irene was an extraordinary nurse pioneer, creative teacher and caring friend. Our student days in the 1960s at UCSF School of Nursing in the master's program were filled with classes and clinical experiences. Yet Irene always had time for friends, classmates, and family at her home in Lafayette, California. I remember taco dinners were a favorite where we all shared cooking and cleanup. Thanks to her family, who included me in their outings, I learned to water-ski at a local lake. There were sad times too, as we each lost family members. Time seemed to fly, and after graduation we both became faculty members at UCSF.

"Later she accepted a position at Ethel Percy Andrus Gerontology Center at USC in Los Angeles, a change for all of us. She engaged her friends and colleagues in the exciting early pioneer days of gerontological nursing to grow along with her in the field. This led to exciting professional experiences. When we taught together, Irene supported my experiential teaching process. Our symbol for learning was the daisy, bright and durable. We introduced the daisy as a symbol of life, learning, and the elderly. Students each were given a fresh daisy at the end of class" (Monea, in Ebersole, 2003, p. 233).

From Sarah Fishman (PhD, RN, adjunct professor at Florida Atlantic University, retired faculty from Rutgers University in New Jersey): "In 1971, when I first started in geropsychiatric nursing, I knew of no nurses writing about mental health nursing with the older adult. . . . Shortly thereafter a nurse guru by the name of Irene Mortenson Burnside, who wrote books about nursing the aged and group work with the aged, was brought to my attention. I needed her knowledge, and I needed it immediately because I had just started directing a geriatric day care center, sponsored by the National Institutes of Mental Health and New Jersey's Trenton Psychiatric Hospital.

"After using her techniques and experiences gained from teaching nursing students, I was able to duplicate some of her efforts in New Jersey. I invited her to Rutgers University to speak at a geropsychiatric conference, and she proved a vital speaker. We got to know each other as she stayed as my house guest. She even put in a request for a clone of my husband, having lost hers long before.

"She influenced so many nurses in the compassionate and creative care of older adults and has left a very valuable legacy" (Fishman, in Ebersole, 2003, p. 233).

From Mathy Mezey (EdD, RN, FAAN, Independence Foundation Professor of Nursing Education, director of the John A Hartford, Foundation Institute for Geriatric Nursing) and Terry Fulmer (PhD, RN, FAAN, Erline Perkins McGriff Professor and Dean of New York University, School of Nursing, recent codirector, The John A. Hartford Foundation Institute for Geriatric Nursing): Irene Burnside "was passionate about promoting interdisciplinary opportunities in education and practice, a commitment that is evident in her early writings and was sustained throughout her career. . . . Her broad approach to promoting interdisciplinary collaboration encompassed both professional and nonprofessional providers."

"Today, the field of geriatric nursing is undergoing a renaissance. Nurse scholars are exploring practice concerns that range from improved management of behavioral alterations that plague people with dementia to understanding the genetic origins of such behaviors. All of us are indebted to Irene Burnside's seminal work and her commitment to both scholarship and practice and promoting a humane and passionate approach to care of older adults" (Mezey & Fulmer, in Ebersole, 2003, pp. 234–235).

From Tonya Thompson (Irene's daughter, a portion of Irene's Ethical Will): "And lastly, take care—exquisite care of yourself, and that means your body, your mind, your soul. Bodies are beautiful; do not deface them. Your mind is better open and constantly learning. And your soul means that deep faith will guide you through the times you think you cannot endure, and your moral code and behavior can influence more than you'd ever dare hope."

Bernita (Bea) Steffl

Bernita Steffl graduated from Ancker Hospital School of Nursing in St. Paul, Minnesota in 1942 (Fig. 2.8). After 4½ years in the United States Army Nurse Corps, serving in the United States, Iran, and Italy, she was

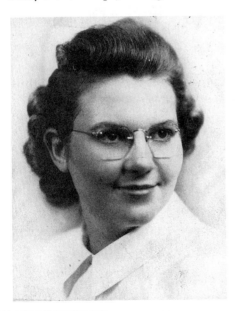

FIGURE 2.8 Bernita (Bea) Steffl on graduation from Ancker Hospital School of Nursing.

discharged as a captain and returned to school. In 1950 she obtained a bachelor's degree, with an emphasis on public health nursing, from the University of Minnesota in Minneapolis and went on from there to earn a master's degree in Public Health Nursing in 1960. In the 1970s she completed post-master's study focused on gerontology and obtained a Certificate in Gerontology from the Andrus Gerontology Center at University of Southern California in Los Angeles. Bea has continued her education through workshops and keeping abreast of research and developments in the field of gerontology (Fig. 2.9).

During the 1950s she worked in a variety of settings after her 4½ years in the Army Nurse Corps, including hospitals, and public health and school nursing. In 1961 she moved to Arizona and began teaching public health nursing at Arizona State University College of Nursing where she remained until her retirement in 1988. She began developing and teaching courses in gerontology in 1971. Early on, she was involved in distance learning about geriatric care to nurses and other health care professionals throughout Arizona.

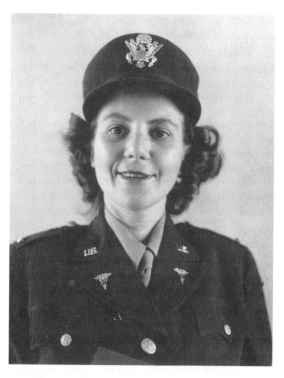

FIGURE 2.9 Bea Steffl in Army Nurse Corps, Iran.

During her years at Arizona State University (ASU) she was instrumental in developing multidisciplinary courses on aging and was one of the pioneers in developing the Certificate in Gerontology Program at ASU. During summers and sabbaticals she obtained the Certificate in Gerontology at the Andrus Gerontology Center and pursued her writing and research interests. Because of her extensive knowledge of public health issues she spent several months in Vietnam as a consultant to the World Health Organization to assess the health status of children after the TET offensive.

Bea Steffl has presented innumerable papers, more than 150 workshops in the United States and taught summer courses in Nova Scotia and Prince Edward Island in Canada. A memorable experience was teaching a series of summer institute classes in Hawaii, which included an ethnic mixture of caregivers in the community and on the island of Molokai. This included a trip by mule to the leper colony to learn about "elder life" and "elder care" there.

Bea has written a dozen chapters in gerontological nursing texts and she has authored several books. In 1984 her text, *Handbook on Gerontological Nursing* (with a heavy emphasis on public health concepts) was selected as one of the outstanding books of the year by *Nursing '84*. Her research interests included: assessment of senior student nurses' interest in gerontological nursing, fall prevention, attitudes toward aging and sexuality and aging. In addition to research and publication she developed two slide cassette programs: *Aging and Sexuality*, was humorous but subtle (1975); another, "The Meaning of Touch" was given second place in the ANA media festival in 1979.

From 1970 until her retirement, Bea received many honors and awards, one of the most significant reflecting her commitment to changing the system encompassing that of geriatric nursing was a Citation of Merit from Governor Bruce Babbit (Arizona) for her work and recognizing her contributions to the Governor's Council on Aging. Arizona has always been considered a maverick state and thus much could be accomplished there that was not necessarily bound in the federal quagmire.

I believe Bea established the Geriatric Nurses Interest Group of the Gerontological Society of America (GSA). As early as 1972, at the annual conventions, she would invite those of us who were interested to her hotel room for wine, cheese, and discussions. Today the Geriatric Nurses Interest Group of GSA is formalized and draws about 400 nurses to each meeting.

Bea was cognizant of the importance of influencing policy and legislation. She was very active as a member of the Governor's Council on Aging and in the Arizona state developments in aging. She supported state and national age-related legislative issues in the implementation of the Older Americans Act and worked on the agenda for the White House Conference on Aging in 1971 and 1981 (Fig. 2.10).

Personal Reflections

"I didn't have a lot of exposure to grandparents in my early life; however, I have vivid memories of old people. My mother was an immigrant, so her parents were in the old country and my father's parents died when I was 5 and 10 years old. My mother died when I was 9 years old and after the war I tried to find her mother in Bavaria, but learned that she had died in 1945. However, I remember a lot of older people being around and they seemed to command respect.

"One incident that stands out in my mind was of my father pointing his finger at my sister and me and saying, 'Don't you kids ever think you are too good to speak to old people.' This came about when, as adolescents, we made fun of 'old man Shreiber,' a friend of his who wore loose fitting overalls, generally needed a shave, and chewed snuff, which sometimes dribbled down his chin and caused him to spit a lot. He used coffee cans for a spittoon. He had a young wife that we thought came from the circus because of her size. When Dad heard our snickers and degrading remarks, he lined us up and said, 'Don't you ever let me catch you making fun of Mr. Shreiber and don't think for a minute that you are any better than he is. When you meet him on the street, you speak to him!' We learned to know the real Mr. Shreiber—a wonderful, loving, and generous man. To this day my sister and I reminisce about his colorful garden and his kitchen where something, usually sauerkraut, was always on the cook stove. A piano and an accordion were in his home because he was, among other things, a musician. I have tried to look beyond whatever meets the eye ever since. There is always an interesting person there, sometimes *locked in the cage of old age*" (Steffl in Ebersole & Hess, 1990, pp. 823–824).

"I trained in a big city county hospital and I remember a lot of the older people, some in big wards. I don't remember one word in the curriculum about geriatrics. We had pediatrics but not a thing about geriatrics, in fact, I don't even remember becoming familiar with the word. I remember two distinct things from old people as patients.

"During the first few months in training an old lady needed a back rest as she had some kind of cardiac problem. We didn't have electric beds in those days so we put a folding metal backrest under the mattress with pillows around her on the bed. I can vividly see her sitting up in her bed, her lips were kind of blue and she told me she was going to die. I was terrified. I didn't really know what to do, I didn't really believe her either. The lady did die shortly after she said that to me. Even though I had

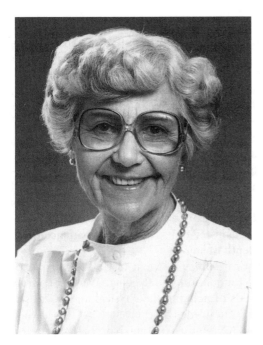

FIGURE 2.10 Bea Steffl.

experienced my mother's death at home and worked up the courage to touch her in the coffin, I needed someone to help me deal with a dying person. No one at the nursing station said anything to me. I went back to the nursing quarters to talk about it with roommates.

"Then there was an old Jewish woman; this was early in World War II and Hitler was in his heyday. She was so sick, dying of pneumonia, I think. This was before we had penicillin. While I was giving her care she said, 'I don't care what happens to me, I just hope I live long enough to see what happens to Hitler.' It impressed me so, the strength of this woman and her interest even as sick as she was. I have often thought of that.

"When I finished my 3-year program I went into the military and could hardly wait to get in because it was a real status symbol, in contrast to the Vietnam War. Everybody wanted to be in action in World War II. I had never before been more than 500 miles from home. I had a very rewarding experience in the service. World War II influenced me heavily as it gave me a broad look at the rest of the world. I will always be thankful for those years. When nurses came back they expected different things and a whole lot of different leadership took place. The GI Bill made it possible for us to go back to school and I did. That opened up so many avenues for me.

"It was a little over 20 years ago (interview took place in 1992, reporting about 1969–1970) that I became interested in gerontology, maybe one reason is because my mother died when I was so young and I have always been searching for a mother or grandmother. I believe it was in March 1970 that I went to a workshop in Santa Monica, California, called, *The RN and the Aged Patient*. That day changed the direction of my career for the rest of my working days and my life. I met and heard some of the great pioneers in gerontology and in gerontological nursing such as Dorothy Moses, Mary Shaugnessey, and Virginia Stone. They talked about developing standards of geriatric nursing, biological research, and needs in long-term care. I met psychologist, James Birren, and an architect who pointed out environmental problems and needs, such as the different riser depth in steps that can be hazardous for older individuals. I think about him and smile in my old age when I experience those hazardous differences in the depth of steps.

"So, I changed my sabbatical plans and went to USC for a year of study to get a real theoretical foundation about aging. We had courses from great leaders in many fields of aging in the physical and social sciences. I was excited with my new knowledge base. From then I was 'turned on' and became active in the ANA and Arizona Nurses Association (AzNA) Councils on Geriatric Nursing. I became involved in the development of community programs for the aged funded by the Older Americans Act and served on the Arizona Governor's Council on Aging. I became more interested and pursued more knowledge and experience in working with feelings and behaviors, basic needs, and sexuality in old age. Over the years I also became interested in the use of music therapy, pet therapy, and the importance of touch in caring for older individuals.

"In my lifetime, nursing leaders have begun to recognize the importance and relationship of the arts and humanities and how they can aid us in helping those for whom we care. Many people are relatively unaware of the value and relationship of music, poetry, and the arts to health. People are also uneducated or miseducated about sexuality and aging. What we see advertised is not true human sexuality. We talk about it a lot but it is so much more than sexual physical contact.

"One summer I taught a course on aging at St. Francis Xavier University in Nova Scotia and was privileged to meet with Sister Michael Guiness, PhD. She had developed the universally used tool to measure attitudes toward aging. We worked together briefly on measuring attitudes about older people and caring for them. When I returned to ASU, I investigated the attitudes and interest of nursing students in gerontological nursing. I was very disappointed. Most wanted something more dramatic, like critical care. Only about 8% to 10% indicated any interest in gerontology. I repeated this 10 years later and it had not changed. . . . I feel one of my major contributions to gerontological nursing was the work with others on developing gerontological nursing essential curricula content, and promoting specific courses in aging in the nursing curriculum at ASU.

"The *Handbook on Gerontological Nursing,* that I edited, was hard work but rewarding when students and those nurses working with the elderly said they found it useful. . . . I learned a great deal more than my students in my classes, but it is very rewarding seeing some of my former students now as leaders and doing a great job in long-term care, teaching, research.

"All my mentors have not been nurses. I will never forget the influence of Alvin Goldfarb, Robert Butler, James Birren, Ruth Weg, and others at USC. Many nurses prominent in gerontology were very helpful to me. I owe the most to Irene Burnside and Mary Opal Wolanin. And, I think I in turn brainwashed my nephew who lived with me for awhile and he has become a respected faculty member at the San Francisco State University Division of Gerontology.

"My vision for the future is that of more work with the legislature and multidisciplines within the community and to promote geriatric nursing content in nursing curricula, for more educated support, and attention to the needs of a growing older population. The whole field of legal and ethical issues in aging is growing. I think we need more geriatric nurse practitioners, family practitioners, adult practitioners, and more geriatric clinical specialists. There needs to be much more attention to the end stages of life—death and dying and the hospice movement. We also need to think a lot more about isolation and loneliness.

"I learned about loneliness from Mrs. Rodgers in Nova Scotia. She had been widowed, didn't have much family, and lived in a very nice residential Catholic retirement home. She said that every time the train came by each evening it seemed to say, 'home, home, home.' She told me about a little frog or toad she would see by a tree each morning. In the fall she placed extra leaves where she thought he might be hibernating to keep him warm. All winter she wondered what had happened to him, and in the spring she looked and looked but did not find him" (Steffl, 1992; Steffl, in Ebersole & Hess, 1990).

"When I get depressed about the future, I console myself with this thought, 'the baby boomers (and boomlets) will solve the problems.' They are smart and educated and I believe they will find solutions to the problems in our society. They have 'had it all' and will not 'go gently into the night.'"

Bea's philosophy: "I have tried to look beyond whatever meets the eye ever since (old man Shreiber). There is always an interesting person there, *sometimes locked in the cage of old age.* I think I have helped at least a few of my students with this approach, 'You see me as I am now, but I see myself as I've always been and all the things I've been—not just an old lady.' . . . For me, the bottom line and greatest need for us to pursue is meeting the basic human needs and understanding the feelings and behavior of older individuals" (Ebersole & Hess, 1990, p. 824).

Laurie Martin Gunter

Laurie Gunter probably is best known and remembered by the numerous geriatric nurses who were first tested and certified by ANA. She laughs, in her exuberant manner, when she tells of the geriatric nurses who had not felt particularly respected in the field of nursing. When the first group was certified in 1968, Laurie with others staged a grand celebration for them; many brought their families, even the children. It was a momentous occasion and carried with it a validation of their work that had not before been noticed (Fig. 2.11).

Laurie Martin Gunter was born in Pelham, Texas, on March 5, 1922. Her parents, Hollie Myrtle Carruthers and Lewis Marian Martin, had three children; Laurie was the eldest. She attended schools in Pelham and San Antonio and graduated at the top of her class in 1940 (Fig. 2.12).

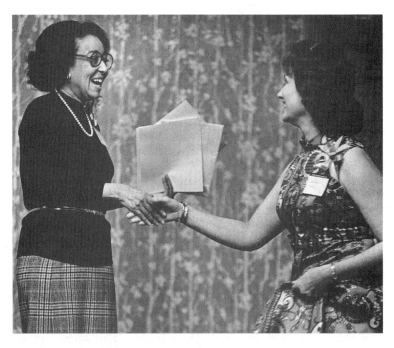

FIGURE 2.11 Laurie Gunter congratulating recipient of ANA Certificate in Geriatric Nursing.

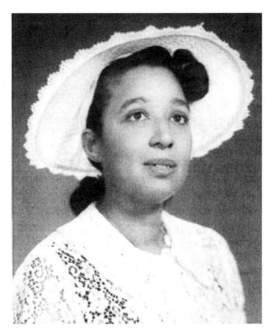

FIGURE 2.12 Laurie Gunter, 1950.

   She graduated from Meharry College School of Nursing in Nashville,
Tennessee, in 1943 and immediately went to work at George W. Hubbard
hospital in Nashville, continued her education, and was awarded a BS degree with a major in home economics from Tennessee A&I University in
Nashville. She persisted in obtaining an education and spent a year at the
University of Toronto with a Rockefeller Fellowship for the advanced
study of nursing. She then returned to Nashville and earned a master's degree from Fisk University and earned a PhD in human development from
the University of Chicago in 1959. She was married and had a 3-year-old
daughter when she entered the University of Chicago. During the first
2 years her mother cared for daughter, Lara Elaine. She had been teaching at Meharry Medical College before 1953 and after 1955 but when
she obtained her PhD she entered the tenure track and was appointed
Dean of the Nursing School. In 1958, she began to specialize in gerontology and served as a Fellow of the Inter-University Council of Social
Gerontology at the University of California, Berkeley. Between 1961 and
1971 she taught at UCLA, Indiana University Medical Center in
Indianapolis, and the College of Nursing at University of Washington. In
1971 she was appointed professor and head of the Department of
Nursing at Pennsylvania State University in University Park and during

the next 4 years she made significant changes in the program. A graduate program and an extended degree program for registered nurses were created. These changes brought the nursing school into preeminence among collegiate schools of nursing. During sabbaticals and leaves she served as visiting professor at the Universities of Delaware, Michigan, Indiana, Tulsa, and UCLA. She retired from Pennsylvania State in 1987.

Laurie was largely responsible for organizing the first International Conference on Gerontological Nursing, held in Los Angeles in 1981. Mary Opal Wolanin and Virginia Stone were two of the speakers who impressed me as they spoke of their own aging.

Among her numerous awards and honors were election to the Institute of Medicine of the National Academy of Sciences, and election as a Fellow of the Gerontological Society of America and the American Academy of Nursing. In addition she was made honorary alumna of Pennsylvania State University and received an award from Sigma Theta Tau for her outstanding contributions to nursing research (Bullough & Sentz, 2002).

Dr. Gunter, with Carmen Estes, was truly a visionary and formulated a conceptual framework of a curriculum for all levels of nursing personnel. Her textbook, *Education for Gerontic Nursing* (Gunter & Estes, 1979), was the first geriatric nursing curriculum text and vital to many nursing schools. In addition, it was in that text that Laurie and Carmen Estes introduced the term "gerontic" as an all-inclusive term that would avoid the constant need to try to discriminate between geriatric and gerontological. In addition to this classic text, Laurie has published nearly 100 papers, journal articles, chapters, and books since 1949. Early publications focused on a broad spectrum of nursing issues with particular attention to cultural needs and differences in health care. By 1971 she was beginning to write about geriatric nursing. The remainder of her publications are almost entirely devoted to the topic.

She lectured, presented continuing education programs, and served as consultant to organizations in the United States, Canada, Japan, and Israel and maintained professional relationships with several black colleges and universities. The department of nursing established a special Laurie M. Gunter Research Fund in her honor (*Penn State News*, 1987) (Fig. 2.13).

Laurie M. Gunter: Personal Reflections

"There is so much history when you live to be as old as I am, maybe I should start when I was a student working on my doctoral degree at University of Chicago, because that got me involved in this particular field. I almost feel as if I have had many lives. Childhood was one, nursing school, young adulthood, professional life and then retirement.

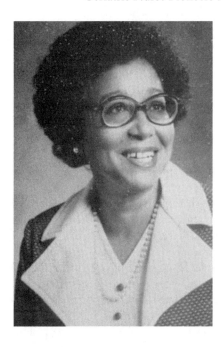

FIGURE 2.13 Laurie Gunter.

"When I began my doctoral studies I was already married and had one child. My mother kept her while I was in school, otherwise I don't think I could have made it. I found it one of the [most] difficult experiences academically that I had encountered in my life but it also provided the most wonderful education. I was working toward a PhD in Human Development. There was little about aging at that time and few textbooks. Cowdrey was the major text on aging and Havighurst was one of our professors. One day I was walking by Judd Hall and met Bernice Neugarten, a professor of human development. She suggested I apply for a Fellowship at University of California in Berkeley. Nashville was so hot and humid in the summer, I told Bernice I would do anything to get out of Nashville for the summer. I applied and was accepted, that was in 1959. This was one month of intensive study with mimeographed articles as texts. Thirty people from medicine, social work, nursing, psychology, sociology and other disciplines were represented. Virginia Stone and I were the ones from nursing. All of the famous names in gerontology were there: Donohue, Tibbits, Busse, and Neugarten, among others.

"When I went to Penn State my purpose was to bring nursing within the framework of the College of Human Development. We were able to develop a very workable curriculum and it may have been the first of its kind. It opened up the view of nursing education to include normal aging and health promotion for the elderly. We tried to establish courses for older people in senior centers. One time we were out in a small community and I was trying to bring my materials to the center; slides, handouts, and A/V equipment. One of the old ladies was talking to a friend who said, 'Here she comes with all that stuff; she wants to teach us about aging. I don't know what she can teach us, but maybe we can teach her something!' . . . It was true that I learned from the participants and now that I am old, I know much more about aging" (Gunter, 2005).

"I became very interested in international gerontic activities. At a GSA meeting I found nurses from other countries would attend the meetings if nursing was on the program, so I always presented a paper so that international nurses could attend with expenses paid. When Bernice (Neugarten) was president of GSA she was always asking me if we wanted to organize a nursing group. There was a difference of opinions among nurses. Some nurses did not want a separate group. From these experiences I became interested in organizing an International Conference on Gerontological Nursing. Fortunately, I was invited to UCLA as a visiting professor. I accepted that invitation for the purpose of organizing an international conference. This was preparatory to the International Council of Nursing meeting in Los Angeles in 1981. This International Conference on Gerontological Nursing was one of my major contributions.

"Another of my significant contributions was the certification of geriatric nurses. This was important for the nurses that were out in the trenches, caring for the old and struggling to increase the quality of care. Even at ANA meetings, some nurses questioned the validity of specializing in gerontic nursing but pediatric nurses and physicians were pushing for certification so it was on their minds. It was geriatrics and pediatrics that established the first credentialing process for nurses. Barbara Davis was a staff person at ANA and gave excellent assistance to the executive committee of the Division of Geriatric Nursing Practice. I agreed to become the chairman. Our criteria were stringent and required a real commitment from these nurses. I was deeply touched by this experience. We were stunned by the number of applicants and had to work over Thanksgiving vacation to process all of the applications. I thought there would be a small ceremony at ANA for those who had completed the process but instead many showed up. Fathers, mothers, sisters, brothers, and children were there, all coming to see their nurses obtain this honor. This was so touching. One nurse later told me, 'I always thought I was a good nurse and performing at a high level of nursing practice but no one ever told me I was a good nurse but after I was certified I felt I could speak for good nursing practice in my agency. I felt I could speak up.' Certification helped these nurses feel that their opinions were respected.

"I don't think my mother or my children ever knew that I was recognized in the profession or were really aware of my accomplishments. They knew I always had my head in a book and that I was gone a lot, even missed some important events in their lives but they never seemed to think my profession took anything away from them.

"I see changes in attitudes toward old people and geriatrics. I see greater emphasis on health and one's responsibility for their own health and development during old age. This is important as in the future there may not be sufficient personnel to take care of us. There are also changing attitudes toward death. I think we are much more comfortable now facing the reality that we can't be rehabilitated all our life. We are now wasting tremendous resources on people in the last month of life. When I grew up we lived for a time in an extended family in a rural area where death was a fact of life. In our extended family we had four generations; my great-grandmother lived a long time and when she became ill I had the opportunity to take care of her and I thought it was wonderful. That is probably why I became a nurse. She died when I was 16 but was not ill for a long time. People were very ill for a week or two. The whole family would have the opportunity to come in and take their turn with the dying person. It was called 'sitting up with a person.' There was someone with them all the time. There was no hospital, no prolonging life or death and there was no isolation. Ethics will become more important in the future but I hope it will be more than just talking people to death about death.*

"In regard to retirement, it seems to me that the need for us to become involved with children supersedes whatever else is going on. Children need the contact with mature adults. When parents are working they may not have time to do all they would like to do with their children. I volunteer at an elementary school. Now I have time to be involved with my younger granddaughter and to teach her reading and arithmetic. We walk to activities when they are close by. I have had many opportunities in the profession of nursing and I have enjoyed it tremendously. I worked hard and I was rewarded with an ample livelihood. I was fortunate to be involved in the development of gerontic nursing. But now that I'm retired, I love that even more!" (Gunter, 1990).

Barbara Helen Allen Davis

Barbara Allen Davis is a renaissance woman. She has participated in the conception of ideas and activities that brought geriatric nursing recognition in theory and practice. As a staff member of ANA some years ago,

---

*This interview took place 15 years ago, long before the emergence of attention to palliative care.

her influence was enormous. She has been on the ground floor of much that has occurred in the advancement of geriatric nursing at ANA and in nursing homes.

Dr. Barbara Davis was born August 13, 1921, in Hicksville, New York, the sixth of 10 children. She remembers wanting to be a nurse when as young as 5 years old. Her childhood was hard and it is evident in reviewing it that her incredible strength of purpose was inculcated by the situations she confronted on a daily basis. When her father lost an arm in a work-related accident, she, as the oldest child at home, became her father's companion, accompanying him and assisting in his daily activity of collecting junk for resale. There was a lot of work to be done around their home, caring for the smaller children and helping her father in the junk business. The children helped their father collect rags, papers, bottles, old metal, and other items for resale. All the children had chores and during the summer worked on local farms (Davis, 2004).

Education did not come easy in that time and place. To attend high school, Barbara walked 4 miles each day, worked in the cafeteria during lunch hour, and frequently did house cleaning in the homes of her teachers. In her home there was no electricity and the kerosene oil lamps were extinguished early in the evening. She and an older sister would do their homework in the light shed by the pot bellied stove in their dining room. She graduated as Valedictorian of her class in 1939. In 1986, Dr. Davis was honored as an outstanding graduate and elected a member of the Hall of Fame at Hicksville High School. Upon graduation she had been awarded a scholarship at a nearby college but, unable to attend because of financial reasons, she entered nursing school.

She graduated from Kings County Hospital Center, School of Nursing, Brooklyn, New York, in 1943. At age 40, in 1961, she was awarded her Bachelor of Science degree in Nursing from St. John's University Jamaica, New York. She was bright and determined to go to medical school but, fortunately for the future of geriatric nursing, the admissions director informed her she had two strikes against her: She was too old and a woman. In 1968 she graduated with a Master's of Science degree in psychiatric nursing from Adelphi University, Garden City, New York, and in 1974 from Teacher's College, Columbia University, New York, with an EdD in social gerontology. In 1971, she was licensed by New York State as a Nursing Home Administrator (Fig. 2.14).

During the years after nursing school she held several positions in New York and in 1967 she became the Program Coordinator for Geriatric Nursing Practice at the American Nurses Association. In 1977 she moved to Los Angeles and became Clinical Nurse Coordinator of Geropsychiatry at the Neuropsychiatric Institute, University of California,

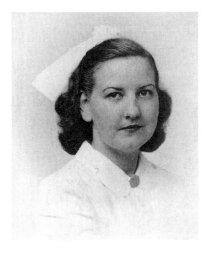

FIGURE 2.14 Barbara Allen Davis, nursing school graduate.

Los Angeles. In 1979 she became the Director of Gerontology Nursing Programs at UCLA and from 1985 until 1994 was the Clinical Nurse Specialist at West Los Angeles Veterans Affairs Nursing Home, Geriatrics and Extended Care.

Her interest in gerontology was developed early in the 1960s and she maintained a consistent focus on publishing articles (34) about gerontological nursing thereafter. Her prolific contributions have advanced the knowledge of geriatric care and its history considerably. Many of her activities and publications were focused on psychosocial aspects of long-term care and nursing homes. She has frequently been called upon for workshops, presentations, consultation, and curriculum development. In 1971 she was an ANA representative to the White House Conference on Aging. Dr. Davis has been visiting faculty at 15 U.S. colleges and universities and in Russia and Israel.

Her interest in the care of the aged began when she was a nursing student and remained throughout her career. While at ANA she helped establish the first standards of gerontological nursing practice. For ANA, she conducted regional hearings throughout the nation on skilled nursing care and nursing homes and presented her findings to the Subcommittee on Long Term Care, U.S. Senate Special Committee on Aging. At one time she was certified simultaneously in three ANA specialties: Gerontological Nursing, Psychiatric and Mental Health Nursing, and Nursing Administration Advanced (Fig. 2.15).

Barbara drafted the original version of a proposal to secure funding for a project to upgrade knowledge and skills of nursing home nurses nationwide. The ANA received federal funds to conduct such a project and

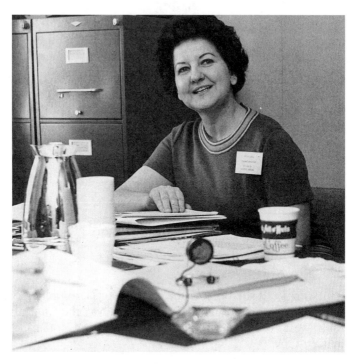

FIGURE 2.15 Barbara Allen Davis at ANA desk, Standards Committee meeting.

Barbara, then a doctoral candidate at Columbia University, continued on the project's advisory committee. This committee devised the strategy to assure the delivery of clinical nursing conferences for nursing home nurses in every state. Barbara acted as faculty for six of the state and regional conferences.

In 1983 she was given a grant to study the history of nursing care of the aged in the United States from 1880 on. Her objectives were to identify events that may have influenced the nursing care of the aged, determine the impact of these events, and formulate hypotheses for further inquiry. Her seminal research on this topic has been integral to this publication and much of it is reported in chapter 1. The impetus for her research was to seek answers to questions about (a) the resistance of nursing faculty in undergraduate nursing programs to the inclusion of gerontic content, (b) the tendency to downgrade the excellence of geriatric nurses regardless of their educational preparation, (c) the dearth of nurses seeking graduate education in gerontology while simultaneously the aged population is on the increase, and (d) nursing administrative resistance to specialized units for the aged.

Her honors are numerous and of special significance are the Gerontological Nurse of the Year Award, American Nurses Association Council on Gerontological Nursing, 1985 and Fellow in the American Academy of Nursing (Fig. 2.16).

Barbara Allen Davis: Recollections

"My interest in the aged began when I was in nursing school as I cared for many aged on medical units. There was no such thing as gerontological nursing. Some time later I was working as a head nurse at a county hospital back East where I had opened a medical unit of 65 beds. We had many elderly patients who were either coming to us from nursing homes or were ready to be transferred to nursing homes. Many of them were very upset about being returned to the nursing home. That triggered something in me to find out just what was going on that nursing homes were 'that way.' Shortly thereafter, I opened a very small nursing home. I converted a private house into a 19-bed nursing home and eventually an

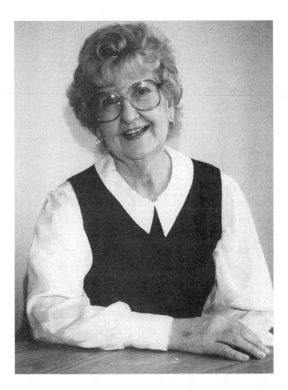

FIGURE 2.16 Barbara Allen Davis VAMC professional photograph.

addition was added and it became a 40-bed nursing home. That's basically where it started with me. . . . This was one of my most gratifying experiences. I was able to put a lot of my talents and skills into play. I also became aware of my lack of knowledge about aging because I carried the acute care hospital model with me. . . . I was doing things like bathing patients daily until the patients themselves told me they didn't want a bath every day so we stopped that. I had learned not to give medications with food; then I found patients who have been taking their digoxin every morning with breakfast for 25 years, and so we just kept that going. After all, if it hadn't done anything detrimental until then it probably never would. . . . To have the nursing home licensed in the State of New York and to be seen as a model in which practices I did were put into action in other nursing homes was very rewarding.

"I have been strongly influenced by groups of aged, especially the old-old aged. . . . I can identify large numbers of them that I cared for in a huge municipal hospital with more than 2,000 patients. . . . They were considered indigent, and they were the kind of patient that I later found in nursing homes. It was that group of patients that influenced me.

"When I review the historic trends which influenced me toward gerontological nursing, I think it was the federal funding of nursing education. . . . I earned a Baccalaureate Degree in Nursing at St. John's University, which was funded by the Nurse Training Act. Later when I studied for a master's degree I was funded by the National Institute of Mental Health. That influenced me tremendously because at the time I was doing graduate psychiatric nursing, there was no specialty in geropsychiatric nursing but I was able to skew all my clinical experiences toward the aged. . . . When we were assigned to the state hospital, I went to the back wards looking for the aged. It was also then I had my first experience with a VA hospital.

"It was during the mid-1960s when I first encountered veterans who had been institutionalized for over 50 years . . . so, once again, I was given the opportunity and the privilege of learning about nursing groups of older persons. . . . I sincerely felt that I had a message to give on aging and I wanted to do that beyond one institution. . . . The American Nurses' Association seemed to be a significant vehicle but I didn't know the strategy.

"It was in the mid-1960s that ANA was wrestling with identifying the areas of specialization within nursing and eventually came up with five divisions: medical/surgical; psychiatric/mental health; maternal/child health; geriatrics; and community health. It's interesting because, I remember the criteria for the formation of a division had to do with whether there was a large number of nurses practicing in that area and whether there was a body of knowledge, and were there issues and problems. I identified nursing care of the aged as an area of issues and problems. . . . Many influential people in nursing were negative about aging. . . . I became the first full-time coordinator for the Division, then called Geriatric Nursing. While I was there the standards were developed. I had experts come in to ANA headquarters and we developed the Standards of Nursing Practice, Certification and so on.

"A public relations specialist at ANA, Katherine Wheeler, helped me to develop the first speeches I gave around the country, reviewed the papers I wrote for publication; she was the one who taught me the need for press releases to get out our stories. One of my roles was to represent nursing at the various national aging organizations: the American Geriatric Society, the Gerontological Society of America, the American Association of Retired Persons, the National Council on Aging, and many others. I became ANA's representative to all of these. . . . The other person whom I identify as my professional mentor was Dr. Ruth Bennett, a social gerontologist from Columbia University. . . . She eventually became the chair of my Dissertation Committee and I followed up on the work she had done in institutions. . . . Those were my two mentors, neither in nursing, unfortunately.

"When I was completing my master's thesis, I could find no one who would be able to guide me on the content of geriatric nursing so I was my own specialist and consultant. The chair of my committee allowed me to go through guiding myself on the geriatric content of my study while I was getting other guidance in handling statistical data from the statistician, and in psychiatric care from one of the psychiatric nursing professors.

"Developing a model nursing home; developing clinical experiences for master's students in geropsychiatric nursing, the ANA Standards of Practice for Geriatric Nursing and certification for nurses in the field, and opening a geropsychiatric unit at the University of California, Neuropsychiatric Institute have all been very gratifying experiences. You suggest that I am a trailblazer in gerontic nursing. As I review it, it appears to be that way" (Davis, 1991).

As a trailblazer Barbara has encountered numerous obstacles along the way. At least six different times she was actively discouraged or questioned about her interest in studying the aged; unfortunately, most of these were from nurses holding influential positions. One prospective interviewer wondered how life satisfaction of the aged was related to psychiatric care and questioned the pertinence of her thesis, *Activities and Life Satisfactions of Aged Female Residents in a Home for the Aged*. Another intimated during the defense of her master's thesis that the topic might influence whether she passed or failed her orals. In another instance she explained to an employer that she had enrolled in a gerontology program and her supervisor asked, "Why would you want to do that?" When Barbara told one dean of nursing that she had entered a doctoral program she was told that was a poor decision, given her background and interest in nursing homes. When she successfully completed her studies and received her doctorate, a leader in the nursing profession said, "Doctoral education is wasted on the middle-aged woman." With her usual aplomb, Barbara replied, "Not on this middle-aged woman!" Another incident, much later (when we would hope gerontology was well-recognized) is worth pondering and came from the curriculum chair of a highly regarded Western university who said a course in the care of the aged was unnecessary, was just a "flash in the pan." A dean in that institution said, "Damn it Davis, if you want it, you teach it yourself!" In fact, through Barbara's professional history it is clear that she received far more support outside of nursing than within it.

I have corresponded with Barbara since first meeting her in my interview and video of her at the West Los Angeles Veterans Affairs Nursing Home in 1991. I was impressed by her in many ways, especially by her dynamic personality and organization. She had carefully prepared for the interview, obtained permission from the powers there, and followed the guidelines I had sent to her. However, I was most impressed when we went to lunch at a nearby cafe. It was a popular and busy place and, as often happens to ladies without male escorts, the maitre d' steered us toward a rather undesirable table in a corner near the kitchen. Barbara said, "This is not acceptable." The maitre d' said, "Well I'm afraid it will be a rather long wait for another table." Barbara said, "We'll wait." We were seated in a view table within the next few minutes. I suspect this is just one instance of how Barbara has impacted so many people in so many places.

Dr. Davis retired at age 73 and now lives in an Independent/Assisted Living Facility, Merrill Gardens in Tamarac, Florida. She continues to use her skills and knowledge of aging as the President of the Resident Council of this facility. Barbara finds her home is in one of the best facilities for the aged and she is expert at assessing such situations.

Barbara maintains her interest in large groups of elderly through volunteer participation in two national endeavors: The Women's Health Initiative, the largest study of older women ever conducted in the United States, and the Medicare Current Beneficiary Survey, one of the primary sources of information about how Medicare affects its recipients.

Mary Starke Harper

Mary Starke Harper has always been politically astute and available for all mental health providers in the Washington, D.C., arena. She began her political career as an infant sitting on her father's lap while he and other African Americans in Phoenix City, Alabama, discussed the formation of coalition groups such as the Black Republicans. She was his adored first child. The Ku Klux Klan were threatened by any organizations of blacks and she clearly remembers hiding in a hay loft for 2 weeks. As a child, Mary occasionally took part in debate clubs at school, but most of her preoccupations were to participate in political and board meetings with her father and in her own entrepreneurship. Mary raised white mice and sold them to hospitals and laboratories. She purchased chewing gum from mail order houses and sold them at church for a big profit. There were eight children and they lived in a two-bedroom house. "We slept two or three per bed or on cots; we had an outside toilet and a big tin tub for bathing" (Harper, 2005).

Dr. Mary Starke Harper, a 60-year veteran of the health care industry, was advisor on Mental Health and Aging to Presidents Carter, Reagan, Bush, and Clinton. Mary is the first nurse in the world to have an entire 220-bed geropsychiatric hospital built and dedicated to her, the Mary Starke Harper Geriatric Psychiatry Center, near the Bryce State Hospital in Tuscaloosa, Alabama. This is a great honor for Mary, who was initially refused entry to a nursing program in Tuscaloosa because she was black, even though she excelled in all the admission requirements (except race).

Dr. Harper has held various faculty appointments in her career at colleges and universities throughout the country, including the University of Minnesota, Minneapolis; University of California, Los Angeles; St. Mary's College, New York; Virginia Polytechnic Institute, Blacksburg, Virginia; and Distinguished Professor in Nursing, Medicine, Psychology and Social Work at the University of Alabama, Tuscaloosa. She has lectured at Yale, Harvard, the University of Pennsylvania, Stanford, and other universities.

She is the author of five books, 82 chapters, and 160 articles on aging and mental health issues, including contributions to *Mental Health: A Report of the Surgeon General* (U.S. Department of Health and Human Services, 1999). In 1991 her book, *Management and Care of the Elderly: Psychosocial Perspectives,* was published by Sage. Earlier she edited a landmark book, *Mental Illness in the Nursing Home: An Agenda for Research* (Harper & Liebowitz, 1986).

Her 30-year career with the U.S. Department of Health and Human Services (USDHHS) included serving as Coordinator of Long-term Care Programs at the National Institute of Mental Health, the National Institutes of Health. During this time she established the first National Research and Development Center in Mental Health for Asian Americans, American Indians, African Americans, and Hispanics as well as the first national fellowships for minority mental health (doctoral and postdoctoral for the disciplines of psychiatry, nursing, psychology, social work, and sociology). In the days of segregation, she was believed to be the *only* provider of psychiatric nursing affiliation for over 25 schools of nursing located in North Carolina, Alabama, Georgia, Florida, Tennessee, and Mississippi (Harper, 2005).

In 1997, Mary was invited by President Clinton to the White House for the ceremony to recognize and apologize to the survivors of the Tuskegee Syphilis Study. Mary, as a young student nurse, had been working in the John Andrews Memorial Hospital in Tuskegee where the study was conducted. She reflected that at the time most were unaware of the ethical implications of this study.

Milestones in Dr. Harper's career (Santo-Novak, Grissom, & Powers, 2004) include the following:

- Co-chair, Clinton Administration's Mental Health/Public Sector Task Force for Healthcare Reform
- Director, Office of Policy and Development and research consultant for the 1981 and 1995 White House Conferences on Aging
- Participant, 1981 World Assembly on Aging in Vienna
- Secretary and a founder of the American Association of International Aging
- Living Legacy Award, National Caucus and Center on Black Aging, and Chi Eta Phi Sorority
- Appointed to serve on the Board of Trustees of the Alabama Department of Mental Health/Mental Retardation by the Governor of Alabama
- Convened the first National Conference on Mental Health in Nursing Homes in 1984
- Member of the Alabama Commission on Aging
- Recognized by the American Academy of Nursing as a Living Legend, 2001
- Co-Founder, National Black Nurses Association
- Nurse representative in the Regional Development of the Southern Regional Board of Education (SREB)
- Conceptualized and implemented the first national fellowship programs for five core mental health disciplines that has produced over 10,000 MDs and PhDs in the fields of mental health

Dr. Mary Harper has been influential nationally and internationally and has influenced so much progress in geriatric mental health and sociocultural issues, that it is not possible in this limited space to recognize all she has done. Additional information can be found in Ebersole (1997d) and Santo-Novak, Grissom, and Powers (2004). But, in addition to her many contributions she is simply a remarkable and most enjoyable human being. I first met her at the Palmer House at a conference and was invited to her room to chat and munch on Cheetos. Later (1992) when I was gathering data about the geriatric nurse pioneers I spent an evening with her at her home on Geranium Street in Washington, D.C. When I arrived Mary was not yet there because she had been in a minor fender-bender on her way home. I wanted to defer the interview until a later time as it was already about 8 p.m. and I suspected she would be rather hassled after a long day and the problem getting home. She wanted to go ahead with the interview but first insisted I have dinner with her and two younger women who apparently were visiting her.

Her house was like a clock museum, with time pieces from all over the world. Many of them had been given her in appreciation for her assistance in various ways. Awards of merit covered the staircase walls of her three-story home. Her entire basement was overflowing with documents she had needed or possibly would need. After a thorough and most enjoyable tour of her home we settled down to videotaping the interview. Mary has a wealth of ideas, energy, and enthusiasm. By 2 a.m. I was flagging, but she was still going strong. She insisted on taking me back to the central city to my hotel and I had my first experience watching the prostitutes in action in Washington, D.C.

What did I learn from Mary? Her life from the beginning has been filled with work, devotion, and opportunities. Great-granddaughter of a slave, Mary's acute awareness of the lack of adequate quality care for many blacks and other underserved people is her abiding concern. Some things she feels have been her major contributions include faculty development awards through the National Institute of Mental Health. As she says, "We want to prepare faculty to teach students (about aging) because you cannot expect students to understand if the faculty doesn't" (Harper, 1992). She also felt that her book with Dr. Liebowitz, *Mental Health and Mental Illness in Nursing Homes: An Agenda for Research,* brought attention to the fact that in spite of the mental health disorders of more than 60% of nursing home residents there are seldom staff with any training in psychiatric or mental health issues. "We need nurses in nursing homes to help staff understand depression, suicide and the wish to die . . ." (Harper, 1992).

How did she get started working with older folk? "When in my graduate studies at University of Minnesota, I specialized in psychiatric nursing and became very interested in the elderly. . . . I concentrated on working with the elderly because I knew that I was going back to the Veterans Administration Hospital and their very large elderly population. . . . As a young nurse I was rather vocal, sometimes asking questions, sometimes dissenting. Next thing I knew, I was placed on a ward where there were all older men, over 150 of them. The average age was 75 years and 80% were incontinent of feces and urine. . . . Well, I realized I was put there because I was not necessarily a 'very good kid' but I was going to make the best out of that and I was going to try and institute some of the things I had learned in spite of the fact that I was not one of their favorite girls. I got together the nursing assistants, and the semi-retired physician that came in occasionally. Actually, he was primarily interested in the stock pages of *The New York Times,* so when I went to him for advice, his feeling was that whatever I wanted to do was OK with him.

"The staff knew only the patients' names and serial numbers, nothing of their lives or their families. So, I started once a week to present case studies: a bit about the patient, his background, family, education, ambitions, illness, pathology, and the like. . . . After a few weeks the staff were given specific training and assignments to do things for their particular patients. . . . After a few months we cut the incidence of incontinence in half. We trained and involved volunteers in corrective therapy as well and patients, with help learned to feed and bathe themselves. . . . After 14 months, believe it or not, we were able to go down to the river and have a picnic with these men with the assistance of staff and a whole bunch of B'nai Brith volunteers. . . . I was a young nurse and this was 1948 (before psychogeriatrics got its name). I saw the results of my work and it was gratifying. When these men were able to shave and feed themselves they began smiling and talking. It was almost a miracle. It was, I think, my most gratifying experience as a clinician." Mary, young as she was and in a bureaucracy, made significant change through her devotion, persistence, and political acumen. With her training knowledge for head nurses and faculty as well as nursing assistants she changed a 60% turnover rate of aides to 10% in 18 months (Harper, 1992).

Her childhood, her young father's adoration of her and his political activities, and her grandparents' influence and the stories of their lives had a profound impact on Mary. She attributes some of her shrewdness to Catherine J. Densford-Greve, her dean at the University of Minnesota. "She was a scholar, a strategist, a leader, a good researcher and she knew how to advance nursing. . . . I shadowed her to see her approach when she met with Governor Youngdahl, and then to see her approach when she went to meet with school deans, to watch her approach when she went out to meet with the leadership in industry, such as Pillsbury & Honeywell Foundation, to see how she went about getting things . . . like a new building. Wherever she went I followed and the black students in junior college used to kid me because I followed behind her carrying her briefcase and books just as a slave.

"Another influence was that of Estelle Osborne. She was a black person and one of the founders of the National Association for Colored

Graduate Nurses and the first black leader in the National League of Nursing. As a young girl from the back woods of Alabama, I would go to the meetings and conventions, not quite sure what to do, what to say, or how to dress. Estelle took me and guided me and ushered me . . . told me when to keep my mouth shut and when to open it and how to dress. Then I was on certain committees and she taught me a great deal about committee behavior and the politics that went on the table and under the table in professional meetings" (Harper, 1992).

Mary had numerous other influential people in her life, including Mary Rockefeller, Rabbi Abraham Heshey, and Dr. Carl Menninger, and learned from each of them. Her history is fascinating and an education to any who listens.

Virginia Stone

Virginia Stone, PhD, RN, FAAN, Professor Emerita of Duke University School of Nursing and pioneer gerontic nurse died December 4, 1993, at the age of 81 years. Dr. Stone began her career in public health nursing after graduation from Stuart Circle Nursing School in Richmond, Virginia, in 1934. At that time the major emphasis was on maternal and child health. During her study for a master's degree at University of North Carolina, Chapel Hill, she became enmeshed in the sociology of aging. Her doctoral dissertation in 1960 was a study of *Personal Adjustment in Aging in Relation to Community Environment*. She held several positions in public health nursing and began teaching nursing in 1959 at University of North Carolina at Chapel Hill. In 1966 she began her teaching career at Duke University, Durham, North Carolina and remained there until she retired in 1978.

Her professional awards, contributions, and recognitions have been enormous. Outstanding among them are the following:

- Fellow, Institute of Social Gerontology, Berkeley, California, 1959
- Development of the first graduate program in the nation in Gerontological Nursing at Duke University in 1966
- Membership in the American Nurses' Association executive committee, Division on Geriatric Nursing Practice, 1968–1976
- American Nurses' Association Honorary Recognition Award, 1974
- Senior Fellow, Center for the Study of Aging and Human Development, Duke University, 1972–1978
- Florence Cellar Gerontological Nurse Fellow, Frances Payne Bolton School of Nursing, Case Western Reserve University, 1986 (Stone, Curriculum Vitae, 1986)

A memorial was established in 1994 to Dr. Stone at Duke University School of Nursing, the Virginia Stone Scholarship in Gerontological Nursing that still continues (Wilson, 1994). The American Nurses Foundation also has established a Nursing Research Grants Program, restricted to gerontological nursing research and funded by a generous bequest from the estate of Virginia Stone, PhD, RN, FAAN (ANF flyer, 1996) (Fig. 2.17).

Among her numerous publications are some that show her forward thinking: The effect of nursing intervention on senility. *Geriatrics*, 68: September 1967; Preparation of the gerontological nurse specialist. *Nursing Home and Extended Care Facility of White Plains, Inc.* 7(1): Spring, 1971; Humanization of the seventh age of man. *Frontiers of Medicine*, pp. 209–222, 1977 (Stone, curriculum vitae, 1986).

Virginia Stone's Recollections

"My early experience with older persons was with my grandmother. I had two grandmothers who lived to be very old. I spent a lot of time with my mother's mother, who lived with us. She was a loving, caring person who had a great influence on my life. Also, my mother and her friends increased my interest in older people. She had to work and the group she worked with sort of grew old together. I think watching them was when I first began to understand older people. They came from a period

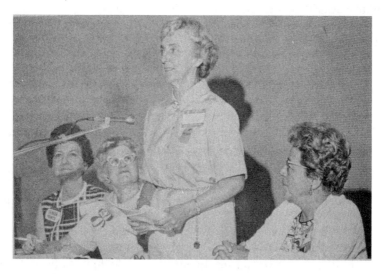

FIGURE 2.17 Virginia Stone presiding at a meeting of Division of Geriatric Nursing Practice.

when people believed in doing things just right, by the book. I learned from these women about aging. Everything had to be perfect so I learned a certain amount of perfection, a certain amount of timing of things, and an appreciation of certain values within people. Actually, I think those have been my strong points" (Stone, 1990).

"I didn't find my interest shifting to working with the aged until in the late 1950s when I went to the University of North Carolina for my master's degree in sociology. I thought about going on for a PhD and that I would need to take a few credits away from the University and a final year on campus. When I was working in Washington at the American Red Cross I took a night course called The Sociology of Aging under Clark Tibbetts. When I left that course I had already decided upon what my dissertation would be. . . . A person who had influence on my decision making was Virginia Lydia Hall. Lydia came down to the University of North Carolina for a summer course. My roommate said to me, 'I want you to meet the most interesting nurse you could ever meet. She's not like most nurses. She wears high heels and dresses fashionably.' What she did that influenced me so much was emphasize the idea that we were into the age of such specialized knowledge that we needed to specialize in nursing."

"I was very fortunate that I came into gerontological nursing at the time when ANA was undergoing a restructuring and, of course, I was part of that conference group that developed the Standards of Geriatric Nursing, and out of that came the Division of Gerontological Nursing. For ANA to have recognized geriatric nursing along with the other four specialties was a major step. I think that I had a lot of influence on that. One of the other things that occurred at that time was the realization that nurses throughout the United States had no background in gerontological nursing. . . . Another thing that happened while I was at ANA; we felt that directors of nursing in nursing homes were not being recognized so we brought directors of nursing together to see what they thought they needed. We at Duke had the first conference for nursing directors of nursing homes.

"The contribution I was known for most of all was in developing the first master's program in gerontological nursing in the country. That has been a real joy and the fulfillment is in what the students who graduated from that program have done." Ruby Wilson notes that Duke University School of Nursing initiated the first Masters in Science Nursing program, developed by Thelma Ingles and Ruby Wilson and graduated their first class in 1960. "I really perceive that as what I prize the most." Sister Marilyn Schwab was one of the most outstanding of my students. She was just tremendous. I'll tell you a story that is very interesting. She did not have a baccalaureate degree in nursing and therefore was turned down by another school. Now I had known Marilyn in ANA and

I had visited Benedictine Center in Mt. Angel, Oregon, and seen her in action. So we took her in our master's program even though others turned her down. She was just wonderful. . . . Eldonna Shields was also one of my students, you know. . . . We also had a grant for a post-master's program in geropsychiatric nursing at Duke in 1967 but it was ahead of its time and we only had one student. But, I think it ought to go down in history that the recognition of the need was there.

"Presently, I am following a small group of people who are 90 years old and over. I have been following some of them for 6 years now. I'm anxious to see what their problems are during this study and how they handle them. I have learned a tremendous amount about their lives. For example, the one who is 106 years old now went to the Kentucky Derby last year. . . . One of the special experiences has been with the lady who thinks she is 112. She gives a beautiful picture of an old black person's point of view. She describes how the 'pipes narrow' and so the blood doesn't go through well. She gives herself oxygen and finds that if she sleeps with oxygen it makes her sleep better. She is only on one medication and does not permit her family to give her medication or monitor her oxygen. One time while in the hospital she thought they weren't doing anything for her and she discharged herself in spite of the doctors. . . . One of the interesting things is that three of the ladies hated giving up the laundering of their underwear. They hated that someone else had to do this for them. I find that very interesting. . . . I don't visit them as a nurse, I visit them as a friend" (Stone, 1990).

"In my own aging process I have developed certain insights: I'm now 77 and I have had cataract surgery; I'm wearing a hearing aid; I'm now going to a wellness program for exercise and so forth. I go three times a week and I have been in it for a year and have already won a tee shirt because I have lost 25 pounds. It was an expensive shirt! This week they are going to recognize me because my cholesterol has come down from 268 to 212. So, I'm taking care of myself and using whatever opportunities are available to keep myself in good health. I had cancer 12 years ago and I have learned a lot about caring for myself. I don't let myself become over fatigued. Like most older people, I have arthritis at times so I found a first floor apartment. I have had to go through a lot of decision making about my future and I think that is rather important for us to do." Virginia says, "Many older people taught me to learn to live from day to day and how to cope and adapt to change. But, I know one must have long range plans and keep in touch with nature" (Stone, 1992, taped interview).

"As I reminisce, I cannot help but think of the progress in gerontological nursing over a span of 25 years. The availability of good textbooks, research studies, standards of practice, certification, and graduate and continuing education have all helped to improve clinical practice. . . .

Already there is a shortage of gerontological nurses in relation to demand. In the future curricula for preparation of nurses to care for the aged will change. All of this change leads to the need for more prepared faculty in gerontological nursing who can attract graduate nurses to the field. The future of the nursing profession can be determined by the quality of services and care available to meet the needs of older people" (Stone, 1990, pp. 816–817).

Reflections of a colleague, Dr. Ruby Wilson: "Dr. Stone spent 10 years in public health nursing, inclusive of Red Cross disaster nursing, and during this time she worked with several nationally known leaders, to whom she gave credit for greatly shaping her career" (Wilson, 1994, p. 180).

"Dr. Stone was awarded a World Health Organization Travel Fellowship to study health facilities for older people in England and New Zealand. In subsequent investigative studies, she focused on the unique health needs of the aged; the health behaviors of older people; personal adjustments of people as they age; and predictors of longevity. Dr. Stone incorporated the findings into her extensive consultation practice.

"Dr. Stone served as an advisor on aging issues to the Kellogg Foundation; the National Joint Practice Commission; the Federal Health, Education, and Welfare Administration (now HHS); and the National Long Term Care Education Center.

"An independent thinker, Dr. Stone described herself as a 'bit of a maverick with a self-styled leadership' that reflected strong opinions and self-confidence. . . . She was a person of warmth and loyal friendship toward professional colleagues and personal friends.

"Dr. Stone will be missed by many people for many reasons—including being a role model of activity and involvement for people of any age, but particularly the aged" (Wilson, 1994, p. 181).

Observations following my interview with Virginia Stone: I had not known Virginia as well as some of the others and always saw her as somewhat aloof and regal but found her pleasant and articulate throughout the interview. Her caring nature emerged as she spoke of her experiences with students and the close relationship with her brother. Her brother died 5 years previously. While she spoke of his death she also talked about her own dying. When she had breast cancer she rebelled against the traditional treatment and began the wellness approach. One of her close friends is now dying and they are planning a trip to the North Carolina coast to spend time in the sun and near the ocean. She said she knows it will be their last trip together. Virginia also spoke of friends in general and how one may become reluctant to make friends in old age as you know they will die.

She has made her specific requests about her own death and has written several pages about how she wants it to be managed. She predicts that active euthanasia will become available in the near future as there are so many old people objecting to the way they are forced to die. Virginia was open in expressing her feelings and especially about the elders she is now studying. Her eyes light up when she speaks of them. She clearly loves them and they her.

Two experiences revealed some of Virginia's special qualities to me. While at Duke I met with George Maddox and asked how he, director of the Duke University Center for the Study of Aging and Human Development, worked with nursing and especially with Virginia. He said something to the effect that she was very strong and reminded him of his mother. In fact, he said, "Sometimes she terrifies me."

Later, at a CWRU reception for her in a posh restaurant in Cleveland we had ordered cocktails. Hers was not quite right. She called the waiter over and he quickly wanted to take it away and replace it with one to her satisfaction. She refused. She only wanted him to know it was not made to perfection.

Virginia Stone was an inspired leader and a true pioneer in gerontic nursing. Yes, Virginia was forceful, a perfectionist and got things done. I have come to believe she quite unconsciously projected a public image of the refined Southern lady stock from which she descended; a steel magnolia. What a treasure it was to discover something of the real Virginia.

Dorothy Virginia Moses

Dorothy Moses was born in Grand Junction, Colorado, in 1914 and died January 15, 1992, at the UCSD Medical Center in San Diego. She was the daughter of a minister. When she was 6 years old her father died, prompting a move to New York City. Her mother began working at a lower East side community center where the family lived in a community house for a while; thus, she grew up in a multicultural setting. When the community house lost its funding, the family moved to Indiana, her mother's home state. Dorothy completed high school in Indiana and then moved back to New York City to attend St. Luke's Hospital School of Nursing (Kelly, 1987). St. Luke's School of Nursing had a reputation as being progressive; nurses were treated with respect and were not required to stand when in the presence of a doctor (Fig. 2.18).

When Dorothy was in the Navy Nurse Corps during World War II, she was stationed in Trinidad and helped take care of survivors of torpedoed ships, many of whom had spent weeks in open life boats (Savage, 1992).

Dorothy wrote, "One of the questions that I am frequently asked is, 'How did you become interested in gerontic nursing?' This is difficult to pinpoint but my interest really came to fruition when I was a graduate

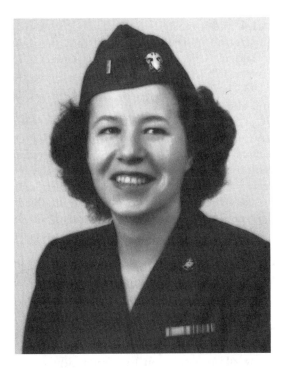

FIGURE 2.18 Dorothy Moses in the Nurse Corps, USN.

student at UCLA (University of California, Los Angeles) in the early 1950s. I had always enjoyed older persons, and I was fortunate to have a large family. One of my most pleasant memories was of visiting relatives in Indiana during summer vacations. I was raised in New York City and always looked forward to those visits. I adored my grandmother, and one of the highlights of those Indiana vacations was attending the family reunions in the local park. The food was great, and the relatives would fondly comment on my growth and my talents. My mother had 96 first cousins and many older great aunts and uncles and so on, who lived on farms, which I delighted in visiting.

In 1941, I joined the U.S. Navy Nurse Corps, since I felt that war was inevitable. I remained in the Nurse Corps through World War II and the Korean conflict until 1952. Late in the 1940s my oldest brother and his wife died, and I adopted their two children, ages 5 and 8. The Navy lifestyle was not very compatible with raising children so I received my discharge and used my GI bill to attend University of California, Los Angeles, completing my B.S. and M.S. degrees" (Moses, 1990a, p. 826).

Dorothy Moses graduated from St. Luke's Hospital School of Nursing, New York City, in 1937. She then earned a B.S. and P.H.N. in

1954 from UCLA and a master's in Psychiatric Nursing and Nursing Service Administration in 1958. Following that she did post-master's work at the Andrus Gerontology Center, University of Southern California, between 1967 and 1973.

Between 1937 and 1941, Dorothy was a staff nurse, private duty nurse, and camp nurse in New York City prior to joining the Navy. In the Navy Nurse Corps she became chief nurse. After her discharge she worked in the Veterans Administration Hospital in West Los Angeles until 1958 and then joined the San Diego State University School of Nursing, retiring in 1980. While there, between the years of 1965 and 1970, she directed a USPHS grant, "Improving Curriculum in Geriatric Nursing" (Moses, 1988). Ms. Moses also was involved with the San Diego State University's College of Extended Studies Educational Growth Opportunities (EGO) for retired San Diegans. After retirement, Dorothy lived in the Wesley Palms Retirement Center.

Dorothy's professional accomplishments, while raising her two adopted children, included numerous awards, honors, activities, and publications. Among these were the following:

- Certificate in Gerontological Nursing for Outstanding Achievement from the Andrus Gerontology Center (1975)
- Certificate of Appreciation for Outstanding Service from the California League of Nursing (1977)
- Gerontological Nurse of the Year by the *Journal of Gerontological Nursing* (1978)
- Edith Moor Copeland Award for Creativity in Nursing, from Sigma Theta Tau (Moses, 1988) (an award she especially treasured)

At the Andrus Center, Dorothy taught the first geriatric nursing course in 1967.

Dorothy was always professionally active and held offices and committee appointments in all of the gerontological organizations of that time: the Gerontological Society of America; the American Geriatric Society; President of the Western Gerontological Society (now the American Society on Aging); the National Council on the Aging; and was appointed by Governor Reagan to the Citizen's Advisory Council on Mental Health of California. She also headed the first ANA Commission on Geriatric Nursing and led development of the Standards for Geriatric Nursing in 1968 at the time Barbara Allen Davis was a staff person for ANA.

She had more than 20 publications in periodicals, book chapters, monographs, and published speeches, and was on the Editorial Board of the *Journal of Gerontological Nursing.* One of the most influential of her articles was published in *Nursing Outlook* in the 1960s. "In a survey of NLN accredited schools of nursing, approximately 150 at that time, there were only eight that taught anything specific to geriatric nursing care" (Moses, 1990b).

One of her most notable pioneering ventures was as hostess/moderator of the TV series on KPBS, San Diego, for 3 years, "Ask the Doctor." This program was focused on seniors' health topics and included time for San Diegans to phone in their health questions. Another pioneering venture was as Director of a Respite Care Program of Fletcher Hills Presbyterian Church and assisting other churches to establish such programs in which volunteers would provide relief in the home to caregivers for short periods of time (Moses, 1988). In her later years she volunteered to work in numerous community service and charitable organizations and established the first Alzheimer's groups in San Diego. "She says it is through these programs that she has become impressed with the work of retired RNs, who make up about half of the volunteers in the state's ombudsman program. . . . It would be difficult to find a health care or social program on behalf of the aged in San Diego that Dorothy Moses has not served as consultant to, been involved on the board, or initiated. At 73, Moses is still pioneering services in the expanding field of geropsychiatric nursing" (Kelly, 1987, pp. 277, 281).

Dorothy Moses Reflects

"While working on my M.S. degree, I was employed at the Veterans Administration Neuro-psychiatric Hospital in West Los Angeles. At this hospital there was an entire building of older veterans, hospitalized from 10 to 30 years. They were labeled "burned out schizophrenics," although some were labeled as senile or having chronic brain syndrome. The positive response of these patients to small amounts of attention was impressive. When I decided to do my master's thesis on remotivation, my academic advisor discouraged me. In the 1950s gerontic nursing was nonexistent. She thought there was no potential and these were old people who were just waiting to die, and that there was not enough literature on the subject. I was so distressed that I changed my major to nursing service administration where my advisor had a little different attitude.

"After receiving my M.S. degree I took a teaching position in psychiatric nursing at San Diego State University. San Diego had an excellent geriatric hospital that evolved from the old 'County Poor Farm.' Other psychiatric facilities were very primitive, since most of the psychiatric patients were sent to the state hospital. I selected the locked wards of the county hospital for student experience with the major goal of attempting to change and to motivate some students' attitudes toward working with the elderly. I was severely criticized by some of my nursing colleagues because they felt it was too depressing for young students. The main advantage of this type of program was that the student could have a long-term relationship with their assigned patients. Students could also plan and participate in group activities. Another advantage was that the student could see how the physical and mental problems of the elderly were interrelated. We were able to introduce many innovative programs and activities in this setting" (Moses, 1990a, pp. 826–827).

"Our older citizens are the ones who have made our country great, and they are living history and fascinating persons to listen to. They deserve all the tender loving care we are capable of giving and are usually most grateful for any attention. They respect nursing and look to us for knowledge and assistance. . . . My own aging experiences have taught me the importance of little things and trying to accomplish at least one important task each day. I still get most impatient when my body will not respond quickly enough to my desires. I have real difficulty in trying to slow down and pace myself and to accept assistance from others. However, I intend to go on giving as long as I am able, since it is in giving that we receive" (Moses, 1990a, p. 828).

One of her most esteemed awards was the Appreciation Award from the Alzheimer's Disease and Related Disorders Association, which she organized in San Diego. The plaque summarizes much of Dorothy's philosophy:

> Presented to Dorothy Moses who dauntlessly blazed trails to teach that dignity and self-respect should forever be the provenance of all life's twilight hours. (Savage, 1992)

My Reflections on Meeting With Dorothy Moses

When I first met Dorothy Moses at a Western Gerontological Society meeting during the early 1970s, I was most impressed by her warmth and willingness to meet with me, a fledgling geriatric nurse still in graduate school. As various people stopped to greet her and chat a moment, I realized she was a figure of significance in the field of gerontology. Later when engaged in my project with pioneer geriatric nurses, she welcomed me into her home at Wesley Palms, ordered a cot brought into her cottage for me, and openly shared her thoughts on videotape (September 13, 1990). One wall of her cottage was covered with awards and plaques from the various groups who have honored her. She dismissed those rather quickly and said she had a whole shelf full in the closet but nowhere to put them. Her dog, Mitzi, was her constant companion, and even through the interview sat on her lap.

As we walked around the grounds I saw the great respect given her from other residents. She had become the resident counselor as she said many had no idea about aging, and often their doctors did not either.

I discovered that she had an avid interest in history, ancient and medieval, demonstrating her innate curiosity and interest in the flow of events and the lives of people. She thought Medicare had been an exorbitantly expensive failure and should be scrapped. The future for elders seemed brighter as so many young people are very conscious of healthy life styles. Her advice to young nurses was to enter the field of geriatrics; the fastest growing field, full of opportunities, satisfactions and gratifications.

It was a gift to spend a bit of time with Dorothy, who has given so much of her's to others.

THE NURSING HOME PIONEERS

Ileta Blanche McFadden Shields

Information and Excerpts From Videotape, 1990

Blanche Shields dropped the name Ileta long ago. She and her daughter, Eldonna Shields-Kyle, were interviewed in their home in Vermilion, Ohio, on Blanche's 86th birthday, October 21, 1990. At 86, she is vivacious, talkative, and has an amazing memory of names, places, and details. Her nails and hair were done beautifully and she was wearing a Kruger Rand on a gold chain that was given her by her children on her 80th birthday. A nicely tailored suit, a corsage, and cream colored boots that came to her calf completed the picture. Her home is full of lovely art pieces, paintings and photographs of old people, many of them collected by her daughter, Eldonna.

Blanche first recognized the need for professional nurses working with older adults, when her mother, Bertha Eby McFadden, opened a "room and board" home for older men in Ashland, Ohio. At the time, Blanche was a new graduate from St. Luke's School of Nursing, Cleveland, in 1924 when she was 20 years old and could not sit for the State Boards until she was 21. From her past experiences with older people, it became her dream to someday own and operate a nursing home. This dream came to fruition in 1945. She had one sister, Marie, who is also an RN and entered St. Luke's the year after Blanche's entry. Marie McFadden Jameson followed Blanche's example and opened a nursing home in Fenton, Michigan.

Shields Nursing Clinic was the first licensed nursing home in Lorain County and she was the first Registered Nurse in the state of Ohio to own and operate a nursing home. She was a charter member of the Ohio

Nursing Home Association and has received numerous honors for her contributions to the care of the elderly and setting standards for long-term care. Blanche was also very active in the American Nurses Association, Ohio Nurses Association, and Lorain County Nurses Association. She joined ANA/ONA in 1924 and remained a member until her death at the age of 89. ANA sent her a dozen roses in honor of her 60th anniversary as a member of ANA. She and her husband Earl always valued education, especially nursing education. They personally financed the nursing education of many of their employees (Fig. 2.19).

Blanche and her husband Earl bought a large old home on 26 acres in 1944, put in a big garden and brought in patients in 1945. They began with seven rooms and 13 residents. At first she did the cooking, cleaning, laundry, and everything else with the help of her children. Soon they were able to hire a cook and a nurse. Earl was an engineer with the B&O Railroad, and so was often gone for several days on train runs. He was an excellent carpenter and engineer so when he retired they really began their expansion program. They kept building, improving, and enlarging, and eventually had 100 patients. Theirs was the first nursing home in the

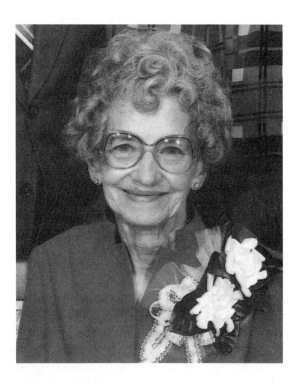

FIGURE 2.19 Blanche Shields.

state to have a sprinkler system; her husband insisted on fire protection. Another aspect of the home that was ahead of its time was nursing care plans and detailed charting. She insisted that each nursing staff had no more than eight patients to care for so they could do a good job. She educated the staff in basic techniques and humane nursing care. She said they were all like family; she never pushed and they always did well. When they left the nursing home there were 50 people on staff. Some of the staff still come to visit her regularly. "We always had a waiting list of staff and patients eager to get into the home." Interestingly, "Grandma Lange," who originally owned the property, came to the home to live and die in her last years.

Blanche's involvement in nursing home care was influenced by her mother who took several "senile people" (the term used in that era) into their home in Ashland, Ohio. They needed care but weren't physically ill. Her mother, Bertha Ely McFadden, a practical nurse, had worked in a state hospital and was appalled by "warehousing"; therefore, she developed her own nursing home. When her mother had a heart attack 3 years later, Blanche took her children and went to take over; the children all helped. Blanche realized special training was needed for the care of people with dementia, and set about to learn. Some were ill and she gave medications and IVs when needed. In addition she tried various methods to stimulate and care for the residents. She joined the groups and organizations that were concerned with nursing homes and attended meetings and educational events. In those years gerontology wasn't a word that was even recognized.

She determined to be a nurse when, as a child with a ruptured appendix, she was in the hospital for a long time as the wound continued to drain. She thought the nurses were wonderful and always loved nursing, caring for people, and making them more comfortable. But the history of her love for nursing goes back to her grandparents, who ran an "old folks home," the county poor farm. She fondly remembers her grandmother, who seemed always to be baking cookies. She says everyone in the family is "implicated." One daughter, Cathleen, runs a dialysis center, another is a nursing home administrator, her son is a thoracic surgeon in Akron, and Eldonna has devoted her life to the care of elders.

Blanche remembers particular patients with great pleasure. One man who had been head of NASA operations was with them for 3 years. She enjoyed him so much because he was "kind, refined, and compassionate." His wife had been an Eastern Star, as was Blanche. He wanted to give Blanche his wife's Eastern Star ring but fearing Earl might not approve, he gave it to Earl to give to Blanche.

They had only one incident in all the years: One resident went down to the "beer hall" and, coming back at twilight, was hit by a car and killed. He had no family and no money, so Blanche and her husband bought his casket and a suit in which to bury him.

She feels pleased with her life and has no important regrets, but said it was the hardest thing to adjust to retirement. She has a portrait of her husband on the wall at the foot of her bed. He died at age 70 but clearly remains much in her thoughts. Together they worked to build a rewarding life that they and their children enjoyed as they were giving comfort and pleasure to countless others (Shields, 1990).

Eldonna Shields-Kyle

As numerous people gathered in the sun room to celebrate her mother, Blanche's, 86th birthday, Eldonna and I sought a quiet corner for an interview. A few times it was necessary for Eldonna to suggest they quiet down a little. The guests and Blanche were having a marvelous time.

Eldonna was born and raised in nursing homes. Some of her earliest memories are of her grandmother's board and care home, working in the garden, weeding, picking strawberries, and feeding the chickens. There was always cooking, cleaning, and laundry to be done. She worked as a nurse's aide while going to high school. When she completed her nursing education at Ohio State University she worked in a Veterans Administration hospital for 3 or 4 years, taught in a diploma nursing program, and then entered the graduate program in gerontological nursing at Duke University; the only one of its kind in the nation, organized by Virginia Stone. This experience launched her professionally. Eldonna had many professional mentors, including her mother, Blanche Shields, Virginia Stone, Lydia Hall, Irene Burnside, and Mary Opal Wolanin.

After graduation from Duke University in 1972, she and Sally Buseck were hired by ANA to staff ANA's first federal grant, a brainchild of Virginia Stone, to conduct 43 3-day continuing education programs throughout the United States on *The Care of the Aged in Nursing Homes.* She and Sally were a team and traveled the nation and U.S. protectorates giving these programs. After the ANA project, Eldonna met Ella Kick, who was a nursing home surveyor for the Ohio Department of Health and came to survey the nursing home. They became close colleagues and worked together at ANA, where Eldonna was Chair of the Council of Gerontological Nursing and a member of the congress on nursing practice. They both represented nursing at the White House Conference on Aging in 1981. Together they co-authored publications and testified about needed legislation for the advancement of nursing home care at the state and national level.

Eldonna has received numerous honors, including the following:

- Gerontological Nurse of the Year Award, American Nurses' Association, Council on Gerontological Nursing
- Outstanding Alumni Award, Ohio State University College of Nursing
- Fellow of the American Academy of Nursing
- Special commendations by the 113th and 115th General Assembly of Ohio for "contributions to the well-being or our state's senior citizens through numerous efforts as a Gerontological Nurse and Educator."

The highlights of Eldonna's experience were when she was named Gerontological Nurse of the Year in 1986; the same year she was inducted into the American Academy of Nursing. Her mother, a member of ANA for 60 years, and her Aunt Marie, a member for 50 years, attended the ceremony, and the Council of Gerontological Nursing sent roses.

Throughout the growth of the geriatric nursing specialty, Eldonna's accomplishments have been notable. She has consulted on and developed innumerable programs to advance gerontological nursing nationwide; designed, developed, and taught gerontological nursing courses in the School of Nursing, Medical College of Ohio, Toledo, in the undergraduate and graduate programs; taught graduate courses at the University of Akron, College of Nursing; developed, implemented, coordinated, and administered the Life Long Learning Program at Lorain County Community College, Elyria, Ohio; and was the Coordinator/Gerontological Nurse Specialist/Therapist of Older Adult Services at the Nord Community Mental Health Center of Lorain, Ohio. She has been heavily involved in the Ohio Board of Nursing and held office as President (1995) and Vice President (1993–1994). Her consultations and presentations to universities, professional organizations, hospitals, and nursing homes throughout the United States and Canada are too numerous to mention. She is also on the committee to advise on the Standards and Scope of Gerontological Nursing Practice at ANA.

Her thoughts about the negative attitudes toward aging arise from several observations: There are fewer close extended families, thus many young people have little exposure to the old; little attention is given to aging in nursing curricula and usually the newest faculty with the least experience are assigned to teach. When gerontological nursing content is integrated into a curriculum, much of it is integrated out. The media and nursing schools tend to emphasize the excitement and challenge of the emergency room and critical care.

Eldonna says there is nothing more exciting than seeing a stroke patient regain function or assisting a person to emerge from the oblivion of an incorrect diagnosis of Alzheimer's disease. Her enthusiasm is apparent when she tells of Benny: On admission to the nursing home he was inert and nonresponsive. With patience and a review of his psychoactive medications it seemed that he had not been adequately assessed. She called in a geropsychiatrist who discontinued all his medications and ordered antidepressants for him. As he improved it was discovered that he was bilingual and very articulate. Soon he was up and doing things; sparkling. He had a life and was no longer vegetating. It is essential that a specialist, of which there are few, assess individuals who are too hastily labeled as demented.

An observation Eldonna has made in several cases needs further study. Old couples often exist in a very fragile system, the delicate relationship is balanced on a "razor's edge." One man who had a stroke, needing almost total care from his wife, began to recover function with appropriate treatment. His wife had problems with alcohol but had been able to care for him. As his independence increased she declined and later died. The tenuous balance had been upset.

With a grant to fund the development of the Geropsychiatric Program at Nord Community Mental Health Center and Lorain Community College, Eldonna and others have established outreach and educational programs within the county for caregivers' groups and Alzheimer's support groups. Initially, Eldonna thought these groups needed more programming that would provide education, knowledge of resources, and facts about aging, but she found many were too tired and stressed to take in such information. It was not a "teachable moment." First they needed the opportunity to talk about their feelings and frustrations. An interactional educational program just before the time of my interview drew more than 100 people, evidence of the great need. Eldonna is deeply involved with a "life-enhancing" educational program for older adults, The Academy for Senior Studies, at Lorain Community College. Eldonna also served as adjunct faculty for the nursing program at the college where she taught gerontological nursing theory and clinicals.

She views herself as moving through the gamut of elder services. In her childhood and youth she was busy in the nursing home. She and the residents would peel potatoes, harvest vegetables and fruit, and set tables. Working in the home and the garden involved residents in useful activities and real, everyday life. Later Eldonna taught and traveled numerous places, giving workshops and lectures. She is still doing these things but is also working with the well elderly (Shields-Kyle, 1990) (Fig. 2.20).

Eldonna married Charles Edward Kyle on June 8, 1985. Eldonna says, "He traveled with me to many meetings, CE programs, and when I

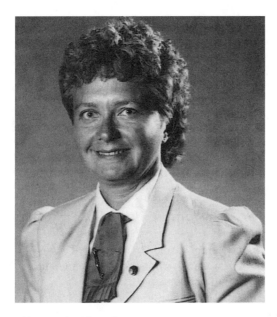

FIGURE 2.20 Eldonna Shields-Kyle.

received honors. He was always proud of my activities and contributions to gerontological nursing and nurse regulation. He died suddenly on August 2, 2001. I treasure my time with him, and will always miss his love, interest, and involvement in my personal and professional life" (Shields-Kyle, 2005, p. 4).

Eldonna's Thoughts About Present and Future Needs

"Nursing homes, for the most part, are based on the medical model, and meaningful daily activities are seldom allowed or encouraged. Nurses in acute care and critical care settings have even greater problems." At the time of the interview, 15 years ago, restraining delirious elders was common practice. Eldonna deplored this and saw this as "subtle professional abuse of older persons" (Shields-Kyle, 1990).

Some of her future hopes and predictions are occurring, but there is a long way to go. She foresaw the need for more nurses in case management, more attention to supportive services that will keep elders in the community, and empowerment of older persons. They may need to be taught assertiveness skills and encouraged to be involved in all decisions affecting them. She doesn't believe "tender loving care" is sufficient; there must be "intelligent loving care."

Her philosophy is taken from that of R.S. Allison, who noted that "whatever may be said of aging, old age is a losing game. We must therefore focus our attention so that the points in that game are not given up unnecessarily."

She believes students and young nurses should be instilled with enthusiasm for geriatric care and recognize the challenges as unique. "Nurses need to value each others' skills; none are better or worse, just different. And to be an effective geriatric nurse one must be caring, sensitive, knowledgeable and have tremendous energy" (Shields-Kyle, 1990). Eldonna exemplifies all these qualities and has been content and gratified in her calling.

Ella Kick

Dr. Ella Kick was born in Wooster, Ohio, on December 14, 1930. She is the daughter of Vincent S. and Agnes E. McClelland Massaro. She married William H. Kick on August 30, 1952, and was widowed February 14, 1967. She and William had two children and she has five grandchildren.

Ella attended elementary and high school in Wooster, Ohio. She earned a diploma from St. John Hospital School of Nursing, Cleveland, Ohio, in 1951. She earned a BSN (1966) and MSN (1968) from Ohio State University. While in the master's program she asked to focus her studies on geriatrics. The dean did not understand why a graduate degree could be of any possible use to work in nursing homes but Ella persisted, and the dean, Wilda Chambers, relented and eventually asked Ella to design the gerontology track in the program. Her thesis topic was a descriptive study of administrative perceptions in nursing homes and her clinical study was of urinary incontinence. Post-master's work was done at University of Cincinnati; Andrus Gerontology Center at University of Southern California; University of Colorado; and she earned a Certificate in Nursing Administration from Wayne State University. In 1986 she earned a Doctor of Science Degree from Indiana University. Since 1966 her activities and professional education have focused on gerontological nursing. Her first faculty position was at the University of Cincinnati College of Nursing and Health (Kick, 1990b).

In 1978 Dr. Kick was awarded a Robert Wood Johnson Faculty Fellowship in Primary Care and worked with Dr. Frank McGlone, a renowned geriatrician at the Denver Clinic (Kick, 1990c). Ella was elected in 1979 by ANA as the first chair of the newly formed Council of Nursing Home Nurses. In that position she had significant influence. Later this was absorbed into the Division of Geriatric Nursing. In 1986

Ella was named the ANA Gerontological Nurse of the Year, and was the recipient of the Ohio State University College of Nursing Distinguished Alumni Award. In 1987 she received the Outstanding Alumni Award from the Ohio State University College of Nursing. In 1990 she was awarded the National HealthCorp Chair of Excellence in Nursing from Middle Tennessee State University.

The National HealthCorp Chair of Excellence in Nursing was endowed in 1990 by Dr. Carl Adams, who opened his first nursing home in 1948 to meet a need that he saw was not being met. Over the years he established a corporation and the numerous nursing homes became a family enterprise. He was very active in the Nursing Home Division of the American Medical Directors Association (AMDA). Because of his deep interest in nursing home care, he endowed a chair at Middle Tennessee State University. In a national search for an occupant of this National HealthCorp Chair of Excellence to honor a nursing home nurse, Ella was selected to hold the chair for a 3-year period. During this time she spent much of her time providing inservice education around the state. She was elected Tennessee Gerontological Nurse of the year during this period at Middle Tennessee State University.

Dr. Kick's work experiences included staff nurse, head nurse, supervisor, and director of nursing in various hospitals and nursing homes. She was a Medicare/Medicaid surveyor and consultant for 5 years and later held university nursing faculty appointments as well as designing the Master's Program in Gerontological Nursing at the University of Cincinnati. She developed and taught the gerontological content. In spite of the program offering stipends and being given wide publicity, there was little interest in geriatric care in 1973 and students selected other specialties that were also offering stipends.

She has consulted in numerous nursing homes and hospitals, acting as legal consultant and expert witness to attorneys investigating problems in the care of older persons. Other consultant activities have focused on gerontological nursing, staffing issues, urinary incontinence, patient care plans, health behaviors, and nursing administration (Kick, 1990c). Dr. Kick was urged by Procter and Gamble to be a consultant on the Attends project but "I had a real dislike for 'diapers' and they were trying to convince me to work for them. I wanted to try the product before I got involved. I wore Attends myself before I agreed to work for them. I made them promise that I could teach bladder retraining anywhere I went for them. They agreed so I had a very good working relationship with them for about 5 years" (Kick, 2004). When giving workshops on the topic of incontinence she encouraged the attendees to wear Attends, all the while focusing on aspects of bladder retraining. She found that in many cases patients were being awakened every 2 hours to use the bed pan or commode and from that her interest in sleep deprivation arose. She asked, "How would you like to be wakened every 2 hours for the rest of your life!" (Kick, 1990a).

Ella firmly believes that new graduates should not be in nursing homes as their first experience. She says they need the hospital experience for at least 2 years: the availability of other RNs with whom to confer, the availability of resources, and the experience to build self-confidence. "In the nursing home they will likely be the only RN, they must function independently, make administrative and staffing decisions. They may have no one to help solve problems with families or staff. They are on their own" (Kick, 1990a).

One of Ella's fascinating experiences was in 1978, working with a family nurse practitioner in a Frontier Nursing Service clinic in Hayden, Kentucky. She saw the older patients and the other nurse the younger ones. She developed "postscriptions." These were compiled after a thorough assessment of the individual and their living situation; a list of things the individual could do to maintain health and function. She was dismayed to discover many of them could not read, but what they lacked in formal education they had gained through life's education and could compensate for their lack of reading abilities by using memory (Kick, 1990c).

She has given numerous seminars, institutes, workshops, and inservice education programs all across the United States. Ella has written many articles and book chapters, most dealing with a variety of nursing home topics.

Ella writes: "What a fortunate teenager I was!! On September 15, 1946, when I was almost 16, I took a job in a small (25-bed) hospital in a small Ohio community. I wanted to get a feel for nursing and to earn enough money for 'nurses' training.' As I think about that experience, I believe, even then, most nurses did not like caring for older people. As a young nurse's aide I was always assigned to the older patients. . . . My favorite patient from those days in the late forties was 'Pop' Mowrer. I heard the doctor call him Pop, so I called him Pop also; I am not sure that I would take that license today" (Kick, 1990c). Ella lived in the basement of the hospital and often spent off hours talking with patients and comforting them. She appreciated the older folk and they loved her.

Pop had surgery on Sunday and on Monday talked to Ella about his fear of dying and leaving his wife alone. She stayed with him, held his hand, and promised to pray for him and his wife, Artie. Several years later, while she was in nursing school in Cleveland, she returned home for the weekend and found that Pop had brought her some wood carvings in gratitude for her caring and also being with his wife when she died. She had not even realized she had attended his wife when she was dying. "This was the beginning of a long relationship—many letters, visits, phone calls, pieces of wood which have a place in my living room, and many discussions that gave me an insight to the lives of older people that would stay with me for a lifetime" (Kick, 1990c, p. 820). Several of the patients she had attended while in the hospital working as an aide sent her money while she was in nursing school. She was very touched by that.

Ella hopes to live long enough to see the following changes: nurses asserting their expertise in the care of the aged; influencing nurses to become political activists, especially to change regulations so that an RN is required in every nursing home 24 hours a day; greater emphasis placed on gerontology in basic nursing education; more attention to wellness and health promotion; and real attention to the effects of drugs on older persons. She firmly believes that much of the decreased mental acuity that occurs with elders results from drugs, dehydration, and sleep deprivation (Kick, 1990a).

In a recent article (Kick, 2003) in the *Online Journal of Issues in Nursing*, Dr. Kick discusses the history of Medicare; healthy old age and quality of life issues; veterans; baby boomers; the need for long-term care options and concentrated planning; the costs of health care; and how far we have come in understanding the care of the aged since the advent of Medicare. She cites studies that address these issues.

Dr. Kick has been an avid activist for the aged for 40 years. She retired from full-time nursing in 1997. Her position at that time was Dean, School of Nursing, Ashland University, Ashland, Ohio. Since that time she continues to be a County Board of Health member, and is a member of the Ohio Nurses' Association and the Ohio League of Nursing. She continues to present continuing education programs throughout the state and volunteers in various organizations related to aging (Kick, 2004).

Her influence has been enormous but most importantly, she relishes each day and her work with the aged wherever they may be. She says she never planned her career but things "just fell into place." Clearly, she is alert to every opportunity to instigate action that will result in an improvement in the situations of the old. In her own aging process she finds herself more flexible, accepting ambiguity and feeling pleased to "pass the torch" to the younger nurses coming into the field. She expects a great influx of nurses and nurse practitioners will enter the field of geriatrics, extended care in nursing homes and the community as it is becoming more prestigious (Fig. 2.21).

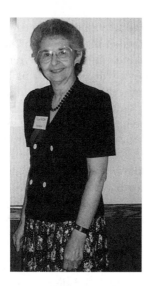

FIGURE 2.21 Ella Kick at workshop.

Sister Marilyn Schwab

Unfortunately, Sister Marilyn Schwab died April 8, 1984, before I had the opportunity to interview her personally. The knowledge of her history and activities has been provided by Lucia Gamroth, a past administrator in the Benedictine Nursing Center (BNC) and some of the staff that worked with her in Mt. Angel, Oregon (Gamroth, 1998); from the biographical notes in her personal journal of the illness experience preceding her death (Schwab, 1984); from the Benedictine Sisters and family members who produced her journal for publication; and from my recollections of working with her on the W. K. Kellogg Foundation Geriatric Nurse Practitioner (GNP) Project in the years 1981–1984 (Ebersole, 2004).

Sister Marilyn was born February 12, 1937 in Silverton, Oregon, lived in Mt. Angel her entire life, and attended the Benedictine Sisters' schools. She began work at the Benedictine Nursing Center as an aide soon after finishing her novitiate. In 1960 she graduated from St. Benedictine's Hospital and School of Nursing in Ogden, Utah. She later earned a master's degree in gerontological nursing at Duke University and became a clinical specialist in gerontological nursing. Dr. Virginia Stone, director of the program, remembered Sister Marilyn as an inspired and outstanding student. She was named Outstanding Alumni, Duke University School of Nursing.

She lectured nationwide and was invited to present a paper at the International Conference on Gerontology in Tokyo, Japan. Sister Marilyn was also a consultant and assistant professor at the School of Nursing,

Oregon Health Sciences University, Portland, Oregon. She served on numerous national committees, including the subcommittees of the American Nurses Association and the U.S. Senate's Special Committee on Aging. In 1980 she represented the Federation of St. Gertrude (of which the BNC is a member) at a worldwide Benedictine symposium in Rome, Italy.

Sister Marilyn was a visionary: She developed a curriculum for aide training that was approved by the Oregon State Board of Nursing to certify nurses aides long before others in the field of long-term care. She was on the ANA Executive Committee of the Division of Geriatric Nursing Practice (DGNP) and assisted in formulating the Standards of Practice in 1973. She testified before the Subcommittee on Long Term Care of the Special Committee on Aging, headed by Senator Frank Moss of Idaho (Gamroth, 1998). Under Sister Marilyn's leadership, the BNC participated in the Kellogg Geriatric Nurse Practitioner/Nursing Home Project Administered by the Mountain States Health Corporation in Boise, Idaho. One of the staff nurses at BNC, Sister James Egell, returned to fulfill the ideal role of GNP within a nursing home: Sister James was a full-time geriatric nurse practitioner within the BNC, conferring with staff and doctors, making thorough assessments of patients, intervening whenever within her scope of practice, developing protocols, teaching staff, and assisting to organize the few GNPs then existing in the western states. The first conferences of GNPs were held at the BNC (Ebersole, 2004; Gamroth, 1998).

Sister Marilyn spoke to many groups, including the American Medical Association, about the role of medical directors and the value of interdisciplinary teams in long-term care (LTC). She spoke to the International Congress in Tokyo about the need for a holistic model not based on a medical model. Marilyn said, "I am less impressed with the nurse who can determine that a patient is 'throwing PCVs' than I am with a nurse who can get a frightened, confused patient to eat" (Gamroth, 1998, p. 160).

Over the years she served the BNC as a nurse, director of nursing, administrator, and consultant. Sister Marilyn then became the Prioress of the Benedictine Sisters of Mt. Angel until in 1983 her illness caused her to resign, although she continued to work on an intermittent basis until her hospitalization (Benedictine Sisters Biographical Note, 1986). Even before Elizabeth Kubler Ross's pioneering work with death and dying, Sister Marilyn was writing and speaking nationally about nursing the dying, gerontology, and long-term care.

"In the mid-1950s, leaders of Mount Angel, a little town of 2,000 people, approached the Benedictine Sisters and asked them to open a home for people who could no longer care for themselves. So the BNC was created in response to a public need and became a community of care for residents and the larger community. . . . Some residents worked in the kitchen, the dining room, or maybe the maintenance shop as a part of their everyday activities. Some residents even had keyed locks to their rooms and decided who would and who wouldn't be allowed to assist them in care" (Gamroth, 1998, p. 160).

Everyone knew everyone else in this small community and the influence of the Benedictine Nursing Center was felt by all. Certain inhabitants of the town were visited in their homes and apartments and given advice and assistance when needed. Some came to the BNC to eat and socialize, even to play pool. On one visit I made, there was a St. Patrick's Day celebration and the people of Mt. Angel were bringing things and avidly participating (Ebersole, 2004). In turn, Sister Marilyn drew on her experience with families, residents, and the community to learn about the many facets of growing old (Smith, in Gamroth, 1998).

"Before working at the BNC, I was very discouraged about nursing. I was being forced to do things that felt contrary to my soul, such as tying people down and shoving tubes down the throats of people against their wishes. When I walked in the door of the BNC, I felt like I had come home. As I was walking around with Marilyn that first day, she introduced me to one person who had been her piano teacher, another who was a relative, and the place had an incredible community feeling about it" (Rader, in Gamroth, 1998, p. 160).

Paula McNeil (McNeil, in Gamroth, 1998, p. 160) writes, "The first memory I have of Marilyn was sitting next to her on a plane on our way to the American Nurses Association convention in 1968. The prevailing notion of the time was that nurses who worked in nursing homes didn't have the skills to be able to work in acute care. Here was this well-spoken, bright, energetic, wonderful person who was saying to me that she believed that nursing's most exquisite skills could be employed in the LTC setting. She thought the profession was overlooking a really important opportunity to demonstrate nursing at its best. I'll never forget how eloquently she stated the role of the nurse and nursing in LTC, and it made such inherent sense to me that it influenced how I viewed gerontological nursing."

"She was known for her warmth, good humor, vision, and care of older people. She believed each person was important, regardless of his or her particular role, and that each had a unique contribution to make to the caring atmosphere of the nursing center. Her interest in the contribution of a nursing assistant or housekeeper was as keen as her interest in a registered nurse or member of the Senate. And she conveyed that equality in ways that staff members believed it and felt valued" (Gamroth, 1998, p. 160).

Many of my memories of the BNC have faded but I particularly remember joining the staff members of the BNC at dinner one evening and was astonished at how openly they discussed ideas and personal problems with each other and how Sister Marilyn made it possible, comfortable, and acceptable. Her love of art, music, history, and nature were apparent as she toured me through the Sister's home and grounds. Being a part of that community on my occasional weekend visits felt natural and very spiritual (Ebersole, 2004).

Her journey through illness and toward death as written in her journal is moving; a remarkable legacy. "I love life and am not depressed but why not welcome release? To know the journey is almost over and one can look forward to eternity—soon! But probably it's not so simple. More likely I will need to learn to be patient with just not feeling good and not being able to enter into life as fully as I have—to watch from the side lines. That would be harder than dying. I can't pray for healing—there are so many more important things to pray for. God, you don't need to take this away—just help me deal with it with aplomb—grace, joy and courage. Help me not to burden others with it" (Schwab, 1986, p. 1).

"I feel blessed with so much. Why should I be angry at this? God doesn't owe me good health! Sickness is part of living in the real world—why should I be spared unnecessarily? There are so many more terrible sufferings people endure this seems so small" (Schwab, 1986, p. 7).

"I was listening to music with the earphones last night (between phone calls!) and went off on this meditation about God's power and presence in all creation—like the wonder of the gift of the composer, the performers, the makers of instruments—the makers of the radio—and the wonder of my own body that I can hear the music, respond with joy and rhythm, even my finger's ability to beat time" (Schwab, 1986, p. 37).

While reading St. Augustine and his renunciation of harmonies, mountains, sunsets, flowers, and worldly things she writes, "I wanted to stand up and say, 'That's crazy!!' It is to like wonderful music and mountains—and friendship and beauty of people. Why would God make all those beautiful things if we are supposed to ignore them or hate them?" (Schwab, 1986, p. 41).

She came to a decision after being told by the doctor that she could and should live in isolation because she was so vulnerable to infection. She writes, "After asking me lots of questions to be sure he really understood me he said thoughtfully that it was reassuring to him to have a patient so clearly choose quality—that usually people will obediently take whatever medicine offers for survival almost no matter the cost" (Schwab, 1986, p. 47).

On April 7, her family and a few sisters were keeping vigil with her as she slipped into a coma. At about 1:30 Sunday morning she woke and asked everyone to gather around her bed and to sing. She then talked about her awe and wonder at facing death and said, "I won't really be gone if you just get in touch with that part of me that is inside of you; and I'll take a piece of you with me" (Benedictine Sisters, 1986, p. 66).

Eldonna Shields-Kyle notes, "Sister Marilyn had been to my home many times. I remember going into the Smoky Mountains with her during weekends at Duke. Her love of nature and music are most memorable. She enjoyed her guitar and taught me how to play a few things and especially taught me to love classical music. She appreciated Mason Williams and his humor" (Shields-Kyle, 2005, p. 5). Eldonna is one of the many that carries a part of Sister Marilyn with her (Fig. 2.22).

Sister Marilyn Schwab's influence on nursing home care, gerontological nursing, and those around her cannot be fully known, much less summarized. However, her life of caring was reflected in her openness regarding her dying experience. Sister Marilyn lived life the way she died. She was truly an inspiration to all who met and loved her. Her legacy is enormous.

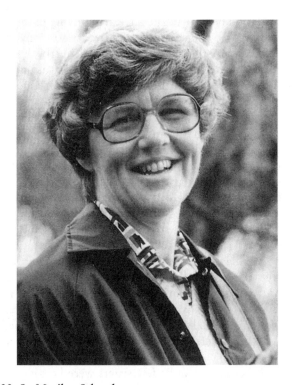

FIGURE 2.22 Sr. Marilyn Schwab.

CONCLUSION

There were many names mentioned during my interviews with these trail-blazing nurses that forged through the jungles of neglect and despair. There were those who had inspired them, assisted them, or discouraged them enough to fortify their determination. Few of those who were help-ful and supportive had any specific knowledge of geriatric care and geron-tology was not yet recognized as a specialty field of study. These geriatric nurse pioneers were winning the war of negligence and ignorance.

CHAPTER THREE

Nurses in Action:
The Second Generation

The nurses of the 1970s through the 1980s saw action! The advent of Medicare in 1965 signaled a new era in the care of the aged. It became profitable for hospitals, doctors, and to a lesser degree, nurses, to focus their attention on the aged. The knowledge base, or ammunition, of caring for the aged was sadly lacking but the territory to be gained was clearly demarcated. The march toward it began in 1966.

I first heard of this amazing plan of action from a wealthy aged lady in a private room, in a luxurious wing of the hospital where I first entered practice. Incredulous, I listened as she explained that Medicare would pay most of her hospital bill. What! And, shortly after that I read Mary Mendelson's analysis: The sick old had not captured the attention of any of the myriad professionals providing health care. Medicare provided incentives that attracted interest in the benefits of the program among health providers at all levels.

Sadly, according to Mary Opal Wolanin, those who thought the benefits would extend to recipients of long-term care discovered it did not, except in cases where Medicare would pay for the first 100 days if the individual was qualified and expected to recover. Doctors seldom crossed the threshold of nursing homes but orders, usually verbally issued on the telephone, ultimately must be signed by a physician. Some budding physicians saw an opportunity for supplementing their income while finishing their residencies. Thus, was born "coat tail" visits in nursing homes.

Walter, a resident in one home, informed me of this system: A doctor would cruise through the building, pop his head in the door of each resident, and then proceed to the charts and sign orders. Walter explained that he didn't have time to grab the doctor's coat tail before he was gone. Walter thought to record this practice but the doctor, whom he tried to detain, found the recorder and reported his paranoia and recommended

he be seen by a psychiatrist. Fortunately, there was no psychiatrist readily available so Walter was not bothered.

Doctors were not the only ones to benefit from Medicare. In my first
6 months of practice (1965) I was given two substantial raises. When I
foolishly questioned this, the director of nurses told me it was correct and
simply to be grateful.

Universities also saw the opportunity and the first, faltering programs in aging began to appear. Some medical schools and schools of
nursing made gestures but, having no qualified faculty or seldom any student interest, the bits of theory that appeared were minimal and "integrated." Some notable exceptions were discussed in chapter 2. In general,
at this time there were far more officers than troops. Terry Fulmer, a
young nurse at that time, said she was pleased to work with the aged as
she had the leeway to try new things and no one bothered her.

In 1969, the Ethel Percy Andrus Center, at University of California
in Los Angeles, was established and became the West Coast mecca of aging studies and research. This center, initially headed by Richard Peterson
and then by James Birren, attracted health care professionals from across
the nation. Someone commented that the aged rats used for research at the
center received more care and attention than most elders in nursing homes.

The enormous network of Veterans Administration facilities also
found they could conduct numerous experimental programs with government support and little interference. In many cases, the Veterans
Administration Medical Centers (VAMC) generated the most substantial
aging research available at the time. Unfortunately, the preponderance of
studies were of male veterans with some disabilities, so they did not represent the aged population as a whole. The Geriatric Research, Education
and Clinical Centers (GRECCs), an arm of the VAMCs, were established
in 1976.

The 1970s through the early 1990s were years of opportunity. The
fields of geriatrics and gerontology were flourishing. Federal and private
foundation funding for research, education, and model projects was
available. By the 1980s, some very good educational programs had been
established and theories about aging abounded. There were several excellent centers throughout the nation devoted to the study of aging. Those
were the golden years for individuals interested in entering the field.

THE SECOND GENERATION

The second generation of leadership in geriatric nursing is not nearly as
circumscribed as we would wish for the purposes of classification. Many,
if not most, are still fervently pursuing their interest and have developed

subspecialties within the specialty. In addition, numerous individuals—to whom we have not had access or whom we do not have sufficient space or information to include in this text—have and are still making major contributions. We recognize that it is simply not possible to include all the individuals important to the burgeoning of geriatric nursing. I have set an arbitrary time line. Those who really entered the field in the 1970s I will consider to be of the second generation. I am one of those.

PRISCILLA EBERSOLE

As many of the extraordinary people who focused their professional efforts on geriatric nursing, I entered a geriatric nursing career quite by chance and have never planned ahead. Opportunities simply appeared in my path. My mentors were Irene Burnside and later, Mary Opal Wolanin. Without their influence I would likely be working as an acute care nurse or in a mental health unit. I enjoyed both of those venues but none would have given the range of experiences I have had in geriatrics and gerontology.

I had two remarkable grandmothers but no contact with my grandfathers. My paternal grandfather died when in his fifties and my maternal grandfather had moved to Florida and remarried long before. However, my exceptional grandmothers were both important in my life.

Grandma Daisy Belle Catherine Brown Pierre Goldsby Ackley outlived three husbands (as you may have guessed) and died when she was 96 years old. Along with her parents and six siblings, she traveled in a wagon train from Missouri to the Washington Territory in 1880 when she was 8 years old. She learned to type and wrote about the experience when she was 80 years old. From listening in awe as she recounted the journey, I learned to appreciate the importance of the life story of older people and the need they have to tell it.

My other grandmother, Kathryn May Shaver Holder, was the quintessential grandmother. She lived on a small farm in the rural community of Liberty (adjacent to Salem, Oregon). Her two sons lived on adjoining property and for a time my parents lived there also. I was the first child of her beloved youngest daughter and the absolute apple of her eye. When I discovered 200 or so letters she had written between 1928 and 1934 to Edna, her missionary daughter in India, I was simply overcome with emotion. I stepped back into their lives as she wrote about daily events, friends, family activities, and hard times. I saw my infant and child self through her eyes, saw the Depression experience as it was for small farmers, experienced my young parents, and learned how individuals and small communities survived those desperate times.

Numerous farms were lost to taxes. She and her two sons managed to keep their farms and sustain themselves. It seemed someone was always "dropping in" on grandma just at mealtime. In letters to Edna, she described in detail each food served at those meals. It became clear to me how important sufficient food was in their lives. She sometimes sent food to friends and neighbors saying in the letters, "We can't let our friends starve." Some excerpts from the letters seem fitting:

"Monday, December 2, 1929: Helen missed her stage so we got her and came back the hill road. We had a nice dinner, Irish and sweet potatoes, roast pork, kraut, cranberries, jam, tomatoes and pickles."

"December 18, 1929: Well, Monday all the folks from Lyons came. Miriam came down and we had the house warm, clean and dinner started. Les and Joe killed the goat so we had some meat."

"April 2, 1930: I sent five bunches of sweet peas to town this morning and Treesa Nilean got $1.70 worth. Mrs. Robbins was here and said Mr. Hammel hadn't had tea or coffee for over a month and was living on 10 cents a day. We can't let our neighbors go hungry."

"May 20, 1930: Times are bad here. I've taken in $90 since the first of March but a lot have not paid yet. Well, I have a good time anyway with my plants. We read something in the papers nearly every day about Gandhi. I hope there will be no serious trouble."

My grandmother had divorced in 1920. There was no government assistance of any kind and she supported herself by selling farm produce and the plants and flowers in her large greenhouse. She was a florist and made flower arrangements for funerals, the grange, and other community events. It seemed there were many funerals.

Thus, I have always had an affinity to old ladies, and there have been special ones in my life for as long as I can remember. One very exceptional lady, Catherine (who died in a nursing home at age 104), taught me most of what I know about aging. She was the one from whom I drew inspiration for the first text that Patricia Hess and I wrote.

I was one of the associate degree nurses who entered nursing at age 35. I had never longed to be a nurse but a new program was established in nearby San Mateo Community College and it seemed like something to do as my children were all in school. Then I was imbued with the desire for more and more education. Fortunately, inexpensive and accessible programs, and some grants, were readily available. San Francisco State University (SFSU) provided an opportunity to earn my BSN and University of California, San Francisco, my graduate degree and post master's work. It was there in 1971 that I met Irene Burnside. As well as a class in critiquing geriatric research, she gave me opportunities to speak and give workshops, some with her and some on my own. I also enrolled in her first class for a gerontological certificate at Ethel Percy Andrus

Gerontology Center, University of Southern California, in Los Angeles. After completing the certificate I taught there for a number of summers. I wrote chapters for Irene's text, *Nursing and the Aged,* and then Pat Hess and I wrote our own texts for Mosby, and Springer Publishing Company.

When I was advised by the Chair at SFSU School of Nursing that I must have a doctorate, I enrolled in an external degree program and focused my doctoral dissertation on the extent to which the nursing students in our "holistic" curriculum retained that orientation as they progressed through the program. As expected, most lost their holistic focus as they experienced the highly technical aspects of care.

From 1981 through 1984 I took a leave from my teaching position at SFSU and was Field Director of the W. K. Kellogg Foundation Geriatric Nurse Practitioner (GNP) Project to recruit nurses from nursing homes in the 13 western states to become GNPs. We arranged for their education in one of the five universities involved in the project and monitored their return to the facilities from which they were recruited. In that position I visited more than 100 nursing homes; most were exceptionally good homes or they would not have welcomed the idea of assisting in the education of a nurse within their facility to become a geriatric nurse practitioner. The Kellogg grant contributed money to their education. In addition to experiencing the best of the nursing homes I was privileged to work with some outstanding nursing faculty: Evelyn DeWalt and Mary Jane Welty (University of Arizona, Tucson); Carole Deitrich (University of California, San Francisco); Carolyn Enloe (University of Washington, Seattle); Jane Swart (University of Colorado, Denver); and a faculty person from the State University of New York (SUNY, Syracuse). I also became acquainted and worked with the leaders in the American Association of Homes for the Aged and the American Health Care Association.

The field was mushrooming and I had numerous opportunities to speak and give workshops across the United States and Canada and attend conferences related to aging and nursing. In 1991 I was asked to become the editor of the *Geriatric Nursing Journal,* then newly acquired by Mosby, which is now edited by Dr. Barbara Resnick. Along the way I have met and worked with most of the people in geriatric nursing and gerontology. I attended the 1995 White House Conference on Aging as a press representative.

In 1988 I was invited to occupy the Florence Cellar Endowed Chair in Gerontological Nursing at Frances Payne Bolton School of Nursing, Case Western Reserve University (CWRU) in Cleveland. Again, I took leave from San Francisco State University. This was an outstanding opportunity to work with May Wykle, Joyce Fitzpatrick, and numerous other exceptional people in nursing and aging. I was also privileged to meet Florence Cellar numerous times and enjoy her life story (Fig. 3.1).

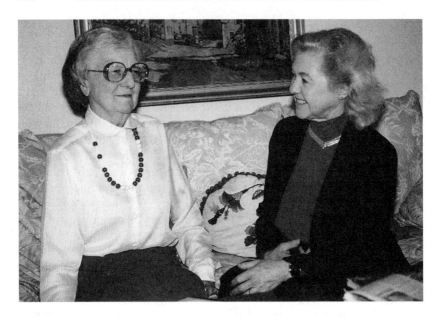

FIGURE 3.1 Priscilla Ebersole (right) interviewing Florence Cellar.

I have asked all of the individuals I have interviewed to tell me about their most gratifying experience in geriatric nursing and now find that I can't define one for myself. Certainly, the opportunity at CWRU was one of the very best and most enjoyable, but the GNP project gave me so much background in long-term care that it was invaluable.

I have been incredibly fortunate and encourage young nurses to be open to all aspects of nursing and keep their eyes and ears attuned to everything that is happening. There are so many outstanding individuals now in various aspects of geriatrics and gerontology that neophyte nurses will find it hard to miss the opportunities to learn about and serve the aged in almost any arena they choose. Also, they will encounter the aged in whatever specialty or subspecialty they select. Maternal and child care has evolved into broader women's issues. Grandmother caregivers have become a major force in shaping pediatric practice. If one is not knowledgeably prepared to work with the aged and their families we are, "professionally negligent, verging on abuse of our position and morally derelict." I don't remember who said that but it is imbedded in my mind.

There were many notable contributors to geriatric nursing theory, research, practice, and education who began their work in the 1970s. I focus on only a few, about whom I have sufficient information, to give a sense of the progress in the specialty. These nurses provide a sampling of the incredible rise of geriatric nursing as a specialty within the past 35 years.

FAYE GLENN ABDELLAH

Rear Admiral Faye Glenn Abdellah, United States Public Health Service (USPHS, retired), has been involved in government policy and planning through the military arm of the USPHS for much of her adult life. She has always been interested in the military and in helping people. An experience significant to her interest in the aged was caring for a professor of health sciences who had Alzheimer's disease. Her influence on quality in long-term care has had far-reaching effects.

Dr. Abdellah graduated from a diploma program at Fitkin Memorial Hospital School of Nursing, Neptune, New Jersey, in 1942. Between 1942 and 1944 she attended Rutgers University, New Brunswick, New Jersey, and took liberal arts courses and chemistry. In 1945 she earned a Bachelor of Science degree at Teachers College, Columbia University, New York City; in 1947, at the same institution she received a Master of Arts degree; and, again at Columbia University, achieved a Doctor of Education in 1955 (Abdellah, 1991b).

As the first and only nurse to serve as Deputy Surgeon General, under C. Everett Koop, and appointed at the military rank of a two-star general, she shared responsibilities for health policy research and development on issues affecting the elderly, such as elder abuse, self-help, incontinence, and standards for nursing home care (Fig. 3.2).

Her interest in expanded roles for nurses generated a study that partially influenced the nurse practitioner movement and from that grew geriatric nurse practitioners and gerontological clinical nurse specialists. She worked with Rita Chow (see later in chapter) to achieve exemplary standards of long-term health care delivery. And, for those of us entering nursing school in the mid-1960s, her text, *Patient Centered Approaches to Nursing* (1961), which focused on 21 nursing problems, became the guide to developing our nursing care plans.

She attributes her desire to be a nurse to an event that occurred when she was 18 years old and living near Lakehurst, New Jersey. On May 6, 1937, the hydrogen-filled dirigible, the Hindenburg, was docking at Lakehurst Naval Air Station after completing the first trans-Atlantic flight, from Frankfurt, Germany. This 804-foot airship was the world's first trans-Atlantic commercial airliner and the pride of Germany. The hydrogen-filled airship ignited while maneuvering to land. Of the 97 people on board, 13 passengers, 22 crew members, and one ground crew member died (http://en.wikipedia.org/wiki/Hindenburg_disaster). Many were injured. Faye and her older brother, Marty, were watching and responded to help the victims.

Lucile Petry (later Leone), director of the Cadet Nurse Corps of the USPHS, inspired her because of her dedication to quality nursing care and

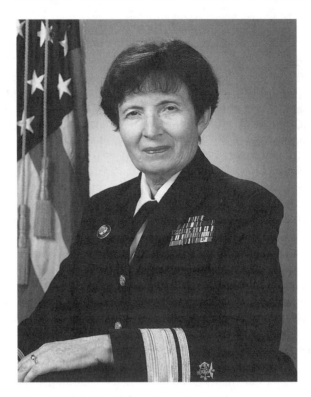

FIGURE 3.2 Faye Abdellah in full regalia and medals.

practice based on nursing science. Casper Weinberger, Secretary of the Department of Health, Education and Welfare under President Nixon, also was very influential in Faye's professional growth and opportunities. In turn, she has mentored numerous Public Health Service nurse officers, and army, navy, and air force nursing students. Many have gone on to leadership positions in nursing (personal communication, 2003b).

Her accomplishments, publications, and honors, which have impacted the care of the aged in the United States and the world, are far too numerous to mention altogether, but include the following: Forty of her 150 publications are directly related to the care of the aged, many to quality issues in nursing homes (Abdellah, 2003a); in the 1970s as director of the Office of Long-Term Care, Public Health Service, of the DHEW (Department of Health, Education and Welfare), now the Department of Health and Human Services, she was responsible for the enforcement and improvement of standards in nursing homes. In this capacity she was able to achieve major reforms in the delivery of services and surveyor practices, introduce the ombudsman concept, and develop federal support of geriatric nurse practitioners. In 1982, by invitation of the Ministers of Health for New Zealand and Australia, Dr. Abdellah participated in a seminar series for nursing home leaders in Australia; in 1989 she was recognized with the prestigious Allied Signal Award for her pioneering research in aging.

In 1994 the American Academy of Nursing honored Dr. Abdellah by presenting her with the Living Legend Award; and in 1999 she was elected to the Hall of Fame Distinguished Graduates and Scholars, Columbia University; in 2000 she was inducted into the National Women's Hall of Fame at Seneca Falls, New York, for her pioneering work altering nursing theory and practice. She developed the first coronary care unit and was the first nurse to hold the rank of two-star rear admiral, and the title of Deputy Surgeon General of the United States. Senator Daniel Inouye (Hawaii) entered a tribute to Faye Abdellah in the congressional record (V 146) (U.S. Department of Defense, Uniformed Services University of Health Sciences, 2003).

In 1993 she established the only military nursing school to prepare advanced practice nurses at the Uniformed Services University of Health Sciences (USUHS). A doctoral program was initiated in 2003. She says, "My champion was Senator Daniel K. Inouye from Hawaii who lost an arm in an enemy ambush during World War II. While recuperating in a hospital, he was so grateful for the nursing care that he received, that he swore that if he lived, he would do whatever he could to help nursing. He attributes his recovery to nurses. His total dedication has been an inspiration to me throughout my entire career. I would love to see the school named the *Daniel K. Inouye Graduate School of Nursing* as a tribute to him, a title which has already been approved by the USUHS Board of Regents" (Military Medicine, 2004).

"My personal development was enhanced by joining the U.S. Public Health Service and rising to the rank of rear admiral and the first woman and nurse to serve as Deputy Surgeon General of the United States. There is no greater reward than to serve one's country and to make a difference in the health care and quality of life of older Americans" (Abdellah, 1991a).

DOLORES MARSH ALFORD

Dr. Alford does not emphasize her credentials, honors, and publications, although there have been many. Her autobiography (Alford, 2004) gives a rousing account of her personal and professional development and other nurses she has regarded highly and influenced along the way. Her unique contribution to geriatric nursing is her venturesome spirit and entrepreneurial success. She was once called a "self-styled iconoclast" by a news report. That appears to be true.

Dolores (Dee) was born in New Orleans in 1928, the oldest of four children. Even though times were difficult during the Depression, her father worked for the railroad, so the family was never destitute. Her family felt it was their responsibility to be generous to those who were less fortunate than they were. She remembers her father "sitting on the curb in front of our house, holding a bottle of wine and crystal wine goblets to ensure that the garbage men had a 'bit of Christmas cheer'" (Alford, 2004). The family read to each other and discussed the books. They were permeated with the desire for knowledge. Dee loved school.

In 6th and 7th grade Dee attended a Catholic school where she won a prize for the best essay, "The Meaning of Democracy to Me." A priest came to the classroom to bestow the prize. All of the students rose as he entered the room except Dee. She refused to stand up, considering it an affront to southern womanhood. The prize, as punishment, was given to a more compliant student.

After high school, her father wanted her to attend business school and become a secretary in one of the rich import/export trade companies of New Orleans. "I wanted an education and I wanted to travel. . . . I lasted six weeks in business school." Dee knew she couldn't afford college, so she attended Charity Hospital School of Nursing, although she really wanted a college-based professional nursing education. Charity Hospital, a 3,000-bed hospital, served the poor but was used as a teaching facility for Louisiana State University (LSU), by the Medical Schools of Tulane University and numerous nursing programs, therapy schools, dietetic internships, and an anesthesia school. Most of her classes were taught by professors of medicine. "I loved working on 'Colored Female and Male' medical units. I found that black patients, especially the elderly ones, were wonderful teachers. What many health professionals still do not recognize is that patients in public hospitals give their most precious possessions (their bodies) to us to learn our discipline" (Alford, 2004).

The Charity Hospital School of Nursing in the 1940s and 1950s required that students provide all direct care to patients, wash beds, clean spills, and rotate through Central Service where they set up equipment trays, autoclaved them, sharpened needles, and packaged syringes. They also spent time in the special diet kitchen under the aegis of a dietitian, who did not like students. She yelled, screamed, and berated them until Dee told her to stop her bad behavior. Interestingly, students did not see this dietitian again during their rotation. As a nursing student, Dee learned about discrimination, voodoo, the beliefs and practices of gypsies, as well as many cultural variations. Dee graduated from the program in 1951.

Fortunately, at the end of her second year at Charity she was able to begin attending the Louisiana State University nursing program part time. She worked at Charity Hospital for 3 years after her graduation from Charity School of Nursing. Her next job was as an instructor in an LPN program until she received a traineeship to finish her senior year at LSU, where she obtained her baccalaureate degree in 1957. She obtained another traineeship for her master's degree from the University of Texas at Austin/Galveston. After graduation, she was education director at Seton School of Nursing. In 1970 she started an independent consulting practice, which she retains to this date. She was also the nursing consultant for a federal grant to the Texas Department of Health to study the feasibility of using federal funds for nursing home care. She was an assistant professor at Texas Woman's University (TWU), Houston, and coordinator of a grant to assist inactive nurses to return to work. She discovered that the main reason individuals left the profession was because it did not offer the satisfactions nurses desired. In 1972, TWU (Dallas) used her consultant services to design and develop a GNP program. She did this and even served as coordinator of the program. After completing the program those students who had been recruited from VA hospitals returned there to work as GNPs, thus making the VA system an early proponent of the value of GNPs.

In 1978, Dr. Alford, in partnership with Janet Moll (one of her GNP graduates), started Nursing Associates, the first independent office practice of nursing in Texas. This office became a place where GNP students could see the GNP role in practice. Dee and Janet also established nurse managed health maintenance/wellness clinics in senior centers, an apartment complex, nursing homes, retirement communities, and churches. The clinics flourished. In 1978 Dee began serving as an expert witness and consultant in cases dealing with mistreatment, abuse, and neglect of the elderly. In that capacity, she worked with a Texas assistant attorney general, David Marks, who insisted she never give up advocating for the elderly. She has heeded his words.

Dr. Alford has had many mentors along the way and has mentored many. One of her mentors, Dr. Cora Martin, mentored Dee as she developed her dissertation proposal that resulted in a doctorate from Columbia Pacific University. Her study, Health Behaviors of Older International Travelers, was chosen for presentation at the World Congress of Gerontology held in Acapulco, Mexico, in 1989. The idea of older travelers and their needs was intriguing for many of the participants. Dr. Alford's study provoked the travel industry to develop a special interest in care and services for older travelers. Thus, "geriatric emporiatrics" was born. From her numerous mentoring experiences she has developed a clear sense of mentorship, the unspoken rules and pitfalls (see chapter 9).

Some of the outstanding pupils whom Dee has helped develop gerontic expertise include: Virginia Burggraf, outstanding author and creative
thinker; Annette Lueckenotte, author of a major textbook and an integral
part of Nursing Associates; and Barbara Dossey, one of the founders of
the Holistic Nurses Association.

Dr. Alford's vision for the future of gerontic nursing includes the expectation that the major portion of primary care of the elderly will be delivered by advanced practice nurses. She predicts there will be an
increased attention to the principles of holistic nursing care as proposed
by Barbara Dossey. Dee also predicts that gerontic nurses will be involved
increasingly in the legal system to help protect their clients and reduce the
litigation presently clogging the court system. Some of her early predictions have occurred, such as the establishment of nurse-managed clinics,
development of institutes of gerontology within universities where the
elderly receive coordinated care by multidisciplinary teams and where research, especially nursing research, provides practitioners with new
knowledge.

Dr. Alford has shown that visions can be realized with diligence and
persistence. She has successfully launched independent nursing clinics
and is a true entrepreneur, one of the few able to sustain such efforts for
decades. She has proved the model and may be the catalyst for other
nurses, not quite as "iconoclastic" as she.

SISTER ROSE THERESE BAHR

Sister Rose Therese Bahr is probably best known for the ebullience that
rises so naturally from her soul; her enjoyment of working with the aged
comes from her family background. Her immigrant Austrian grandparents were a vital part of her home life and she fondly remembers her grandmother making wonderful pastry delicacies, especially the "kuchen." They
lived in a large farm home in Albert, Kansas. Her father raised diversified
crops, cattle, hogs, sheep, and chickens. Sister Rose was the first daughter and fourth child in a family of five. Her younger sister also became a
religious nun (Bahr, 1998).

Dr. Bahr was valedictorian of her high school graduating class in
Olmitz, Kansas, and entered the congregation of the Sisters of the Most
Precious Blood of Christ in 1948. She became interested in gerontologic
nursing when she worked in a Catholic nursing home for a summer be-
fore entering nursing school. She attended Sacred Heart College in
Wichita, Kansas, to fill the liberal arts requirement of St. Francis Hospital
School of Nursing. She then attended Catholic University of America
School of Nursing in Washington, D.C., and obtained a baccalaureate

and a master's degree. She earned a doctorate from St. Louis University in Missouri (Bahr, 1998).

She also received a Senior Research Award (1982), a monetary award from the University of Kansas that allowed her to conduct research in European countries. She and Sister Mary Balthasar of Niagara University developed a qualitative questionnaire to study the health practices and lifestyle of ambulatory older adults in Madrid, Spain; Stuttgart, Germany; Vienna, Austria; and Schaan, Lichtenstein. She was fascinated with their diversity of lifestyle and their definition of health and health beliefs (Bahr, 1990).

When asked the major gerontologic accomplishments of her life, she cites the planning and implementation of the gerontological nursing track in the master's nursing program at University of Kansas, Kansas City (1981–1984). It was the first in a five-state midwest area.

Her status as a Fellow with the American Academy of Nursing, the Gerontological Society of America, and the American Geriatric Society, and service as chair of the ANA Council of Gerontological Nursing, have all given her great satisfaction. She has been a member of the Catholic religious order entitled Adorers of the Blood of Christ for more than 40 years (Bahr, 1990; Ebersole, 1997a) (Fig. 3.3).

I first met Sr. Rose in Chicago at the second annual NGNA convention held in the Palmer House, Chicago, in April, 1987. I was on a panel discussing ethics and Sr. Rose welcomed us to the stage as if we were long-lost friends. Many professionals wore a cloak of dignity, and sometimes seemed unapproachable; her inherent friendliness captivated me immediately. Sister Rose was the program coordinator and planned the entire 2-day conference with guest speakers who were gerontological nurse experts with national renown and pioneers in the field.

Extrapolations From the Interview with Sr. Rose

The family met every Sunday after mass at the maternal grandparents' home, where her aunts, uncles, and cousins gathered to discuss the work week and make family decisions. Her grandmother, the matriarch, was greatly respected and in turn she respected the others in the family and their opinions. This laid the foundation for Sr. Rose's appreciation of elders. "At an early age I was introduced to aging and its inherent beauty" (Bahr, 1990). This was affirmed when she worked in a Catholic long-term care facility before entering nursing school in 1951. From this experience she learned the value of the history of each aged person and how it was often ignored by the family and society in general.

While attending the Catholic University of America (1958–1960) she came under the tutelage of Sister Lucille Kinlein, PhD, RN; the first

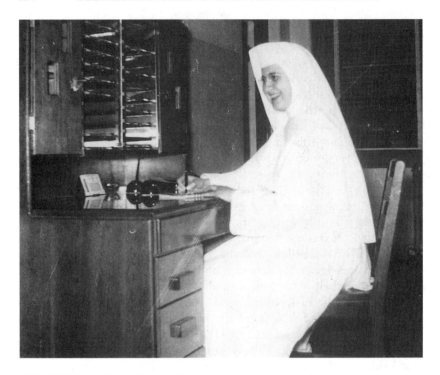

FIGURE 3.3 Sr. Rose Therese Bahr at desk.

independent nurse practitioner. Her courses were grounded in a philosophy of the uniqueness of each individual, based on culture, lifestyle, and
work history. Upon graduation with a BSN degree in 1960, Sr. Rose became immersed in gerontological nursing from a holistic perspective.

Another important time was spent with Lucille Gress, MSN, RN,
Kansas University School of Nursing faculty member, at the 1976
International Conference on Gerontology in Hawaii where, "there was a
group of older adults from China, the Philippines, Taiwan, Portugal,
Poland, Germany and other countries. It was like a microcosm of the
world." There she met Irene Burnside and discussed the psychological
and social dimensions of aging. Sr. Rose brought up the spiritual component and Irene said, "Absolutely, the interactions that I have had with
older people demonstrate that the spiritual or inner spirit component is
very important to their survival and, in a sense, motivates them to continue on" (Bahr, 1990). In 1977 Sr. Rose and Ms. Gress began publishing
articles about curriculum development for gerontological nursing to assist other nurse educators in course development on aging. They stressed
the appreciation of older adults and individuation of their care.

Sr. Rose sees that some of the problems with elders that are specific to the United States arise from our orientation to individualism and productivity and a lack of awareness of the reservoir of wisdom and experience that could be tapped to mentor the young. Somewhat akin to that is her concern about the suicide rate and the unavailability of a suicide assessment scale appropriate for older adults. She cites the example of a 64-year-old man who had risen from broom boy to an executive in a corporate structure. He had been with the company for 49 years. He was called into the president's office one morning, thanked for his wonderful contribution to the company, and told to clear his desk. He was a potential candidate for suicide. His work was his life.

Dr. Bahr's work has been accomplished in numerous venues and her influence is both broad and deep. She has worked within ANA as the Chair of the Council of Gerontological Nursing; NGNA as Conference Program Coordinator for 7 years; AARP; the Catholic Golden Age Foundation; and remains an active Fellow of the American Academy of Nursing. She feels she has been successful in achieving most of the objectives she has set out to accomplish. She sees a bright future in geriatric nursing specialties and says, "At present, we as nurse gerontologists, are building on the shoulders of giants in the field; those who were willing to be very assertive visionaries" (Bahr, 1990). All her published work, including, *The Aging Person: A Holistic Perspective* (1984, and with translation into Japanese) is archived within her religious community, Wichita Center, Wichita, Kansas (Fig. 3.4).

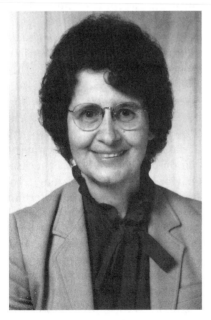

FIGURE 3.4 Sr. Rose Therese Bahr.

BEVERLY BALDWIN

Dr. Beverly Baldwin's untimely death at the age of 53 ended her prolific career at its peak. At that time Dr. Baldwin was a professor of nursing at University of Maryland, Baltimore. One of her nurse proteges, Barbara Resnick, provided the following information about her.

Beverly Ann Baldwin was an early leader and visionary in the area of geriatric nursing. Dr. Baldwin started her nursing career after graduating from a diploma program at the Charity Hospital School of Nursing in New Orleans in 1965. She went on to get a bachelor's degree in nursing from Northwestern State University in 1966 and a master's degree in psychiatric-mental health nursing from the University of Iowa in 1970 as well as a master's degree in sociology at the University of New Orleans in 1975. She completed traditional studies when she earned her PhD in sociology at the University of Kentucky in 1984. Her research in geriatrics focused particularly on older adults with cognitive impairment, particularly to help formal and informal caregivers provide the best possible care to these individuals.

Just before her death in 1995 she was the coinvestigator on a National Institute of Aging grant to study the impact of an intervention that focused on reducing disruptive behaviors in cognitive impaired residents in long-term care settings. This study was developed to compare the effectiveness of a psychosocial activity intervention, an activities of daily living intervention, and a combination of the two interventions in decreasing the frequency, duration, and intensity of disruptive behaviors in cognitively impaired older adults in long-term care facilities. A longitudinal component of the study also was built in to describe the relationship between disruptive behaviors and psychological, cognitive, and functional status of older adults over time.

"Well recognized for her research work, Dr. Baldwin was the recipient of many honors. She was inducted as a Fellow into the American Academy of Nursing in 1991 and a Fellow of the Gerontological Society of America in 1992. She was also a Maryland Higher Education Eminent Scholar. Dr. Baldwin's extensive research on dementia and other mental health issues, caregiver stress, and behavior management in long-term care institutions has provided, and will continue to provide, an important service to the field."

"Dr. Baldwin was also a wonderful mentor and example for nursing students interested in geriatrics. Her door was always open and usually very well decorated for whatever holiday was upcoming. Moreover, she always had kind and encouraging words to say and was dedicated to helping nurses develop their research and/or geriatric focus. She worked closely with 20 predoctoral students, and many of these students went on to take positions at universities where they could emulate her caring and teaching. She provided students with experiences in research and helped them to not only understand what they were working on and working with, but also encouraged them to share and publish their findings in the area of geriatrics. She inspired a new generation of geriatric nurse researchers" (Resnick in Ebersole, 2002b, p. 100).

Among the individuals she mentored are the presently well-known experts in geriatric nursing: Joyce Rasin, Sandra Picot, Marcella Griggs, Dorothy Herron, and Barbara Resnick. Barbara writes of Beverly, "Beverly left me with help to carry on . . . when rejections came whether it be from a paper or a grant, Beverly's response was, 'The world just isn't ready for you yet.' No one was ever wrong or stupid. We were all just out there in front . . . thinking and bringing new ideas to practice and that is how the helix grows. She was just amazing. Tonight I was actually thinking of her. She was a wonderful mentor and role model and someone I still think of often and hope I can make her proud as she watches from above" (Resnick, 2005).

H. TERRI BROWER

Dr. Terri Brower has spent much of her professional life in education; focused on curriculum development, especially for geriatric nurse practitioner programs; attempting to facilitate gerontologic content in undergraduate programs; and working toward adequate licensure testing for geriatric knowledge.

Her early life, like many of the geriatric pioneers, was hard but the difficulties encountered gave her the strength and flexibility to overcome obstacles, and venture to accomplish things she saw that needed to be done. She remembers her first six grades spent in a two-room school with an outhouse (Brower, 1990). She has survived an incredible number of traumas in her life and not been "bowled over" (Brower, 1991a). She was a first-generation American; her parents were immigrants from Sweden and England, so she had no contact with an extended family or grandparents. However, she remembers certain old people who impacted her life.

One, the neighborhood children called "grandma," eagerly welcomed them into her home and made them sodas with ginger ale and ice cream, a very special treat. They often went to her house as she was so warm and loving. She was an alcoholic but Terri says, "That didn't stop me from loving her." There were also the two Potter sisters, neighbors who really became surrogate extended family for her (Brower, 1990). The family moved from New Jersey to South Florida when she was 15 years old.

For a while during her educational experience at Columbia University Terri worked part time in a nursing home on Long Island and had a "dreadful experience." This undoubtedly influenced her belief that nursing students should not be in nursing homes as their first clinical experience, because facilities are not good models in many cases and the experience can be "horrifying." She notes that it is much better for them to learn from the "worried well" in the community and to make a functional assessment of their instrumental activities of daily living (IADL) and their living environment (Brower, 1990).

Her professional education began in 1957 in a community college in Florida, from there she went to Teachers College, Columbia University in New York City, and graduated with a bachelor's degree in 1966 and a master's degree in 1968. In 1973 Terri earned a Family Nurse Practitioner Certificate at the University of Miami School of Nursing, Florida. Her doctoral studies were completed in 1978 at Nova University in Ft. Lauderdale, Florida, with a focus on curriculum and instruction (Brower, 1991c).

Dr. Brower's nursing and teaching experiences have been diverse. She taught primarily at University of Miami School of Nursing, and Auburn University School of Nursing, Auburn, Alabama. She has almost 50 text contributions, journal articles, monographs, and books to her credit and has presented more than 100 papers and workshops; many of them on topics related to the geriatric nurse practitioner movement. These have been given nationally and internationally.

She developed Florida's first and (at that time) only geriatric nurse practitioner certificate program in 1975 and the first graduate GNP program in 1980. In 1976 she began consulting with educational programs about establishing gerontological content in nursing programs and developing geriatric nurse practitioner curricula (Brower, 1991c). Terri served as a consultant for ANA's certification examination for gerontological nurses from 1979 to 1982, and the American Association of the Colleges of Nursing (AACN) project on graduate Gerontological Nursing and Nursing Services Administration. She was a delegate to the 1980 Governor's Conference on Aging in Florida and was the first chairperson of the steering committee for the self-support groups for Alzheimer's disease in Dade County, Florida (Brower, 1991b).

Dr. Brower is highly recognized as a geriatric nursing expert witness, having served on more than 60 cases. She feels that one of the ways to make an impact on the care of long-term care residents and patients is through the legal system. Although, she strongly supports tort reform, she states that it has been through legal cases that nursing has become more cognizant of the special needs of older persons (Brower, 2005).

She has had many awards and recognitions but enjoys knowing she was the first nurse from southeast Florida to achieve fellowship in the

American Academy of Nursing (AAN) and one of the first three nurses to be awarded fellowship in the Clinical Medicine Section of the Gerontological Society of America (GSA).

Dr. Brower has considerable research experience and is best known for several studies on aspects of nurses' attitudes toward older persons. Speaking of the attitudes toward the aged she cited a speech she heard by Barbara Silverstone, an early geriatric social worker. Barbara said, "We all have gerontophobia. We must each confront our own fears and biases" (Brower, 1990).

A Delphi Study of Research Priorities for Long-Term Care Nursing, a project supported by grants from Sigma Theta Tau and the Department of Health and Human Services (DHSS) Division of Nursing, revealed numerous items deemed extremely important for patient welfare, nursing education, and nursing practice. From these were generated methods to have maximal impact on education, nursing practice, and patient welfare (Brower & Christ, 1982).

Insights From the Videotaped Interview

In 1971, Terri heard Barbara Allen Davis speak and was thrilled with the possibilities in the field of aging. She says of that experience, "I first experienced Barbara Davis, whom I see as a real pioneer, not myself, at a conference when she was working on her doctorate at New York University (NYU) and I was just enthralled with what she had to say about gray power and caring for older people. She had very different experiences and perceptions of the nursing home than I did" (Brower, 1990). Later, one of Terri's most satisfying experiences was functioning as the first ombudsman in Florida's Long-Term Care Ombudsman program. She was also the first nurse on the appointees committee in that program.

Shortly after meeting Barbara, Terri found her niche and began her commitment to encouraging the placement of geriatric content in undergraduate nursing programs. The problems she experienced convinced her that testing for RN licensure gave far too little attention to geriatrics and most to pathophysiology and critical care. She feels there have been some improvements but still a lot more is needed. She believes there is so much not being done in baccalaureate programs because most teach to the test, even though few nursing schools admit that. Another problem in these programs is the need to include community health and administration. This content is not included in associate degree (AD) programs; therefore, it seems to her, there is more opportunity in the AD programs to provide geriatric nursing content.

When asked how we can attract students to geriatric nursing, Terri thought it essential that they have a desire to serve, and a strong, instinctual caring motivation. She felt the "driven nurses" seldom embody these qualities. One of the most important things is having faculty who are informed and enthusiastic about aging. As few have learned that in their own education, they must make additional efforts to achieve that knowledge. Perhaps it should be a requirement that they pursue information about geriatric care. Students learn from faculty models.

Terri feels that much has been accomplished in the last few years. A "rich array" of excellent texts are available. Research into aging has increased at a phenomenal rate and the political scene has been conducive to support this. At present there is "a wide field of opportunity."

In the future Dr. Brower expects more long-term care accountability, because the rate of growth in that field has been incredible. Nurses will need to be much more involved and influential in policy development on state and national levels. More undergraduate programs will have a serious commitment to teach geriatric content. She cites the success of the Community College and Nursing Home Partnership (CCNHP), funded by the Kellogg Foundation. Staff from nursing homes and educators in community colleges met together regularly, and participated in geriatric educational events that fostered the mutuality of their concerns. "The *entire* faculty was gerontologized. This provides an excellent model that has been replicated across the United States (see chapter 8 for further discussion). There will be many more graduate programs focused on gerontology and geriatric nurse practitioners" (Brower, 1990).

RITA CHOW: A TAILOR'S DAUGHTER

Rita Chow may be best known for her adaptability and serenity. She has a holistic and spiritual approach to geriatric nursing and to life. Rita says, "The starting point of my journey toward caring about the aging happened at an intersection in an unexpected career opportunity in the USPHS. In April 1974, when I was serving as Deputy Chief Nurse Officer of the USPHS in Rockville, Maryland, I also was named to be the Deputy Director of the Office of Nursing Home Affairs (ONHA) in the Department of Health, Education and Welfare (DHEW). The staff was responsible for coordinating and directing nationwide nursing home affairs and long-term care. This significant mission was carried out in two phases. The first was a Long-Term Care Improvement Campaign that surveyed a national sample of 288 nursing homes to assess quality of care. Each was visited by a team composed of eight professional disciplines. The data were reported through multimedia and in the department's ONHA publications, including the *Long-Term Care Facility Improvement Study: Introductory Report*, July 1975. The second phase focused on helping nurses carry out systematic patient care evaluation in approximately 188 skilled nursing and intermediate care facilities" (Chow in Ebersole, 2002c, pp. 43–44).

When in 1979, Rita was reassigned as the Chief of the Quality Assurance Branch of the Division of Long-Term Care in the Office of Standards and Certification, she was able to help the Health Care Financing Administration (HCFA, now CMS) to reshape regulations and achieve more standardized inspections of facilities. Simultaneously, she began studying for gerontological certification at George Mason University in Virginia.

Dr. Chow's history is fascinating. Her father arrived from China when he was about 12 years old but his vital records were destroyed in the San Francisco earthquake of 1906. This occasionally presented problems, but none that were insurmountable. He was industrious and became an apprentice tailor and later a successful independent tailor and manager of his own "Peter's Jacket Shop" in the San Francisco Mission District (Fig. 3.5). His wife, May Chan, was the eldest of 12 children. They had limited education and thus Rita's parents placed a very high value on education of their two daughters and son. Education, religion, and spirituality were integrated into their everyday life. They lived in the rear of the tailor shop and the children performed some of the simpler tasks. Rita studied art, psychology, and nursing and graduated from the baccalaureate program at Stanford in 1950 (Chow, 2004b).

In 1954 she was selected for the Army Nurse Corps RN Student Program to complete a master of science degree. Following graduation she was later promoted to first lieutenant and had several assignments. She was the youngest officer teaching large classes of medics at Brooke Army Medical Center, San Antonio, Texas. When her U.S. Army active duty was completed she remained in the army reserves but continued her education at Teachers College, Columbia University, New York City. Her doctoral dissertation focused on the postoperative care of cardiac patients. Her findings were published in *Nursing Research* and the textbook, *Cardiosurgical Nursing Care: Understandings, Concepts and Principles for Practice* (Chow, 1969, 1975).

By 1968 she had achieved the rank of major in the Army Nurse Corps Reserves and chose to transfer as a nurse officer to the commissioned corps of the USPHS. During her 27 years in the USPHS she had many unusual assignments and in each found very satisfying activities. Interestingly, at one point she was assigned to the USPHS Indian Health Service in Rosebud, South Dakota, where she met tribal elders and learned the "enchanting folk stories, revealing one way in which Native Americans transmit their mores through myths. . . . I realized that my experience on the reservation was a memorable blessing that supplied many new insights" (Chow in Ebersole, 2002b, p. 44).

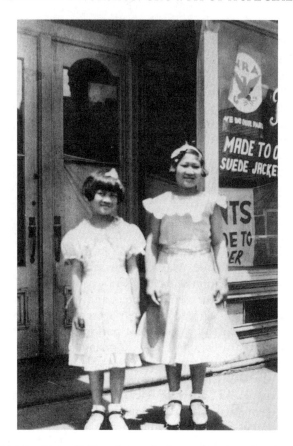

FIGURE 3.5 Rita Chow (left) and sister in front of Dad's tailor shop.

In 1971 she staffed the committee meetings headed by Dr. Roger O. Egeberg that studied and produced a federal "white paper" exploring extended roles for nurses that gave impetus to Primex programs such as the one at Cornell University (see Schwartz, chapter 2) (Chow, 1972; USDHEW, 1971). Their work was the genesis of the nurse practitioner movement (Chow, 2004b).

Dr. Chow says the years 1971 to 1977 were remarkably dynamic gerontological experiences for her and the country. "Not only because President Nixon made a rallying announcement of August 6, 1971, to improve the quality of life and care of older adults, but also because the federal staff response to his nationwide initiative entailed so much to be accomplished so quickly. Originally, the ONHA was created in November 1971 with Marie Callendar named as its first director"

(Chow, 2004b, p. 6). Later Assistant Surgeon General Faye Abdellah was named director of ONHA.

From 1984 to 1989 Rita worked with older persons at the National Hansen's Disease (leprosy) Center in Carville, Louisiana, and also served as adjunct faculty at Louisiana State University School of Nursing, New Orleans. These experiences provided new insights and opportunities for teaching that impacted patient care and staff education. The history of the center in Carville is remarkable.

The center originated in 1894 in the abandoned Indian Camp Plantation (sugar) as the Louisiana State Leprosarium. Dr. Isadore Dyer, President of the Louisiana Board of Control for the Leper Home, realized the dire need for nursing care, so on March 25, 1896, he contracted with the Daughters of Charity of Saint Vincent de Paul to serve and receive $100 per year for clothing and incidental expenses. Their responsibilities were to:

> have full charge of the domestic management appertaining to the servants, kitchen, household and detail of nursing, which last shall be at all times under the direction of the resident physician. (Hannefin, 1981; Ross, date unknown, p. 11)

Many sisters from that order volunteered; four were chosen. On arrival they found their 20 patients housed in seven dilapidated old slave cabins. Nearby, the sisters settled into two habitable rooms of the 30-room mansion that was in disrepair. Water moccasins, bats, rats, and lizards were everywhere, so the sisters kept an ax and lantern by their beds. Progressively, through the years, through extraordinary vision and exertion by an interdisciplinary staff, the site became renowned for quality care and medical research.

The first historical step was made in 1914 when Congressional Bill 1751 was introduced to establish the National Leprosarium. However, from a personnel perspective, a crucial turning point was the 1916 policy toward professionalism—that all sisters at Carville would be registered nurses or certified in their respective fields. Another significant change occurred on February 3, 1917, with the enactment of the national legislation to provide for the isolation and treatment of persons with leprosy under the administration of the USPHS, followed by the federal purchase of the Louisiana Leper Home and the approximately 337 surrounding acres on January 3, 1921. Subsequently, the USPHS ensured that the Daughters of Charity became salaried federal civil service employees.

In retrospect, numerous pioneers in the health field enabled the National Hansen's Disease (HD) Center to become one of the foremost sites for medical and physical therapy; rehabilitation; eye, hand, and foot surgery; scientific research; and professional education. Pharmaceutical discoveries, such as the sulfones, even thalidomide for erythema nodosum leprosum reactions of lepromatous HD, helped reap therapeutic benefits for patients. Effective combinations of diagnostic tests, antibiotics, monitored pharmacotherapy, and the establishment of Regional Hansen's Disease Centers in several states, including Hawaii, California, New York, and Texas, have enabled patients to receive clinic care and be at home with their families. Also, the National Center's patient education program (1984–1989) emphasized disability prevention, health promotion, and self-care (Chow, 2004a).

During the years 1984 to 1989, as Director of Patient Education, Rita went to Israel and New Zealand to present information gained from her experience at Carville. She also went to Australia, where HD has been found among the aborigines. Subsequently, the need for a large national center diminished. The federal government has now closed most of the center at Carville, and returned the land to Louisiana for such purposes as Job Corps training.

The care of individuals with HD has largely been relegated to clinics. However, some people who have grown old while in isolation from society remain at Carville and at the Father Damien Center on Moloka'i because they have nowhere else to go.

Rita's final experience in the USPHS was to be Director of Nursing of the Fort Worth, Texas, Federal Correctional Institution (FCI), under the aegis of the Federal Bureau of Prisons. Her task was to administer the nursing services for ambulatory, subacute, and long-term care for approximately 1,400 inmates. "This 6-year gerontological experience (1989–1995) required high energy, patience, and imagination at the FCI that was successfully converted into the first fully accredited Federal Medical Center for Long-Term Care by the Joint Commission on Accreditation of Health Care Organizations (JCAHO)" (Chow, 2004b, p. 10). Many of these men had grown old serving their sentences and developed chronic disorders that needed special attention. In addition to establishing facilities for their care, palliative care for terminal inmates was added. She participated in the planning and design of this first long-term care prison facility and also was responsible for medical and nursing staff continuing education in addition to the entire nursing services.

After retiring from the USPHS Commissioned Corps in 1995, Rita became a nurse consultant in Singapore, Japan, and Taiwan. She also was invited to give a presentation in Thailand. Her broad range of experience gave her invaluable insights to share that have international significance. Subsequently, she took on the directorship of the National Interfaith Coalition on Aging (NICA), a constituent group of the National Council of the Aging (NCOA).

Dr. Chow is a credentialed nurse educator, certified gerontological nurse, and advanced practice holistic nurse, and has more than 100 publications in nursing and related areas to her credit. She has received many honors, including a Distinguished Service Medal of the USPHS from the DHHS; the Special Act Award from the Federal Prison System; the Commendable Service Award for Outstanding Service to the Federal Bureau of Prisons; the Holistic Nurse of the Year Award by the Holistic Nurses Association (2001); and the USPHS Chief Nurse Officer Award in recognition of her outstanding contributions to nursing. In addition to being a fellow in the American Association for the Advancement of Sciences (AAAS), American Academy of Nursing (AAN), and the GSA, she also became a fellow in the American Association of Integrative Medicine (AAIM), and Diplomate of the AAIM College of Nursing; and a fellow of the NGNA.

The one award that speaks most to her outstanding attributes and contributions is the "Artist for Life" First Prize in New York City from the International Women's Writing Guild given for "one who combines the qualities of wisdom, maturity, vision, resourcefulness, stamina, hopefulness and the ability to inspire others" (Ebersole, 2002b, p. 44).

Rita's professional life has taken her all over the world, involving her in many facets of nursing practice, research, education, and administration. The Center for Nursing Historical Inquiry at University of Virginia has archived a collection of her papers, photos, and artifacts (Fig. 3.6).

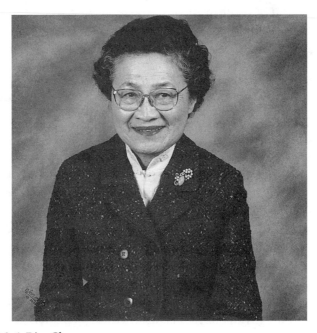

FIGURE 3.6 Rita Chow.

LOIS EVANS

Lois Evans and Neville Strumpf began working together more than 20 years ago, inspired by Doris Schwartz, to investigate the common practice of restraining the elderly. They were an ideal team, as Lois' background was in geropsychiatric care and Neville's was in adult and gerontological nursing. Their complementary strengths contributed to their robust research into the problem of restraining the frail elderly, which resulted in more humane and individualized care that ultimately produced changes in the standards of practice.

When they first met in the early 1980s, Lois was the principal investigator and Neville Strumpf a consultant on one of the Teaching Nursing Home Projects funded by the Robert Wood Johnson Foundation. Lois joined the faculty of University of Pennsylvania (Penn) School of Nursing in 1984 and there reconnected with Neville Strumpf. The results of their first study of the perceptions of nurses and patients about restraint use were published in *Nursing Research* (Strumpf & Evans, 1988). They then undertook a thorough review of the literature on the subject and found that little was actually known about the realities of physically restraining elders (Evans & Strumpf, 1989). Subsequent studies of restraint use in nursing homes shed further light on the problem in the United States. These studies and reports stirred public and professional interest in the problem, including hearings by the U.S. Senate Special Committee on aging, at which they testified in 1989. Investigating the use of restraints among European nurses revealed methods that were used to care for frail elders without the use of restraints and side rails. This led to their investigation, funded by the National Institute on Aging (NIA), of methods that effectively reduced restraint usage (Evans & Strumpf, 1997; Sullivan-Marx, Strumpf, Evans, et al., 2003) in nursing homes and hospitals. Their findings were widely publicized and a national effort to try alternative methods of safe care was established.

Lois grew up in a rural area of northern West Virginia in a "hollow" named Plum Run for the wild plum trees that lined the creek when the first settlers arrived in the late 1700s. Throughout her childhood, her grandparents lived nearby and were closely involved with her family and the community. A great-grandfather was particularly respected and was a model of aging well for Lois. From her early experiences she learned about growing old and also about caregiving, including caring for her grandmother after a hip fracture. Her grandparents were wonderful teachers about life, love, relationships, family, and hard work.

Lois was active in 4-H and won state championships with her sewing. An excellent student, she graduated first in her high school class and was the only girl among her classmates to attend university. She loved music, and studied the piano and French horn; however, she had always wanted to work with people, so she followed her instincts into nursing. Exposure to a public health nurse during the early polio immunization clinics influenced her career choice.

She was awarded a scholarship to study nursing in a progressive program at West Virginia University, in Morgantown. Gerontology and research were integral to the program and Lois became "hooked" on both. In her senior leadership course she studied the food intake at mealtime among residents in a home for the aged.

After graduation she took a position as a public health nurse in Washington, D.C., and reveled in the captivating stories of the older adults she served. She then entered graduate school and studied psychiatric and mental health nursing at the Catholic University of America. She then began teaching at Georgetown University and was appalled when she took students to the federal psychiatric hospital and found that elders were merely "housed" and lacked attention or stimulation. This led to Lois's doctoral studies about isolation and how it affected institutionalization. Her dissertation research focused on *The relationship of need awareness, locus of control, health state and social support system to social interaction as a form of self-care behavior among elderly residents of public housing.* In 1980, post doctoral geriatric nurse practitioner studies at the University of Rochester, New York, piqued her awareness of the sociocultural similarities among institutions for the mentally ill and nursing homes and she resolved to find ways to create a therapeutic milieu in long-term care.

While at Georgetown, Lois developed and implemented its first graduate program in gerontological nursing and subsequently was awarded one of the Robert Wood Johnson Teaching Nursing Home Project grants. This enabled her to launch an important nursing home model based on humanistic management principles and represented an important connection to Mathy Mezey and Joan Lynaugh, at University of Pennsylvania (Penn), who directed the national project for the foundation. This project was carried out at the Health Care Institute, a subsidiary of Greater Southeast Community Center for Aging.

Her milestone study of sundown syndrome (confusion most apparent in the evening) and her finding that those individuals restrained in the morning were much more likely to be agitated and confused in the evening had extensive implications in the care of the aged (Evans, 1987).

At the Penn School of Nursing, Lois was greatly influenced by Dr. Claire Fagin, then dean, Ellen Fuller, director of the center for nursing research, as well as Drs. Mezey, Lynaugh, and Strumpf. Her activities at Penn School of Nursing included the development of a geropsychiatric nursing track in the graduate program; leadership of the Nursing

Academic Practice Initiatives, including establishment of a day hospital; the creation of a Program for All-inclusive Care for Elders (PACE); implementation of nursing consultation services; and creation of a nurse managed continence care program, and a community-based nursing center that provides comprehensive primary care for all ages.

Dr. Evans serves as Associate Director for the School of Nursing Center for Gerontologic Nursing Science at Penn, and the John A. Hartford Foundation Center of Geriatric Nursing Excellence. She spearheads the Hartford Center's dissemination efforts, including web-based products and guideline development, and works closely with pre- and post doctoral scholars as they develop their own lines of inquiry.

Lois's research activities have come full circle, from changing the practice of restraint usage to examining the results in long-term care of conventional versus humanistic care. Her great desire to make the nursing home a place where people who live and work can flourish has never wavered.

TERRY FULMER

Terry Fulmer is most notable for her groundbreaking work in elder abuse and her generosity of spirit. In the early 1980s she began her foray into gerontology at Beth Israel Hospital, Boston, and steadily rose in responsibilities as well as pursuing her interest in elder abuse. In 1988 she was on the Board of Directors of the National Committee for the Prevention of Elder Abuse. She has conducted research, made numerous presentations, consultations, major contributions, and notable publications in this area of interest. Other research interests have included acute care of the elderly and alternative medicine. She has served as director of NYU's Center for Nursing Research and is the director of the New York Consortium of Geriatric Education Centers.

Her energies extend to the community and the profession but Terry's family comes first. Each year I can expect a photo and update on the progress of her two daughters and son. In spite of her commitments in numerous directions she served in 1991 to 1992 as president of the Rye Presbyterian Nursery School Board.

Terry is the dean of the College of Nursing at New York University, was the co-director of the John A. Hartford Foundation Institute for Geriatric Nursing and in 2005 was the President of the GSA. Terry is the first nurse to occupy this leadership position in the largest gerontological organization in the nation. This signal honor is well deserved and demonstrates her active involvement in GSA for several years as well as the esteem in which she is held by her colleagues. She is a fellow of the GSA and the American Academy of Nursing (Fulmer, 1999).

When asked why she became a nurse, Terry said it was because her mother and eight of her aunts were nurses. Her mother died quite young but "was a wonderful role model and inspiration." It is worth noting that her mother, Margaret Flynn Thomas, graduated in 1944 from the U.S. Cadet Nurse Corps Program as did Margaret's twin sister, Kathleen. Terry says, "Mother was so proud of her status in that important program! She was a major influence in my life and I was so very proud of her pride in her profession as well as her remarkable talent as a nurse. My older sister, Kathy, and my nieces Bridget and Carolyn are also nurses. Finally, my daughter, Holly Fulmer, is currently a nursing student at the University of Vermont. I think it is fair to say nursing runs in my family! This does not even begin to mention my cousins. . . . My grandmother was born in 1897 and wanted to be a nurse, but her Victorian mother was concerned about the image of nurses and would not let her pursue nursing as a career. You can see how my grandmother kept her passion alive! . . . I love nursing and can think of no other path that would have served me as this one has and does!" (Fulmer, 2005, p. 1).

"The real reason I became interested in geriatric nursing is because on my first job at Beth Israel Hospital in Boston, fresh out of nursing school, I found that nurses for the most part were kept busy following the orders of doctors. Beth Israel was a Harvard Medical School teaching hospital and had an excellent staff, but when I would ask what to do about one of the aged patients who was not eating or developing a pressure sore, they would say, 'Do whatever you think best.' Doctors were neither educated toward nor interested in the daily supportive care of the aged. I soon realized that, in the arena of caring for the aged, I could have an autonomous nursing practice that would make a real difference in medical outcomes. I could practice the full scope of nursing. It gave me a great sense of freedom and accomplishment" (Fulmer in Ebersole, 1999, p. 107).

Terry has at last count received more than 50 honors and awards, been principal investigator of 15 grants, published more than 90 articles and 6 books, contributed chapters to 40 books, and has held academic appointments at nine universities. Her faculty experiences began at Salem State College at Salem, Massachusetts teaching rehabilitation nursing in 1977. From there she taught at Boston College, Harvard, Yale, Columbia, and finally New York University. She also has occupied the Florence Cellar Chair in Gerontological Nursing at Case Western Reserve University (Fulmer, 1999) (Fig. 3.7).

Terry's philosophy of nursing, "evolves from the interdisciplinary centeredness the professional nurse serves on the health care team for the benefit of the patient. I am devoted to the patient as the driver of the health care plan with all of us constantly coordinating and supporting the

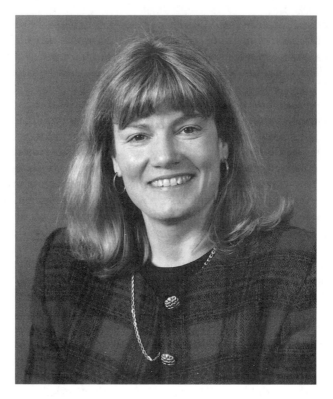

FIGURE 3.7 Terry Fulmer.

goals and objectives of the patient. My crystal ball indicates that there will be more interdisciplinary requirements for contemporary health care systems and nursing will be a central feature for cohesion of the team" (Fulmer, 2005, p. 2).

MAY FUTRELL

Dr. May Futrell grew up in Waterbury, Vermont, a town of only 3,000 people, and some say that sturdy New England strength is evident in all she does. In this small town everyone was well acquainted and helped each other, giving a strong sense of community. May was from a large extended family, including four healthy grandparents who dearly loved her and her sister. This undoubtedly influenced her wellness approach to the aged. One grandfather had a profound influence on her life and professional career.

We first met at the Andrus Gerontology Center while she attended geriatric nursing classes given by Irene Burnside and me. She was in the middle of completing her doctoral dissertation and I was astonished at her ability to simultaneously concentrate on studies in two important areas in her life. She also brought to my attention that someone at the center was drawing from the work of Irene and myself and not giving appropriate credit. I was grateful to be made aware but even more impressed by her integrity and sense of professional ethics. These qualities are apparent in everything May has accomplished.

May Futrell considers her greatest contribution to gerontic nursing to be the planning, implementation, and evaluation of the Gerontological Nurse Practitioner program at the master's level at University of Massachusetts, Lowell (UML). Her program was the first graduate program in the United States to educate primary care gerontological nurse practitioners, able to function in both wellness and illness situations. The model became a template for numerous other such graduate programs and is still being used. The model incorporates five principles:

1. The attitudes toward aging held by care providers are important.
2. Wellness and health promotion are basic concepts preceding the progress to illness.
3. Psychosocial and mental health wellness are as important as physical health.
4. Political, social, and policy issues are important parts of GNP education.
5. The GNP role is complementary and independent and is not that of a physician substitute.

May earned a bachelor's and master's degree and MA in nursing from Teacher's College, Columbia University in New York (Fig. 3.8). She began teaching at Boston University in 1961, where she became interested in the gerontology courses being offered to psychology and sociology students. She took these courses and decided she wanted to pursue knowledge in this "new field" (Futrell, 1991). After that, in 1976, she earned a doctorate in Social Policy and Social Gerontology from Brandeis University. She began teaching at Lowell in 1970 and became project director of the Gerontological Nurse Practitioner program in 1975, and was director of the Professional Nurse Traineeship program from 1981 until 1987 .

In the fall of 1987 she was a visiting scholar and postdoctoral fellow at the University of Edinburgh in Scotland. She has numerous awards and honors; outstanding among them are: fellow of the American Academy of Nursing; fellow of the Gerontological Society of America; co-leader of

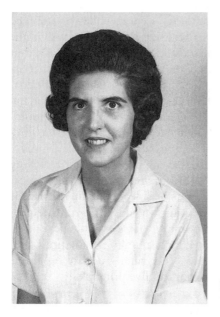

FIGURE 3.8 May Futrell in the early 1960s.

the Soviet American Geriatric Nurse Study Tour to the U.S.S.R. in 1983; selection by the National Institute on Aging to participate on a panel of experts for the preparation of the House Appropriation Bill for Training in Geriatrics and Gerontology; honored by the Futrell Award established by Eta Omega, Sigma Theta Tau; and selected to attend the Conference of National Experts, held at Georgetown University, to determine gerontology curriculum in baccalaureate nursing programs (Futrell, 1991). Recently, May was featured in *A Special Celebration at UML, Honoring Individuals Who Are Making an Impact* and was given the Francis Cabot Lowell Faculty Award.

May has received innumerable research and project grants, published prolifically, provided consultation services to numerous nursing schools, and has given papers and workshops across the nation. Some that have had particular significance is the publication of *An Evidence Based Protocol: Wandering* (Futrell & Melillo, 2002); the publication of wellness papers with Dolores Alford; and those of the Expert Panel on Aging, American Academy of Nursing; and the publication in the 1980s of the first textbook for GNPs, *Primary Health Care of Older Adults* (Futrell, Brovender, Mullett, & Brower, 1980).

She has been at the University of Massachusetts for 35 years and is presently chair of the Nursing Programs, a University Scholar, director of Professional Nurse Traineeships, and Graduate Coordinator (Fig. 3.9).

May Futrell: Reflections and Insights From the Interview

"I have learned the importance of genetics and the part that biology plays in aging. I have watched what happened in the family and to me based on my own biology. . . . I think our program at Lowell is attractive to students because we instill the idea that well elderly are the major portion of the population and their needs are important." Another factor in the program success is that "We did not 'farm' the students out to agency people. The faculty went with the students. . . . From the experiences at Andrus Gerontology Center, with Irene Burnside and Priscilla Ebersole, we brought group work into our curriculum and it is still a part of the curriculum that faculty and students enjoy. We also have a wellness clinic at the University where we do physical assessments on faculty, students, and university personnel" (Futrell, 1990).

"I am interested in people, I love different cultures, I like people who are different and do different things, who are creative. The elderly certainly bring new situations to the forefront in conversation. . . . I see a very hopeful situation, I think the client, the older adult, is going to be better off economically and healthier. It's probably nursing care of the oldest old that is going to be very important." As for nursing students, "I have a feeling that 18 year olds still want to master the technology or

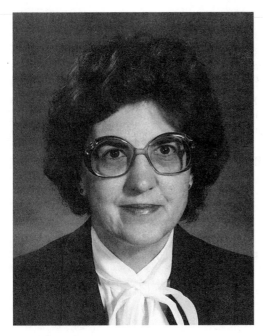

FIGURE 3.9 May Futrell.

whatever it is that gives the excitement of illness and cure. . . . I think there is some maturing that goes along with liking (to care for) older people. . . . I found in my doctoral dissertation that the older you were as a nurse, the more interest you had in older people" (Futrell, 1990).

Some of the younger students, who seemed interested in their own aging or that of their parents, had held two or three jobs in nursing and later called her to express their growing interest in the field of aging, saying, "I should have paid more attention to some of the things you said." "I had one student from last year's class come to my door last week asking me about recreational therapy for the elderly" (Futrell, 1990).

"When I graduated there really was not 'care of the aged.' . . . I can remember physicians saying that for anyone over 60 with a fractured hip there was not much hope. We will spend our time with younger clients. . . . My first experience caring for an elderly patient as a young nurse was very negative. I think it was at the end of my first year in the diploma program and I was asked to go into a room and clean up a woman who was literally covered from head to foot with feces. The floor nurses were so tired of cleaning her that the students got stuck with it (Futrell, 1990)."

"My dissertation research was on attitudes of physicians, nurses, and social workers toward the elderly. The social workers had a more positive attitude and I think part of the answer was that they were in 'well' situations and they did not constantly see sick older people" (Futrell, 1990).

"I think in the future geropsychiatric nursing will be an important focus, and international nursing will become more important because most of the countries are 'aging' and some have aged more rapidly than the United States. We can learn a great deal from Europe and Japan and in turn we can help them" (Futrell, 1990).

"I have enjoyed my 30 years in nursing and especially the last 20 in the field of aging. I have combined two disciplines and I would go that route again because I am not only using my nursing in gerontology but I am using gerontology expertise in nursing. Three special people that I have mentored, Karen Mellilo, Susan Houde, and Diane Mahoney, I believe are making an impact in health care because they have both fields. Mentoring young graduate students is a very satisfying experience" (Futrell, 1990).

JEANIE KAYSER-JONES

Dr. Kayser-Jones began her activities in gerontology in 1975 and is still a major contributor to research and education as the director of the John A. Hartford Center of Geriatric Nursing Excellence (HCGNE) at the

University of California, San Francisco, and as dissertation chair for numerous doctoral students and mentor for postdoctoral fellows. There are only four other HCGNEs in the nation: University of Pennsylvania, Director Neville Strumpf; University of Arkansas, Director Claudia Beverly; Oregon Health Sciences University, Director Patricia Archbold; and University of Iowa, Director Meridean Maas. These Centers are discussed further in chapter 7.

Jeanie's autobiography is inspirational. As the sixth child in a family of seven children born on a farm in Nebraska, she remembers learning at a young age the necessity of hard work, responsibility, and respect for elders. Her father, a strict disciplinarian and a member of the school board, expected his children to take their schooling seriously, and they did. She writes of a charming anecdote: "In the evenings, he would line the seven children up against a wall in the kitchen. First he would give us mental arithmetic problems, then we would have a 'spelldown,' and finally, under his supervision, we sat at the kitchen table and practiced our penmanship" (Kayser-Jones, 2004, p. 1).

Her father wanted to keep the children near home but an older brother, Loran, had left home to pursue higher education at the University of Nebraska. He encouraged Jeanie in her pursuit of education away from home. She says, "I worked for a year, saved every penny that I could and at age 17 went off to nursing school" (Kayser-Jones, 2004, p. 2).

She found St. Elizabeth's School of Nursing, a diploma school in Lincoln, Nebraska, an excellent experience and her fellow students very supportive. "Our nursing instructors were superb! They took a personal interest in each one of us, and they were wonderful role models. They taught us not only how to care for our patients, they also taught us ethics, professionalism, and the importance of discipline, integrity, responsibility, and respect for everyone, regardless of their status in life" (Kayser-Jones, 2004, p. 3).

Soon after graduation, Jeanie had the opportunity to go to Denmark as part of the ANA's Nurse Exchange Program. She and a classmate went to work at Bisbebjerg Hospital in Copenhagen. This experience influenced her decision, much later, to obtain her doctoral degree in medical anthropology. After her return from Europe she met and married H. William Kayser while working at Baylor University Hospital in Dallas, Texas. Unfortunately, he was killed a month later in an auto accident. She returned to her roots in Nebraska and worked in a large hospital in Omaha. Later she went to the University of Colorado in Denver to obtain a bachelor's degree in nursing and then immediately after, went to the University of California, San Francisco, School of Nursing to earn a master's degree. She met her present husband, Theodore Jones, while in her first teaching position at the University of San Francisco (USF). In this

Jesuit university she found that most faculty had doctorates and realized the need for one. "While teaching undergraduate nursing students, I saw many clinical problems, and I realized that while I could alleviate the problem for one patient, without a research degree I could not bring about change on a larger scale" (Kayser-Jones, 2004, p. 4).

Her interest in gerontology began while teaching at USF and discovering that her students were working in nursing homes as jobs were always available but said that after graduation they would never work in a nursing home. Jeanie investigated students' interest in working with older people and found interest sadly lacking (Kayser & Minnigerode, 1975).

She soon entered the doctoral program in medical anthropology at the University of California, Berkeley. When planning her doctoral dissertation she heard that the United Kingdom had an innovative approach to long-term care, and remembering the distress and depressing surroundings when her beloved grandfather died in a nursing home, and her students' feelings about nursing homes, she decided to do a cross-cultural comparison of long-term care in the United States and Scotland. This landmark study was the first of its kind, a full-scale anthropological study of nursing homes (Kayser-Jones, 1981, 1990).

Jeanie's interest in nursing homes led her to study the oral health status of residents. There were many problems and nurses usually were minimally aware of them. Dentists were seldom available and dentures were ill fitting or lost. With the help of a colleague, Dr. William Bird in the UCSF School of Dentistry, Jeanie designed a useful tool for oral health assessment, the Kayser-Jones Brief Oral Health Status Examination (BOHSE). This has become a highly regarded assessment tool, and is still being used in nursing homes throughout the United States and abroad (Kayser-Jones, Bird, Paul, et al., 1995).

Jeanie considers her most significant contribution to be the investigation of myriad factors that influence eating behavior in nursing homes. The results of this research were widely published and resulted in an invitation to be the lead panelist at a congressional forum on "Malnutrition in Nursing Homes." After her presentation to the U.S. Senate Special Committee on Aging, the General Accounting Office, the investigative arm of the U.S. Congress, investigated the extent of dehydration and malnutrition in nursing homes. Jeanie was asked to assist in the investigation and from that it was found that "more than half of the 'suspicious deaths' in California nursing homes were probably due to neglect, including malnutrition and dehydration" (Kayser-Jones, 2004, p. 10). As a result, surveyors' guidelines and protocols were revised to identify the problems. Jeanie says, "One of the most rewarding moments in my career occurred after I gave a keynote address to a large audience of personnel from state Departments of Health. An official from the HCFA, now the

Centers for Medicare and Medicaid Services (CMS), came up to me and said, 'You have touched the lives of more than a million nursing home residents'" (Kayser-Jones, 2004, p. 10).

Another especially significant moment in Jeanie's life occurred when she received the prestigious Doris Schwartz Research Award, presented in 1999 by the Hartford Institute for Geriatric Nursing, New York University, and the Gerontological Society of America.

Through it all she says, "No story of my career could be complete without mentioning my husband, Dr. Theodore H.D. Jones, who has been my colleague, mentor, and best friend for the past 28 years. Nothing would have been possible without his ongoing support and love" (Kayser-Jones, 2004, p. 16).

MARY LUND

Mary Lund is the first geriatric nurse ethicist of whom I am aware. Her insights and commitment are beacons in this field, which is becoming more perilous with each new technologic possibility. At this time when there is so much that can be done, the pertinent question is, should we? How did Mary become so committed to ethical approaches to health care and particularly to the care of the aged?

Mary was born in a small town in Wisconsin, the fourth of eight children. Those of us who have studied the effects of ordinal placement in the family believe that these middle children are the practical, stable ones; the negotiators between the powerful and the more dependent. Mary demonstrates these qualities. Mary was always engrossed in reading from the time she was a child. She was not particularly drawn to nursing but remembers walking across the field to summon Mrs. Hall, the local midwife, to attend her mother in childbirth. Mary thought of her as a nurse. The doctor in this small town performed everything from surgery to dispensing eye glasses, and posted quarantine signs on the door of homes where a communicable disease was found.

Her commitment to humane concerns may have come from reading about the Maryknoll missionary sisters and desiring to join them. The Franciscan sisters taught at her parish school and she joined the order because they were accessible. They needed nurses to staff the hospital and that is how she became a nurse. There was no recognition at that time of special needs of the elderly but she often wondered what happened to older people when discharged. How did they manage their illnesses and chronic conditions?

Mary left the order after 15 years and entered graduate school at the University of Wisconsin, Madison. There were no courses in nursing specifically focused on geriatrics. She sought knowledge from the writings of sociologists such as Anselm Strauss, Marcella Davis, and growth and development experts Robert Havighurst and Bernice Neugarten, and social gerontologists, Vivian Wood and Jaber Gubrium. These became her mentors in various ways. She was full of questions.

When she finished her graduate work she wasn't sure where to go with it. She taught briefly at the University of Milwaukee School of Nursing but was then offered a position at a community hospital as a clinical nurse specialist, managing the entire medical nursing service. In addition, this hospital had a skilled nursing facility and that appealed to her. Joint appointments were in vogue then and she taught at University of Wisconsin, Milwaukee, carried on her responsibilities at the hospital, and managed to spend time in the nursing home. Mary "soaked in" all she could from these varied settings and became ANA certified in gerontological nursing. The dean at the University encouraged her to get a PhD, so she began studies in sociology at Marquette University, with the guidance of Dr. Jay Gubrium. When a doctoral program in nursing opened at the University of Illinois, Chicago, she joined the first class.

The geriatric nursing field was developing: Virginia Stone wrote *Give the Old Person Time* for the *American Journal of Nursing;* Burnside's text, *Nursing and the Aged,* appeared in 1976; ANA Standards for Geriatric Nursing Practice were developing; and Mary Opal Wolanin was speaking out about digitalis and tranquilizer dosages in nursing homes. Mary's communication with Virginia Stone and Mary Opal developed into long and fruitful friendships. Throughout these few years, Mary Lund packed in experiences whenever an opportunity arose. One of the first seminars she attended, in 1972, was presented by Eldonna Shields under the aegis of the ANA.

While still a doctoral student and with her usual chutzpah, Mary spoke to the dean of Marquette University Medical School about the need for geriatric content and, like most nursing school administrators, he countered that there was no room in the curriculum. Three years later she obtained a joint appointment at that medical school, now called the Medical College of Wisconsin. She began teaching in the geriatric section. Eventually a minimal amount of time was allotted to geriatrics in the medical school curriculum. She wrote a paper on drug therapy and elders for the *State Medical Journal* but, when published, a geriatrician colleague was named as first author. Even though nurses no longer rose when a physician entered the room, doctors were still given preferential treatment.

Mary believes the years 1980 to 1990 were her most productive. While holding a joint appointment between the medical center hospital and the geriatric section of the medical college, she planned and directed the multidisciplinary Geriatric Assessment Team, edited the campus newsletter, *Agelines,* and developed and coordinated a campus-wide multidisciplinary geriatric interest group.

She was called on to consult and teach about geriatric care. Mary found acceptance among all disciplines but was often disappointed in the receptivity of nurses. It was unusual to have a PhD nurse in a clinical setting. The director of nursing in the hospital in which she worked at the time thought Mary's position as nurse gerontologist expendable, so she resigned and began teaching at the Medical College of Wisconsin, which had opened a school of nursing.

Dr. Lund had been interested in ethical issues for some time and established a good relationship with two lawyer/ethicists who had established a bioethics center at the medical college. She joined the center and became an unpaid postgraduate fellow. Bioethics was in its infancy and "it was a heady time." In this phase she was given numerous opportunities for public speaking, research, and consultation. One of her projects was reported in *Geriatric Nursing* (GN) (Lund & Wei, 1990) and for a short time she wrote an ethics column for GN. Because of her knowledge of bioethics she was offered a position by the Health Education Network as consultant in ethics, aging, and geriatric nursing. She continues to do this, although her responsibilities for her husband's health needs require that she use available technology and accomplish this from her home.

Mary writes, "Before me as I write are letters from Mary Opal Wolanin and Virginia Stone, dated 1976 and 1977" (Lund, 2004, p. 15). These were important among her many mentors and encouraged her to continue in her study of aging, and offered criticism and suggestions for improvement of her doctoral dissertation. There is also an encouraging letter from Irene Burnside and an autographed copy of Laurie Gunter's, *Education for Gerontic Nursing.*

"How can I give credit to all the academics, clinicians, and elders who by word and example taught me to 'do geriatrics?' . . . I was very lucky to be in the right place at the right time, just as the field was starting to life . . . . So, there you have it, the story of a working class girl, dreaming of becoming a foreign missionary, who joined an order of mainly teaching nuns, selected (in reality ordered) to become a nurse, and in the broadest of definitions of a missionary, became a propagandist for the cause of elder care. What a ride it has been!" (Lund, 2004, pp. 15–17).

MATHY MEZEY

Dr. Mathy Mezey is to geriatric nursing as was Peter the Great to Russia, tugging and dragging the care of the aged into the 21st century. This has not been caused by her alone—the field was plowed by numerous pioneers—but her vision knew how, when, and where to plant. When one thinks of strengthening tender tendrils with proper feeding and cultivation, one must think of Mathy.

I first met Mathy when she was the director of the Robert Wood Johnson Foundation Teaching Nursing Home program. This program linked schools of nursing and nursing homes in order to improve the care of the aged. A geriatric nurse practitioner was placed in each nursing home involved in the program.

In the 25 years of our association I have been astounded by her accomplishments and those of others that she has assisted, supported, and encouraged. Through awards, grants, and fellowships she, with the endowments of the John A. Hartford Foundation, has made excellence in geriatric practice and research visible. Specific activities of the Hartford Institute for Geriatric Nursing include developing geriatric curricula for schools of nursing; providing models for developing and disseminating best practices in acute and long-term care; developing and distributing practice guidelines, assessment tools, and materials for the advancement of geriatric nursing practice; creating partnerships with staff developers in health facilities to infuse best practices into work settings; providing faculty training programs; periodically conferencing with national geriatric nurse leaders; providing a resource center; and being present and giving presentations related to the care of the aged at specialty nursing association meetings and gerontological conferences. The Hartford Institute was the first national program of what is now a $35 million investment in geriatric nursing on the part of the John A. Hartford Foundation, including the establishment of Centers of Excellence at five universities. The overall goal of the Hartford Institute is to improve care received by older adults by stimulating best practices in nursing education, clinical care, research, and public policy.

I have dubbed Mathy Mezey and Terry Fulmer the Dynamic Duo. Together they have made the nurses of the nation aware of best practices in geriatric care. In 1996, she and Terry became the directors of the John A. Hartford Foundation Institute for Geriatric Nursing in the Division of Nursing at NYU. Mathy is also the Independence Foundation Professor of Nursing Education at NYU and directs the GNP program (Fig. 3.10).

Mathy's roots in gerontology sprang from an intense interest in the care of the aged as she worked in the New York Visiting Nurse Service, early in the 1960s. She experienced the potential of nursing to alter and enrich the daily lives of the elders she served. One must remember that elders of that era had often emigrated in their youth and were a diverse group. She especially enjoyed the ethnic and cultural differences and histories of these individuals. She fell in love with the work and, as her husband is a pediatrician, she believed that serving the opposite ends of the

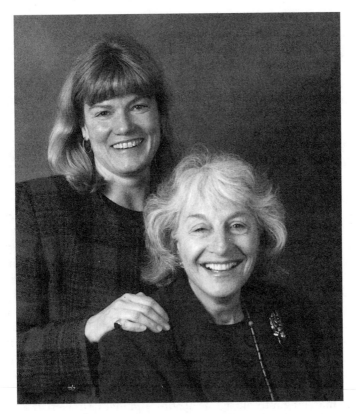

FIGURE 3.10 Terry Fulmer and Mathy Mezey, the Dynamic Duo.

life cycle provided an interesting contrast of professional interests in their marriage (Ebersole, 1999c).

Mathy received her undergraduate and graduate education at Columbia University in New York City. Her early nursing background included working as a public health nurse, and as a staff nurse on the medical surgical units at Jacobi Hospital, an acute care facility that was part of the New York City Health and Hospitals Corporation. For 10 years Mathy was a professor at the University of Pennsylvania School of Nursing and directed the geriatric nurse practitioner program.

Dr. Mezey has earned many honors and is a Fellow of the American Academy of Nurses; the Gerontological Society of America; and was a Board Member of the American Federation of Aging Research (AFAR). She is a board member of the *Geriatric Nursing Journal;* and on the board of the Visiting Nurse Service of New York. Mathy was also a member of the Ethics Group of Hilary Rodham Clinton's Health Care Reform Task Force.

Dr. Mezey has authored 12 books and over 100 publications that focus on nursing care of the elderly and bioethical issues that affect decisions at the end of life. She is series editor of the *Springer Series in Geriatric Nursing* and has twice received the American Journal of Nursing Book of the Year Award in Geriatrics. She is presently a trustee of Columbia University, her alma mater.

Mathy's current research and writing focuses on the role of the advanced practice nurse in the delivery of care in hospitals and nursing homes.

Mathy's accomplishments and contributions to geriatric care cannot be sufficiently summarized in limited space; however, her guiding philosophy is most important.

Before coming to the United States when she was 10 years old, Mathy lived in England where her mother worked in the laboratory of a hospital. She dates her early interest in nursing to seeing the English nurses at the hospital with their wonderful red-and-blue capes that they hung elegantly slung over their shoulders. She believes that nursing has been an extraordinary career choice. "Nursing allows you to be very clear every day as to what you have accomplished in helping others, and where you have fallen short. Nursing is extraordinarily flexible; it allows you to re-invent yourself every few years: clinician, educator, administrator. Because geriatric nursing especially offers nurses the unique opportunity to dramatically impact people's lives for the better and for the worst, it demands the best that you have to offer. I am very optimistic about the future of geriatric nursing. Increasing numbers of older adults are interested in marching into old age as healthy and involved. Geriatric nursing offers a unique opportunity to help older adults meet these aspirations, while at the same time maintaining a commitment to the oldest and frailest in our society" (Mezey, 2005) (Fig. 3.11).

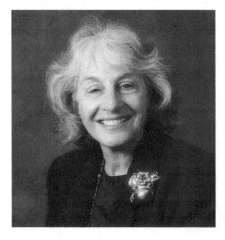

FIGURE 3.11 Mathy Mezey.

NEVILLE STRUMPF

Dr. Neville Strumpf was influenced toward nursing and the care of the aged by both parents who were nurses and by loving and beloved grandparents. Their influences and her origins, in a small town outside of Albany in upstate New York, gave her security and a stable sense of self. Frequent visits to her grandparents, at their farm in the Shenandoah Valley of Virginia, imparted a solid sense of the wisdom, strength, and resilience of older adults. Neville remembers many occasions of simply sitting quietly with her grandmother, swaying gently in their porch rockers, telling stories, watching fireflies, or listening to the silence of the country night beneath a canopy of stars. Such moments gave to her an appreciation of older adults and the desire that all should have the opportunity for a "good old age."

Neville's most notable contribution to geriatric nursing was in response to Doris Schwartz's call for investigation of the nearly ubiquitous practice of restraining the elderly, commonly thought to be for reasons of safety. She teamed with Lois Evans to conduct scrupulous research about when and how restraints were used and for what reasons. This was over 20 years ago when they were relatively new faculty at University of Pennsylvania School of Nursing (Penn). Their proposal to conduct a pilot project, submitted to Penn's Center for Nursing Research, was rejected for "lack of significance and unlikelihood of further funding." This rejection only increased their determination. They persisted and received grants to study the problem, then published numerous articles, as well as testifying to a U.S. Senate Select Committee on Aging, that heightened public and professional awareness and influenced policy changes about elder restraints. They found that restraints were actually hazardous in many situations (Fig. 3.12).

Their research has been influential throughout the United States and markedly changed the standards of practice. Benchmark studies showed that with appropriate staff education and consultation, decreased restraint usage could be accomplished without increases in staffing, psychoactive drugs, or injurious falls (Evans et al., 1997; Strumpf et al., 1992). These findings influenced the Federal Nursing Home Reform Act.

Dr. Strumpf has earned numerous awards for her contribution to nursing practice such as: Baxter Foundation Episteme Award, Maes-MacInnes Award for Outstanding Singular Contributions to the Nursing Profession, Sigma Theta Tau Cameo Research Award, and the Doris Schwartz Gerontological Nursing Research Award bestowed by the John A. Hartford Foundation Institute for Geriatric Nursing and the Gerontological Society of America (Ebersole, 2003b). Neville has been a fellow of the American Academy of Nursing since 1987, and has occupied

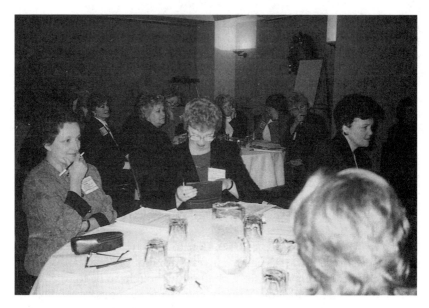

FIGURE 3.12   Neville Strumpf (far left) at NLN meeting, 1995.

the Doris Schwartz Term Chair in Gerontological Nursing at the University of Pennsylvania, now held by Sarah Kagan. In 1994 she was named the American Nurses Association Gerontological Nurse of the Year.

Presently, Neville is the Edith Clemmer Steinbright Professor in Gerontology at the University of Pennsylvania School of Nursing, Director of the Hartford Center of Geriatric Nursing Excellence, and Director of the Center for Gerontologic Nursing Science at the School of Nursing.

Neville earned her baccalaureate degree in nursing at the State University of New York, Plattsburgh, in 1969. She continued on toward a master's degree at Russell Sage College in Troy, New York, and earned a doctorate at New York University in New York City in 1982. The subject of her doctoral dissertation was *The Relationship of Life Satisfaction and Self-Concept to Time Experience in Older Women* (Strumpf, 1982).

She began teaching nursing at Hartwick College, Oneonta, New York, in 1973 and from 1977 to 1982 taught in the Department of Nursing at H. H. Lehman College, City University of New York, before going to the University of Pennsylvania, School of Nursing in Philadelphia. She was the director of the Gerontological Nurse Practitioner Program at Penn from 1985 to 2000. This program was rated number one in the *U.S. News & World Report,* 1998 and 2001.

In 1998 she was appointed Faculty-Mentor for Seminar/Fellowships in Gerontological Nursing for Post-Doctoral Fellows by the John A.

Hartford Foundation Institute for Geriatric Nursing, at NYU, and is a past director of the Hartford Center of Geriatric Nursing Excellence and now the director of the Center for Gerontological Nursing Science at the University of Pennsylvania School of Nursing.

Neville has authored or co-authored more than 50 refereed journal articles, four books, four monographs, and 30 book chapters. She has been awarded, as principal investigator (PI) or co-PI, more than $10 million in federal, foundation, and other funding for her research, as well as for program projects improving geriatrics education and practice. Her current interests include palliative care in nursing homes and the historical underpinnings of the field of gerontology. She has several research interests, most focused on considerations of safe and humane care, particularly for frail elders. She was on the task force of the American Nurses' Association to revise the *Statement on the Scope of Gerontological Nursing Practice* in 1986 and 1987. Neville has given numerous speeches, consultations, and legal testimony regarding geriatric nursing (Strumpf, 2003a).

As with many of the second wave of gerontological nurses, Neville has accomplished much more than seems possible to upgrade and influence the care of the aged. She and others at the University of Pennsylvania have, and are having, a great influence on progress in geriatric nursing. They have produced an excellent "crop to seed the third generation." Many of them are making marked contributions at present: Liz Capezuti, now at New York University, made a distinct contribution investigating the safety of side rails (Capezuti, Talerico, Strumpf, & Evans, 1998); Mary Beth Happ, at the University of Pittsburgh, is known most for her focus on voiceless older adults in critical care units; Meg Bourbonniere, at Yale University School of Nursing, is known for her research on transfer of care of older adults across setting. There are many others that have been mentioned throughout this text in conjunction with their contributions.

Neville's philosophy "remains deeply rooted in individual choice, comfort and dignity, especially for frail, older adults. I fervently hope that the future will be characterized by a health system capable of supporting these values throughout a person's life, and that we shall someday see the routine application of evidence based practice to the care of all older adults, whether they are in the community, a hospital or the nursing home. We have not yet achieved that dream" (Strumpf, 2005, p. 1).

ANN WHALL

Dr. Ann Whall has been in the forefront of much that has happened in geriatric nursing within the last two decades, particularly in geropsychiatric research, dementia, and aggressive behaviors. Her early work with

Dr. May Wykle and Dr. Kitty Buckwalter led to cooperative ventures among them over the years.

Ann Louise (Flanagan) Whall is a native of Michigan. Her education from BSN, MSN, to PhD, was accomplished at Wayne State University (WSU) in Detroit. While persuing her graduate degree and working in public health nursing, Ann was stirred by the elderly urban poor people who lived alone, were often ill and in desperate circumstances. These experiences led her to pursue geropsychiatric nursing as a specialty.

After her doctorate, Ann was given two postdoctoral fellowships, funded by NIMH, at which time she began working with May and Kitty. After her second postdoctorate she moved to University of Michigan and began working with Dr. Thelma Wells.

Her accomplishments are numerous and include Distinguished Visiting Professorships at Iowa, Tennessee, Oakland University in Michigan, and from the University of Ulster in Northern Ireland.

Ann's joint work across disciplines, universities, and nations resulted in well over 100 publications, Fulbright Awards, and many honors. Her emphasis on the importance of collaboration and interdisciplinary research was an important consideration in her selection for the 2003 Doris Schwartz Gerontological Nursing Research Award.

THELMA WELLS

Dr. Thelma Wells is Professor Emerita of University of Wisconsin-Madison, School of Nursing. Thelma's consuming passion has always been, since her earliest days in nursing, astute bedside clinical nursing care. Her extensive research (22 published research papers) has constantly been directed toward clinical problems that needed attention. Her energy and enthusiasm are infectious. Every student entering nursing should have the opportunity to see or hear Thelma.

Thelma entered the diploma nursing program at Massachusetts General Hospital in 1959, graduating in 1962, and while there developed curiosity about the older patients and their needs. During her baccalaureate education at Boston University (1965–1968) she asked to visit the state mental hospital where she was appalled to see elders in "such desperate, tragic" situations. One of the nurses told her that conditions were much better; that is, the wards were cleaner than they had been. She became so angry and shocked at the warehousing of the old that she channeled her energy into action. Seeking more knowledge and credentials she entered the master's program at Frances Payne Bolton School of Nursing, Case Western Reserve University, in 1968.

All along her clinical research path Thelma has operated under the assumption that "sticking your neck out means it may get cut off." But, her sense of commitment to changing the conditions of geriatric nursing care motivated her. She tells the story of Sophia, a patient in an old converted hotel nursing home, who was the genesis of Thelma's study of incontinence. This lady "an impoverished seamstress of Russian heritage fought to keep her pride amid dreadful circumstances. After some months of regular contact, she whispered that she had an awful secret to tell me. Unable to imagine what this could be, I listened as she, in great shame and dismay, told me that she wet her pants—to her a fatal loss of self-control and adulthood. I assured Sophia that surely something could be done" (Wells in Ebersole, 1998, p. 103).

Thelma, still in graduate school, immediately searched the literature in order to help Sophia with her incontinence. She could find no literature at that time and was dismayed that no one seemed to be interested in this massive problem. She heard that a lot of interest in the problems of aging people was being expressed in England, so, after graduation (1970) she went to England to learn more. She intended to stay for 6 months but remained for 5 years working with a highly skilled team of geriatricians, social workers, nurses, occupational therapists, and physical therapists. She worked in an acute assessment ward at Crowley Road Hospital in Oxford and with Professor John Brocklehurst, MD, at the University of Manchester Department of Geriatric Medicine. Awarded a 3-year fellowship to study with Dr. Brocklehurst, she received her doctorate in 1975. In her heart she still feels much like a British nurse.

When she sees problems, Thelma attacks them. She began focusing on the environment of nursing in her doctoral work and how that influences patient care, the ease or difficulty of responding to patients by the very nature of the environment. She says, "How we deliver care, our perception of the problems, are all influenced by how we set up and use the environment; there are subtle influences of environment that we seldom notice."

Thelma became concerned about chairs. Large groups of institutionalized aged simply sit in chairs; none designed for their individuals needs. "Whenever there are pillows, restraints for positioning, or footstools, it is an indication that the chair is not suitable for that individual. A chair should be a therapeutic tool!" When Thelma sees such a problem she looks for whatever needs to be done; counts, measures, documents, studies, labels. These are the tools of her research.

As a young graduate nurse, she experienced an epiphany while working in a very good ICU. A very old man said, "Nurse, I'm dying." She went into action with all the equipment at her disposal. He died. She had wanted to stay with him and provide comfort rather than following protocol but did what she was trained to do even though in her heart she felt that it was wrong. She became convinced that nurses should listen to their feelings as part of clinical decision making and take greater responsibility in changing care practices.

When asked about her mentors, Thelma says there were so many who influenced or challenged her in those British team conferences and elsewhere, but the patients were her real mentors; "That little incontinent seamstress, and memories of many interactions with patients." She tells the story that before the NASA invention of female urinary collection devices for astronauts, Dr. Brocklehurst wanted to evaluate one that had been designed in England. The device offended the nurses because of its appearance but one patient said she wanted to try it because, "Dearie, you don't know what its like until you wet your shoes." This listening to patients is a core value for Thelma.

In 1981, Thelma, Carol Brink, RN, MPH, and Ananias Diokno, MD, established the first continence clinic in the country (Wells, 1994). A year later this team began serious study of the problem of incontinence, working with older women living in the community. They had found six studies of incontinence in the relevant literature, and these were vague, generalized, and lacking in specificity. So they set about careful assessment and testing specific behavioral treatment interventions in the first nurse-directed incontinence research funded by the National Institute on Aging (AGO 3542).

In 2002, Thelma Joan Wells and Carol Brink were selected as the recipients of the Doris Schwartz Gerontological Nursing Research Award, given in recognition of visionary and exemplary contributions advancing the field of geriatric nursing research. Their presentation at the Nurses Interest Group of the GSA included their comments about looking back and looking forward. "Looking back 20 years ago, the GSA's annual meeting was held in Boston. Joe Ouslander, MD, organized a symposium on incontinence. I believe it was the first-ever urinary incontinence themed session at a GSA meeting. Carol and I presented a paper, *Nursing Interventions for Urinary Incontinence in the Elderly*" (Brink & Wells, 2003). They also contributed to the second (1981) and third (1988) editions of Burnside's book, *Nursing and the Aged,* and found that in the intervening 7 years between those editions, there had been much progress in nursing's understanding of urinary incontinence.

Thelma says, "I love clinical research; it's like riding a roller coaster. There are always problems to solve and excitement in discovering your own and others' strengths. There is a thrill a minute." Carol says, "Thelma was always eager for problems. She used to say, 'If we don't have problems doing this research, we're not paying attention'" (Brink & Wells, 2003).

Other recognitions that have been most significant include Fellowship in the Royal College of Nursing (1987); the 1991 Episteme Laureate (Baxter Foundation/Sigma Theta Tau International); the 1997 NLN/Ross Laboratories Long-Term Care Award; and in 2003 the establishment of the Wound, Ostomy, and Continence Nursing Association Annual Thelma J. Wells Continence Lecture.

Some of Thelma's interest in aging came from her mother's father, the only grandparent she knew, as the others died young. He was a stern New Englander but wise. She developed the habit of listening to old people because they are "great repositories of wisdom."

What has she learned about her own aging? Middle-aged at the time of the interview she said, "I've learned resilience, surviving the downs of the roller coaster. I have lots of energy but there are always ups and downs. In my heart, soul, and head I'm a clinical bedside nurse" (Wells, 1990). In 2002, Thelma said, "I'm looking forward to retiring this May (2003). I've loved my nursing career but I'm ready to savor my senior years." Carol said, "I know Thelma will be working with Chris Kovach, RN, PhD and her research program at the University of Wisconsin-Milwaukee for a few years" (Brink & Wells, 2003, p. 5).

Immediate issues in nursing that Thelma saw in 1990, "Basic gerontic nursing must be at the base of nursing education. Some see gerontic nursing as a narrow, limited, specialized field, mostly acquired in graduate school. I don't believe this. If interest is not captured at the base level, it may be too late. We need to recognize the reality of nursing today. We cannot deny the tidal wave until it is upon us. The cadre of early geriatric nursing leaders is retired. We need their sense of drama and the excitement of those early days. We are the group coming up and part of the approaching tidal wave (Wells, 1990). Looking forward in 2002, both Thelma and Carol know that gerontological nursing will survive and the students coming into the field are an energetic and committed group (Brinks & Wells, 2003) (Fig. 3.13).

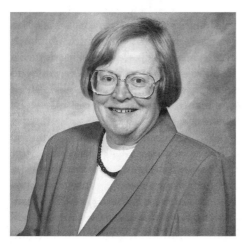

FIGURE 3.13 Thelma Wells.

MAY WYKLE

Dr. May Wykle seems to be present everywhere, touching lives world-wide, always seeking to contribute more to the profession of geriatric nursing and creating opportunities for nurses from impoverished backgrounds. Her enthusiastic mentorship has moved many nurses forward until they gain their own momentum. Dr. Wykle is the dean of nursing at Florence Payne Bolton School of Nursing, CWRU, Cleveland, and occupies the Florence Cellar Chair in Gerontological Nursing. Cellar endowed the chair for perpetuity in 1984, and Dr. Wykle is the first full-time occupant. She was greatly influenced by Doreen Norton, the first occupant of the Florence Cellar Chair in Gerontological Nursing. May says, "I was fascinated by her knowledge of everyday problems confronting older adults, from the type of furniture they need to the amount of medication they receive" (Wykle in Ebersole, 1999b, p. 51).

Dr. Wykle is the director of the CWRU University Center on Aging and Health, a fellow of the American Academy of Nursing, as well as the Gerontological Society of America. In 2000, Dr. Wykle received the Doris Schwartz Gerontological Nursing Research Award from the John A. Hartford Foundation Institute for Geriatric Nursing and the Gerontological Society of America. The award was presented to honor her outstanding contributions to the field of gerontological nursing research and specifically her work with minority caregivers. Most recently, in the summer of 2004, she became the third woman and the first nurse to be awarded the prestigious Frank and Dorothy Humel Hovorka Prize.

Wykle grew up in rural Ohio and graduated from Mount Pleasant High School, where grades 1 through 12 were housed in the same building. As a young woman, she intended to be a physician but an experience as a nurse's aide and encouragement by nurses changed her direction toward nursing. However, she was refused admission to several nursing schools because of her race. She was accepted at the Ruth Bryant School of Nursing in Martins Ferry, Ohio, and became the first African American to attend that school. May's professional accomplishments are awesome and prodigious. From that first struggle to gain acceptance in nursing school, one cannot help wondering how much the geriatric nursing specialty would have been lost had she not been accepted.

After graduation from the Ruth Bryant School of Nursing, May continued her education at Case Western Reserve University, obtaining a BSN when it was still called Western Reserve University. While raising a family, caring for elders of her extended family, and working as a nurse in several settings, she continued her education until she achieved her PhD in 1981.

May learned about old people when she was very young. She remembers as a fifth grader feeding her grandfather, who had a stroke, coffee through a glass straw. She also helped her grandmother care for May's godmother, who incidentally had been a slave, and often told stories about her experiences as a slave. Her grandparents lived with the family and her grandmother, active in charity organizations and in the community, was her role model. Her mother and grandmother cared for elderly friends and neighbors in their home, as well as her ailing grandfather. Now, May is a grandmother and carries on the family traditions of caring for others. She cultivates and treasures the intergenerational connections with her grandchildren.

However, May is not focused only on family, community, and university, though that seems sufficient. She has also developed a commitment to international nursing that began when she attended the 12th World Conference on Health (1985) in Dublin, Ireland, and discovered worldwide problems similar to our own: caring for dependent elders and ensuring financial and functional capacity.

Dean Wykle has been a professor at Frances Payne Bolton School of Nursing, CWRU, since 1986 and dean since 2001. She began her nursing career at Cleveland Psychiatric Institute in 1958 and throughout her pursuits she has been involved in psychiatric, geropsychiatric, and ethnically oriented care and education. She has served as chair or on dissertation committees for more than 50 students toward achieving their PhDs. During her early faculty tenure at FPB, May headed one of the first geropsychiatric graduate nursing programs in the nation. This program provided an opportunity for many students to become geropsychiatric nurse specialists, including a cadre of African American nurses. The influence of Mary Starke Harper in finding federal funding for this program made it possible. Mary Harper is discussed in chapter 2.

May has been especially interested in caregivers, both formal and informal. Her involvement with the Teaching Nursing Home project at Margaret Wagner House/Benjamin Rose Institute in Cleveland was a means to influence the standards of care and to promote an inspiring and growth environment for caregivers in the institution.

Among numerous honors and special recognitions some of the most recent include Visiting Professor at the University of Zimbabwe, Nursing Science Department, Harare, Zimbabwe, Africa; Pope Eminent Scholar at the Rosalynn Carter Institute, Georgia Southwestern State University, Americus, Georgia; Estelle Osborne Distinguished Lecturer, New York University School of Education, Division of Nursing; Doris Schwartz Gerontological Nursing Research Award, Gerontological Society of America and the John A. Hartford Foundation Institute; Lifetime Achievement Award, National Black Nurses Association, Inc.; and a Certificate of Special Congressional Recognition as a Council of Black Nurses Hall of Fame Inductee (Fig. 3.14).

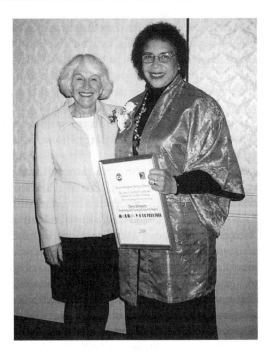

FIGURE 3.14 May Wykle receiving the Doris Schwartz Gerontological Nursing Research Award.

Professional activities of recent significance include: president of Sigma Theta Tau International (2003), and member of the Board of Commission on Minority Health appointed by Governor Taft. She has served as consultant nationally and internationally on a broad range of nursing and educational concerns. May has served as editor, coeditor, and reviewer for a number of publications and is a member of the Advisory Board, *Springer Series on Adulthood and Aging*. Her research projects are extensive and have contributed greatly to the understanding of black caregivers, formal and informal. In addition she has served on training grants and educational program development nationally and internationally. Recently she has been codirector of several projects to further the development of gerontological nurse practitioner programs. May has written nine books, contributed chapters to 32 books, and written over 60 journal articles, as well as many commentaries on published articles. She has produced a dozen videotapes focused on a wide range of issues from caring for stroke and Alzheimer's patients to developing a PhD program of health research in aging.

May was invited to present a series of lectures on enhancing the care of the elderly in Kenya. "The problems of caring for elders in Africa is an emerging issue not unlike the problems of caring for older adults in rural United States. Elders often are left alone in rural areas when their children go off to find work in the cities; subsequently, no one is left to provide for them. The health ministries of African countries are quite worried about how to treat the health problems of an increasing number of old people. This concern was echoed in Botswana, Zimbabwe, Uganda, and South Africa, countries where I was privileged to interact with public health nurses. In Zimbabwe, research in the care of elders and their unique needs has begun in the medical school and now in the school of nursing, in which the FPB (Frances Payne Bolton, CWRU) School of Nursing, supported by the Kellogg Foundation, helped establish a master of science nursing program" (Wykle in Ebersole, 1999b, p. 51).

Dr. Wykle also traveled to China, Taiwan, Hungary, and Slovenia to teach and investigate the needs of elders. "Clearly, the quality of care for aged people is an international challenge to nursing" (Wykle in Ebersole, 1999b, p. 51).

A Nordic Conference on Aging in Denmark that May attended included individuals from Norway, Sweden, Finland, Denmark, and Iceland. These countries have formalized comprehensive systems of care to address the problems elders face.

Her myriad world experiences have reinforced her belief that care of the aged must be an international, interdisciplinary effort. "Our most important goal in nursing is to promote the creativity, health, and independence of older people and provide an appropriate infrastructure if we are going to live in a responsible, worldwide aging society" (Wykle, 1999, p. 51).

In keeping with her development of global linkages, during her regime from 2001 until 2003, as president of Sigma Theta Tau International, Dr. Wykle facilitated the inclusion of 12 new honor societies from Canada, Mexico, South Africa, and the United States. Her leadership resulted in board approval for 12 joint research grant partnerships and a formalized relationship with the International Academic Nursing Alliance; guidelines for collaborative international research; and development of a strategic plan for 2005. In addition, a white paper on diversity is in development that includes working definitions for global diversity (Wykle, 2003). A prominent experience during her presidency was the opportunity to present Her Royal Highness Princess Anne, the United Kingdom, with a Lifetime Achievement Award for her global humanitarian endeavors and contributions to health care. Nancy Dickenson-Hazard, CEO of Sigma Theta Tau International, was the co-presenter of the award.

Most outstanding, in my opinion, among May's many attributes is her warm acceptance of people and her down-to-earth approach to problems. She reaches out to everyone in her path with honesty and generosity.

May believes that the future of geriatric nursing is critical and needs to become an essential part of all nursing education programs. Competent geriatric education will contribute to the quality of life for all persons across the generations.

CONCLUSION

The individuals discussed and quoted throughout this chapter are representative of the vitality, leadership, and range of directions that geriatric nursing has taken in the last 30 years. There are many other remarkable geriatric nurses, less well known to me but no less important. I wish all could be included.

CHAPTER FOUR

Geriatric Nurse Leaders Today

At present, the tempo of progress in geriatric nursing is exponential and the numerous participants cannot possibly be individually addressed. The once-faltering steps of geriatric organizations have become giant leaps. The influence of these and so many others cannot be contained within the limitations of this text. The following individuals serve to exemplify some of the movements that are occurring in the field but are only the tip of the iceberg. Geriatric nursing is flourishing.

CORNELIA BECK

Dr. Cornelia Beck is best known for her prolific research studies. Her interest in the care of elders began while she was with the Visiting Nurses Association in Conway, Arkansas, and was further stirred while supervising students in nursing homes. She observed the decline in function of elders, particularly those with Alzheimer's disease, which occurred soon after admission to a nursing home and speculated that some of the deterioration was iatrogenic and could be curbed with appropriate interventions. This led to pilot projects, which eventually launched her research career. She says Beverly Baldwin, PhD, RN, University of Maryland (see chapter 3) taught her how to frame the clinical issues that she was passionate about into fundable proposals and to "dream the impossible" (Beck, 1999, p. 7).

Dr. Beck's fundamental goal is to influence caregivers to preserve the highest level of independence of elders by appropriate interventions. Her research has generated a standard set of behavioral strategies that can be prescribed after conducting an assessment of an individual's cognitive and functional abilities and disabilities. Caregivers can use these prescriptions when helping persons with activities of daily living.

Dr. Beck is currently a professor in the College of Medicine, Department of Geriatrics; College of Medicine, Department of Psychiatry and Behavioral Sciences; and College of Nursing, at the University of Arkansas for Medical Sciences, Little Rock.

Dr. Beck has earned numerous state and national awards including the University of Arkansas for Medical Sciences, College of Nursing, Excellence in Scholarship Award (1992); Fellowship in the American Academy of Nursing (1994); Distinguished Contribution to Nursing Science Award, American Nurses Foundation (1998); National Gerontological Nursing Association Lifetime Achievement Award; and the Nursing Competence in Aging Writer's Award in 2004 (Beck, 2005).

She was the first recipient of the prestigious Doris Schwartz Award for Gerontological Nursing (1998). When receiving the award she spoke of the need for personal, social, and creative courage, life-giving play, and authenticity as fundamental to growth, personally and professionally. "The quality of our research and what we choose to research will be greatly influenced by who we are and who we become as persons" (Beck, 1999, p. 9).

Cornelia wrote, "With personal, social, and creative courage, each of us can contribute to the synthesis of both humanistic and scientific knowledge. My challenge to you is to work toward understanding yourself and your emotions more fully, to be authentic and generous in stimulating and supporting one another, and to allow yourself the discomfort and joy of creative change" (Beck, 1999, p. 9).

KATHLEEN (KITTY) BUCKWALTER

Dr. Kitty Buckwalter is a highly respected leader in nursing, an excellent educator, a clinical practitioner, and a meticulous researcher. She says, "For as long as I can remember, I enjoyed being around older people. As a child, my fondest memories are of times spent with my grandparents, who lived in an older Czech neighborhood in Iowa City where activities revolved around St. Wenceslaus church and polka dances at the social hall across the street from their home. My grandfather, Ed Shea, was a red-headed Irishman and blacksmith who used to take me to play among the old tires and rusting vehicles in a salvage yard while he 'jawed' with his cronies. My parents would never have permitted these outings had they known the locale, but we always had a wonderful time" (Buckwalter, 2002).

"During my undergraduate nursing program at Iowa, I always sought out clinical experiences with older adults and chose to work as a nursing home aide (a role I reprised in a volunteer capacity for 6 months in 1991 and still found enjoyable!). As if to foreshadow my ultimate career path, in 1970, as a senior nursing student, I took an independent study course exploring the 'new' concept of senile dementias" (Buckwalter in Ebersole, 2001, p. 93).

Dr. Buckwalter has produced a prodigious amount of nursing research on an ongoing basis for over 20 years. She has developed models for delivering mental health services to the elderly and has mentored numerous colleagues as they developed studies, projects, and dissertations (Buckwalter, 2000). She was instrumental in the development of the well-respected master's and doctoral program in gerontological nursing at the University of Iowa, as well as a post master's specialization in geropsychiatric nursing. In addition, she has convened major clinical and research conferences, and served on the governing boards and advisory councils of numerous research societies, professional organizations, and federal agencies (Buckwalter, 2002).

One of her greatest contributions has been the dedication with which she has researched models for the care of persons afflicted with Alzheimer's disease and similar dementias. There has been an overabundance of descriptions of Alzheimer's disease and its effects on functions and families, but a paucity of investigations of clinical interventions that modify and assist in the management of the difficult behaviors that so often accompany dementias. For nearly two decades, Kitty has worked with Dr. Geri Richards Hall, who developed a model to address these clinical and management issues: the Progressively Lowered Stress Threshold (PLST) Model. The PLST model provides a workable framework for interventions with the cognitively impaired. Research using this model has consistently documented important care recipient and care provider outcomes in a variety of settings (Hall & Buckwalter, 1987; Smith, Gerdner, Hall, & Buckwalter, 2004). There is no question that in this respect she has contributed a great deal to the ability of nurses everywhere to manage disturbed behaviors with aplomb, fewer medications, and the maintenance of dignity for the afflicted person. Dr. Buckwalter has led the field in applied research, integrating her research into patient care and nursing education. She has developed and evaluated widely used conceptual frameworks that guide patient and family care and provide theoretical grounding for research and innovative models of health care delivery for the elderly, particularly high-risk, underserved groups and those without access to care (special dementia care units and rural outreach projects). The national influence of her work extends in many directions and has dramatically changed the nature of geropsychiatric nursing practice.

Kitty is proficient in several arenas: She has obtained funding for 34 research grants totaling nearly 13 million dollars; published over 300 articles, book chapters, monographs, editorials, and policy papers; and received national recognition for her seminal research and scholarly works. In addition to publication of the PLST model in 1987 (Hall & Buckwalter, 1987), and a recent article in the *Journal of the American Geriatrics Society* that chronicles 17 years of testing of the model (Smith et al., 2004), other publications of particular importance follow: *Mental Health Services of the Rural Elderly Outreach Program* (Buckwalter, Smith, Zevenbergen, & Russell, 1991); *Caregiver Training for People With Alzheimer's Based on a Stress Threshold Model* (Gerdner, Hall, & Buckwalter, 1996); and *Access to Health Care Resources for Family Caregivers of Elderly Persons With Dementia* (Kelley, Buckwalter, & Maas, 1999).

In January of 2005 she returned to the faculty of the College of Nursing at the University of Iowa, having completed 7 years as associate provost for Health Sciences, while continuing as editor of the *Journal of Gerontological Nursing*. In these positions her influence is vast. The *Journal of Gerontological Nursing* has reached new levels of professional respectability under her editorship.

Kitty quotes Pasteur and tells students, "Chance favors the prepared mind." We believe she has developed a prepared mind and will encounter numerous additional opportunities to enhance the care of the aged through her various activities. Her contributions have been instrumental in moving geropsychiatric nursing into the forefront and bringing it to the attention of nurses throughout the nation. Dr. Buckwalter remains on the cutting edge of geriatric science and practice issues.

VIRGINIA BURGGRAF

Dr. Virginia Burggraf is what I consider a "mover and a shaker." She likes to say she "thinks out of the box" and in the 15 years I have known her that has certainly proved to be true. She was an original member of the National Gerontological Nursing Association (NGNA) and has been instrumental in forging a memorandum of agreement between the NGNA and the Canadian Gerontological Association (CGNA). She has served on most of the NGNA committees at one time or another. She was also the long-term care representative for ANA staff for 10 years, focusing her attention on health promotion and lifelong personal development.

She is one of the most generous of geriatric nurses. She has been instrumental in establishing a Mary Opal Wolanin Scholarship fund at NGNA; made major financial contributions to AAN; and hosts an annual "mentoring luncheon" at the Gerontological Society of America annual convention. Her graduate students, funded by the John A. Hartford Foundation, lunch with gerontological nurse leaders and discuss their current research and projects. This expands their horizons so they can begin to see themselves as prospective leaders. See chapters 9 and 10 for additional discussions of Virginia's contributions.

Virginia is a Sigma Theta Tau Henderson Fellow and a fellow in the American Academy of nursing. She is on the editorial review boards of numerous journals, including *Geriatric Nursing,* and has over 60 publications and two textbooks, one of which received an *American Journal of Nursing* Book of the Year Award.

It is not surprising that Virginia is interested in caregivers and caregiving. A child of immigrant parents, she lived in a three-generation household in Brooklyn, New York, until she left for college. Living with grandparents instilled her love for older adults. "They never seemed to get older." Named for her French grandmere, Virginia speaks of her often as a prime mover and independent person.

Early on, her father planned for her to attend Cornell University, because the daughter of his boss went there and he was her dad's role model. After graduation from Cornell University New York Hospital School of Nursing, she married and had six children. In between working and raising children, she obtained a master's degree at Seton Hall University, South Orange, New Jersey, which had a U.S. Department of Health, Education and Welfare (DHEW) grant to train gerontological nurse practitioners. Virginia was one of the student recipients of this grant.

In 1979, she moved to Louisiana and served on the faculty at the Louisiana State University School of Nursing where she developed the gerontology curriculum and simultaneously held a clinical position at the Veterans Administration Medical Centers in New Orleans. Her husband, Tom, died at an early age. After his death she went on to doctoral education and her career took a different path. Her doctoral dissertation, earning a PhD from Louisiana State University, addressed *Caregiver Burden, Health, Depression and Social Support in Employed and Unemployed Caregivers of Older Adults.* Her dedication and commitment to caregivers is not surprising as she was caregiver to Tom before his death. Her four living children have produced seven children of their own. The family is close and Virginia thoroughly enjoys her grandchildren. At present her research continues to address caregiver health. She presently directs a caregiver support group for faculty and staff at Radford University, Virginia, with the assistance of her graduate students.

Virginia's philosophy of aging is the metaphor of a wagon wheel: It has traveled far with detours, bends, and dents along the way. It has become slower, a little rickety, but is still capable of reaching its destination. The older adult is similar, bearing the marks of a lifetime but still alive and useful, even though frail and impaired.

KATHLEEN FLETCHER

Dr. Kathleen Fletcher constantly broadens her horizons. "Kathleen Fletcher has been an exemplar clinician in providing services for frail and underserved older adults. As the director of Senior Services at the University of Virginia (UVA) Health Systems in Charlottesville, Fletcher has developed, implemented, and evaluated interdisciplinary geriatric services throughout a continuum of care" (Mezey, 2002, p. 164). She is particularly aware of the needs of rural communities.

Kathleen was the second oldest of 10 children of an economically, although definitely not psychologically, impoverished family. She always dreamed of being a nurse, although she did not believe it would be possible; but her determination and her mother's fortitude made her dream a reality. Allegheny General Hospital, in Pittsburgh, where she and her siblings had been born, responded to a compelling request from her mother and in 1968 Kathleen became the first nurse to be funded by the hospital auxiliary to attend Pennsylvania State University.

After graduation she worked as a staff nurse, head nurse, and supervisor at Temple Hospital in Philadelphia. Later, while working as the Public Health Nurse Coordinator at the Veterans Medical Center in Prescott, Arizona she discovered the challenge of working with elders and sought graduate education at University of Massachusetts, Lowell (UML), and became a geriatric nurse practitioner in 1982.

Her major contributions have been in creating innovative health care programs and disseminating knowledge to nurses and older consumers. Kathleen has developed and taught national programs in physical and symptom assessment, crises and emergencies, medication management, and laboratory values related to geriatric care. A video series on geriatric symptom assessment and management that she developed, marketed by Mosby, continues to be used in educational programs. A textbook she coedited, *Management Guidelines for Gerontological Nurse Practitioners*, is in its second edition and recently was translated and released in Italy. With a grant from the American Association of Colleges of Nursing (AACN) and the John A. Hartford Foundation, she and a UVA faculty member developed a post master's gerontological nurse practitioner program at UVA.

Her interest in rural elders and their families has led to her appointment to the Jefferson Area Board of Aging, becoming an active member as well as a speaker for the Alzheimer's Association in her rural county. She also writes a monthly column for her local newspaper that provides health advice for seniors and their caregivers. She currently serves on three governor's boards in Virginia: the Board of Nursing Home Administrators, Future of Nursing, and the Aging Action Agenda.

The range and impact of Fletcher's activities have been broad; if she sees a need she tries to do something about it. For example, she developed a four-bed respite unit at the VAMC Hospital in Wilkes Barre, Pennsylvania for caregivers needing a break from arduous care and was given a grant by the hospital auxiliary to provide geriatric educational resources for employees at UVA who were caregivers of aging family members.

Kathleen teaches at UVA in nursing classroom and clinical settings. The benefits to her students and the residents, in a high-rise housing facility, of providing health services for low-income elderly were considerable, but Kathleen was concerned about the lack of such services when students were not available during school breaks, summers, and holidays. She was instrumental in obtaining a $3.5 million grant to extend the health services in this setting and initiate similar services for elders in other low-income housing sites. She now has developed a cadre of more than 60 expert nurses with geriatric skill, knowledge, and ability to serve as geriatric resource nurses in settings ranging from the hospital emergency department to geropsychiatric and home care at UVA.

She is devoted to improving the care of elders as a clinician, educator, researcher, and administrator. Her active involvement in these aspects of gerontology on a state, national, and international level was recognized and in 2001 she was awarded the Nancy Vance Award by the Commonwealth of Virginia for her selfless devotion and exceptional service to older adults. In 1996 she was given the Outstanding Employee Contribution Award at the University of Virginia and in 1997 was named Outstanding Nurse by the Beta Kappa chapter of Sigma Theta Tau. In 2002 she was elected a Fellow of the American Academy of Nursing (FAAN).

MARQUIS (MARK) FOREMAN

Dr. Mark Foreman is best known for his research in delirium. He has consistently pursued this interest and produced an algorithm that established his status as the leader of investigation into this common and distressing condition, which is so prevalent among the aged, particularly when hospitalized.

Mark had two important experiences that directed his interest toward care of the aged, particularly those who became confused as a result of morbid conditions, environmental factors, and mental frailty. When Mark completed high school and was still uncertain what direction to pursue, he took a position as a psychiatric aide in a state-run psychiatric institution. He was assigned the night shift on a unit to provide custodial care for 70 older men. He and the three other staff on the unit had a wide range of responsibilities, including managing incontinence, wound and skin care, behavioral disorders, and cleaning the unit and the equipment. Medications and restraints were used when necessary but little was done for the patients' mental health or psychosocial needs. This experience was pivotal in his decision to become a nurse and in his appreciation of the needs and challenges in caring for the old. He worked on this unit for 2½ years before entering nurses training at St. Vincent Hospital School of Nursing.

The second important experience occurred after he became a registered nurse. For the first 4 years of his nursing career he worked in high tech units: the emergency department, intensive care, trauma, and vascular intensive care. The majority of the patients were elderly and he felt unprepared to take care of them. He found that strategies that worked with younger adults failed with them, and many more of the older patients became acutely confused or delirious. He decided to go to graduate school and specialize in the care of older people. In 1980, he was one of 10 students who were in the first class of the MSN program in the School of Nursing at the Medical College of Ohio in Toledo. As a class assignment he attempted to synthesize the literature on how to prevent or treat confusion. One of his teachers shared his paper with Mary Opal Wolanin who encouraged him to publish it. It became his first publication, titled, *Acute Confusional States in the Elderly: An Algorithm* (Foreman, 1984). His study of acute confusion continued through his doctoral studies at the University of Illinois Chicago (UIC) College of Nursing, where, in 1987, he earned a PhD in Nursing Science. He joined the faculty there in 1989 after completing a 2-year postdoctoral fellowship. He continues to study the delirium of hospitalized older people. Additional discussion of his research can be found in chapter 8.

SUSAN CROCKER HOUDE

Dr. Susan Houde, a protege of May Futrell, is a tenured, associate professor of nursing at the University of Massachusetts, Lowell, where she serves as director of the master's program in nursing. She has made significant contributions to research and the gerontological nurse practitioner program at the university. Her involvement in a nursing home demonstration evaluating the effective use of nurse practitioner-physician teams served as a model that influenced development of beneficial legislation about the role of nurse practitioners in nursing homes. While a Gerontological Research Scholar at the Hartford Institute of Geriatric Nursing at New York University, she explored research ideas related to self-care of family caregivers of functionally impaired older adults in the home. She is also a co-investigator in a research study related to the prevention of age-related macular degeneration in the older adult. The study explores the effect of egg consumption on blood levels of lutein, zeaxanthin, and cholesterol levels. She has published articles related to the nurse's role in the prevention and treatment of age-related vision loss in the older adult (Houde, 2001; Houde & Huff, 2003). She also has studied gender differences in family caregiving (Houde, 2000), and physical activity and the older adult (Houde & Melillo, 2000). She and Dr. Karen Devereaux Melillo have co-edited a text titled *Geropsychiatric and Mental Health Nursing* (Melillo & Houde, 2005).

Dr. Houde earned a PhD from Brandeis University in social policy and aging. Her dissertation focused on predictors of the use of formal services in the home by family caregiver/care recipient dyads (Houde, 1998). Her master's degree is from the University of Massachusetts, Lowell in gerontological nursing.

She is an active member of the National Organization of Nurse Practitioner Faculties (NONPF), where she has served on the Educational Standards Committee and the Educational Resources Committee. As a member, she worked on a team that developed a preceptor manual for nurse practitioner faculty (McAllister, DiMarco, Houde, & Miller, 2000). Dr. Houde is a public policy editor of the *Journal of Gerontological Nursing* and a reviewer for several other nursing journals. She has published and presented widely on topics related to the care of older adults.

Recently she was appointed associate director of the Division of Aging, Center for Health and Disease Research at UML. She also is in a private practice, providing primary care to older adults. We expect that her continued devotion to gerontological nursing research and education will have a positive effect on the future of gerontological nursing practice.

ANN SCHMIDT LUGGEN

Dr. Ann Luggen is a leader and an organizational person. Wherever she is involved she takes on the tasks of the group, brings in others to participate, and establishes herself as a major contributor. Coming from a close family of five sisters, one might partially account for this by her family background. Her interest in gerontology began with intimate connections to great-grandparents, grand aunts and uncles, and grandparents. In addition, her own mother provided a model of aging well and coping with Parkinson's disease before her death.

Ann Schmidt Luggen is a tenured professor of nursing at Northern Kentucky University and is certified through the American Nurses Association as a Clinical Specialist in Gerontological Nursing (APRN, BC). She has been the NGNA's section editor of *Geriatric Nursing* and the editor of *New Horizons,* the NGNA newsletter, and also has served as president of NGNA. Throughout her affiliation with NGNA she was a driving force in the growth of the organization. Ann's visible as well as supportive activities helped move the organization forward and strengthened it as she immersed herself in its goals and directions. Presently Ann is a section editor of the NCGNP portion of *Geriatric Nursing.* Ann unstintingly gives of herself and is committed to professionalism, insisting on excellence.

Ann's professional activities include numerous papers, presentations, research projects, and two edited core curriculum volumes for gerontological nurses and advanced practice nurses (Luggen, 1996; Luggen, Travis, & Meiner, 1998). These texts provide information for nurses and advanced practice nurses seeking to be certified as gerontological specialists on general and advanced levels. They are also excellent resources with extensive information for faculty involved in curricular development. She coauthored a third major textbook, *Handbook for Care of the Older Adult With Cancer* (Luggen & Meiner, 2000). Ann is immersed in gerontological professional organizations in Ohio and Kentucky.

Ann's research interest in cancer and the elderly began some years ago when caring for a patient with myelocytic anemia and continues to be an important concern of hers. Of course, this led back to her interest in pain management. Other research interests have included loneliness, cultural diversity, and staff development.

Ann says, "I believe the future of gerontological nursing is tied to the development of professional organizations. Gerontological nurses are going to become more and more important as a larger portion of the population becomes elderly. The gerontological nurse needs to become increasingly professional, needs to take a strong leadership role in the care of older adults. We need to strengthen the professional gerontological nursing role in long-term care" (Luggen in Ebersole, 1999a, p. 217).

DIANE FEENEY MAHONEY

Dr. Diane Feeney Mahoney was prepared as a gerontological nurse practitioner in 1980 at UML in the program established by May Futrell (see chapter 3). Soon after graduating, she established a nurse managed health center in the Riverside Towers elderly housing complex. From that base, through innovative health programs and community screenings, she was able to reach out to medically underserved adults, in churches, clubs, and even in a laundromat, to cross over racial and ethnic divides then present in the community. In 1988 she received the Syntax Nurse Practitioner Award for her work with elders in the community. Futrell recruited Dr. Mahoney back to UML to develop the role of the community nurse practitioner in the curriculum and to involve GNP students in outreach home visits and assessments.

Diane's dissertation research investigating prescribing practices of GNPs and physicians showed that NPs were often more judicious than physicians in prescribing appropriately for older persons. Publications from this work were used across the country in support of changing state policies that barred nonphysician prescribing. Mahoney received the Gerontology Society of America (GSA) Social Policy and Practice Award for the best research paper and the VA Health Services Award for her dissertation research. She has been honored with numerous awards since that time.

Dr. Mahoney is recognized nationally and internationally as a pioneer in the emerging field of gerotechnology and computational sensor home monitoring, and is the Director of Gerotechnology and Enhanced Family Caregiving at the Hebrew Rehabilitation Center for the Aged in Boston. Her numerous research publications are found in nursing, gerontology, and technology journals. She presently chairs the GSA Nursing Special Interest Group (Mahoney, 2003) (Fig. 4.1).

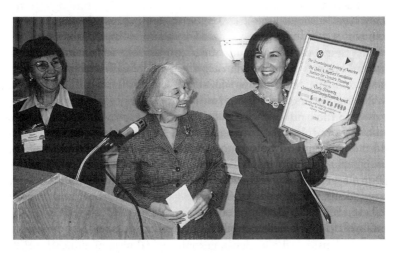

FIGURE 4.1 Diane Mahoney and Mathy Mezey giving Cornelia Beck the Doris Schwartz Gerontological Nursing Research Award.

MARIANNE LAPORTE MATZO

Dr. Marianne Matzo is most notable for her interest in and contributions to end of life (EOL) care. She is the first nurse to be funded individually by the Soros Foundation Project on Death in America Faculty Scholars Program, and one of the first nurses to direct research about the individual's experience of dying. She is devoted to developing pedagogical methods that can be used to teach care of the dying patient to all nursing students.

When Marianne was in high school she joined the "Legion of Mary," a Catholic service group in Michigan. Her assignment was to make a weekly visit to an older adult in her parish. The woman had no indoor plumbing, was nearly blind, and had numerous physical challenges, but never complained. Marianne listened to her talk about growing up in Maine and about her family, and she grew very fond of her. She realized that her presence with this older lady made a difference in both their lives.

Later, while attending Worcester State College School of Nursing, she was especially attracted to caring for difficult older patients. Vito became a favorite, even though he threw his dentures at her when they first met. Her successes with these patients challenged her to become a gerontological nurse practitioner (UML) and ultimately to obtain a PhD in gerontology at the University of Massachusetts, Boston. Her 1996 dissertation topic was "Registered Nurse's Attitudes Toward and Practices of Assisted Suicide and Patient Requested Euthanasia." She found that nurses were seldom asked how they felt about these issues and generally their attitudes were influenced by religious beliefs. The findings from her dissertation led her to the desire to educate nurses about the care of the dying person.

The first 9 years of her nursing career were spent working in mental health and later in geropsychiatric nursing. In 1987 she was hired at Saint Anselm College (New Hampshire) to direct a federal grant from the Division of Nursing, U.S. Health and Human Services, to integrate gerontology into their nursing curriculum and help faculty and students learn about older adults. During this experience she learned that students needed actual clinical experience in working with the older adult in order to spark the necessary empathy and interest to provide excellent gerontological care. She developed curricula, lecture materials, and clinical experiences that have been disseminated nationally. She also developed innovative models to deliver EOL nursing care and empower nurses to change this care in acute care settings. Largely because of her work, Saint Anselm is considered a leader in gerontological nursing education.

In her professional development she especially appreciated the mentorship of Dr. Lillian Goodman at the start of her nursing career, Dr. Terry

Fulmer in gerontological nursing, and Dr. Betty Ferrell in EOL care. She says, "They are such outstanding nurses and mentors!" (Matzo, 2004). She believes that without the support of these mentors she never would have felt empowered to do the work she has done.

Throughout her career Dr. Matzo has taken an innovative approach to patient care, an interdisciplinary focus, and creative curriculum development. She has coedited two textbooks about palliative care nursing. Both were awarded an American Journal of Nursing Book of the Year award (Matzo & Sherman, 2001, 2004). Recently, Dr. Matzo has been named to occupy the Frances E. and A. Earl Ziegler Endowed Chair in Palliative Care Nursing, College of Nursing at the University of Oklahoma, Oklahoma City. This is the first endowed chair in palliative care nursing to be funded in the United States.

Marianne writes, "I have always believed that our work in gerontological nursing should focus on productive and healthy aging and hated when gerontological content was grouped with death and dying. That said, older adults live so long with nondramatic, terminal illnesses the care of which is primarily palliative. My current mission is to facilitate nurse's knowledge not only in the provision of excellent gerontological nursing care, but also in excellent gerontologic palliative care" (Matzo, 2004).

GRAHAM McDOUGALL

Dr. Graham McDougall, Jr. is most notable for his research into cognition and particularly for developing strategies to enhance memory, reflecting both his interests in research and practice. He created a new paradigm, the Cognitive Behavioral Model of Everyday Memory (CBMEM) in which self-efficacy theory is applied to the cognitive difficulties experienced by older adults (see chapter 8).

Graham says, "Having three sets of grandparents while growing up in New Orleans created an age-friendly environment for me. I spent lots of time with the grandparents and thought it was only natural to surround myself with older adults. They were an integral component in all family decisions" (McDougall in Ebersole, 2000, p. 261).

While attending Louisiana State University Health Sciences School of Nursing his studies led him to pursue advanced practice specialization in geriatric psychiatric nursing. After graduate school he organized and chaired a committee of the Louisiana Mental Health Association, emphasizing mental health concerns of older adults and provided leadership for a newly formed committee on Mental Health Issues of the Elderly for the New Orleans Health Department. An outcome of this community organization was the development in 1983 of a new in-home mental health treatment service provided by advanced practice nurses and reimbursable under Medicare; a new model at that time, although quite common now.

His nursing experience includes geropsychiatric care in the home; clinical nurse specialist/education coordinator; private practice as a psychotherapist; and nursing supervisor. His faculty appointments from 1985 until 1991 were as a research/teaching assistant at the University of Texas, Austin. In 1991 Graham joined the faculty of Frances Payne Bolton School of Nursing, Case Western Reserve University, Cleveland, and remained there through 1998 until moving to his present position as a tenured professor in the School of Nursing at the University of Texas, Austin.

Because only 7% of registered nurses in the United States are male, Graham's activities are particularly visible and have enhanced his leadership opportunities.

Graham has achieved various honors and awards. Especially significant are his selection as a Fellow of the American Academy of Nursing (2001) and the Springer Publishing Award for Applied Gerontological Nursing Research in 1999 (Fig. 4.2).

His numerous professional activities include research and leadership activities with NGNA; membership on the advisory group for the Robert Wood Johnson Teaching Nursing Home Project; and positions on the review boards of several journals. Graham is an active and valued member of the advisory board of *Geriatric Nursing,* contributing research briefs, manuscripts, reviews, and suggestions of individuals who have developed manuscripts suitable for publication. We have been fortunate to have his diligent and consistent involvement in the professional development of the journal.

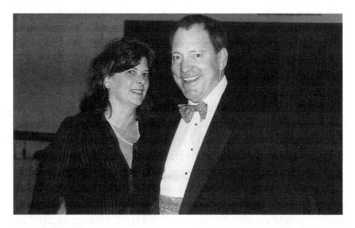

FIGURE 4.2   Kathleen (Kitty) Buckwalter with Graham McDougall when he was inducted into the American Academy of Nursing.

KAREN DEVEREAUX MELILLO

Dr. Karen Devereaux Melillo is a much-esteemed protege of May Futrell, achieving her GNP education at UML, and subsequently accepting a faculty position there. She earned her PhD from Brandeis University's Florence Heller School for the Advanced Study of Social Welfare in 1990.

In 2001 she was selected as a Fellow in the American Academy of Nurse Practitioners, received the Distinguished Alumni Award from Massachusetts Bay Community College, and was the Francis Cabot Lowell Outstanding Alumni Award recipient for the College of Health Professionals at UML.

Dr. Melillo is actively involved in research investigating the use of nurse practitioners in institutional long-term care, for which she received the Long Term Care Research Award from the American College of Health Care Administrators.

Karen has more than 50 peer-reviewed publications in nursing journals and is coeditor with Dr. Susan Houde of the text, *Geropsychiatric and Mental Health Nursing* (Melillo & Houde, 2005). She is active in a number of professional organizations and serves on the board of several. She has researched physical fitness and exercise activities of older adults; nurse practitioner counseling interventions in primary care to increase physical activity and exercise among Latino elders; as well as the use of a wandering technology device for older adults with Alzheimer's disease (Houde & Melillo, 2000; Melillo & Futrell, 1998; Melillo et al., 2001). She is a coinvestigator of a 5-year, $3.5M National Institutes of Health, National Institute for Occupational Safey and Health (NIOSH) funded study of *Health Disparities Among Health Care Workers,* in which she leads the Long-Term Case Study Team involving two partnering nursing home facilities.

May Futrell's 27-year relationship with Karen has grown from that of mentor/mentee to one of collaborative contribution. Both have grown in this relationship; the essence of good mentoring.

ROBIN REMSBURG

Robin writes, "confessions from an old young geriatric nurse" (Remsburg, 2005). Her geriatric nursing career began during her doctoral studies at the University of Maryland when she took part in a research study at Bayview Medical Center's General Clinical Research Center (GCRC). Before that she had been a clinical maternal/child nurse and educator. Her doctoral studies were geared in that direction until working with two outstanding physicians, Rick Bennett, a young man in a geriatric fellowship program engaged in studying pressure sores, and William B. Greenough III, working on a rehydration project. These physicians were concerned with the whole patient, not just their particular research. Robin's input was welcomed and valued. She developed insight into the major issues facing adults in nursing homes and found the joy of working with elders.

Opportunities opened up for her at Johns Hopkins Bayview Medical Center and the Johns Hopkins Geriatrics Center. Her skill as a recruiter of older research participants was recognized as well as her research design expertise. Her research mentors included those physicians previously mentioned; Jonelle Wright, in the Division of Geriatric Medicine and Gerontology; and Karen Armacost, expert in nursing home care, with whom she conducted studies of staffing problems in nursing homes. Together they studied restorative care also.

In 2002, Robin joined the National Center for Health Statistics as the long-term care statistics branch manager. Recently they have planned and conducted the first-ever National Survey of Nursing Assistants. Robin has published more than 30 articles, contributed chapters to several books, garnered many research grants, achieved various honors, and mentored other nurses entering the research arena and doctoral studies. As a latecomer to geriatric nursing, Robin has developed an outstanding geriatric nursing career. Her clear ideas of how to recruit nurses into geriatric nursing are discussed in chapter 9 (Remsburg, 2005).

BARBARA RESNICK

"My interest in becoming a nurse started when I was in middle school, despite encouragement from my father to go to medical school. At this time I volunteered as both a candy striper and research assistant, learning more about the role and assuring my father that nurses take care of people and physicians take care of diseases. A nurse is what I wanted to be! I really started my career in nursing as a nurse's aide in a nursing home while in high school. I had the opportunity to provide hands-on care to older adults and knew that I had found my place in the profession. I was quite comfortable in the nursing home environment as I had spent a good deal of my time while growing up visiting grandparents in a nursing facility. I fondly remembered going for rides in wheelchairs while sitting on their laps and visiting other residents" (Resnick in Ebersole, 2002a, p. 101).

"The focus of my undergraduate work was the care of the older adult, and I graduated with distinction for doing a special project entitled, *The Effect of Touch on Disoriented Elderly.* Knowing that I wanted to pursue my career in geriatrics, I explored a master's degree in geriatric nursing. The University of Pennsylvania provided what I wanted and I graduated from their Gerontological Nurse Clinician/Nurse Practitioner program in 1982. I successfully passed the American Nurses Association certification examination to practice as a GNP, and worked with older adults in a variety of settings, including a continuing care retirement community, long term care, outpatient care, and acute inpatient rehabilitation" (Resnick in Ebersole, 2002a). In 1996 Barbara completed doctoral studies at the University of Maryland School of Nursing.

Dr. Resnick was involved in the development of the geriatric nurse practitioner program at the University of Maryland, and has continued to teach in the program since its inception more than 10 years ago. She has consulted with numerous other universities on their geriatric nursing programs and helped to establish a master's program with a geriatric track at Hebrew University Hadassah Hospital School of Nursing.

Dr. Resnick has received numbers of honors, including commendations for contributions to nursing practice and Nurse of the Year Award (1980) from the National Institutes of Health, and the 2004 Springer Geriatric Research Award. Dr. Resnick is a Fellow in the Fellowship of the American Academy of Nurse Practitioners, and a Fellow of the American Academy of Nursing (Resnick, 2005) (Fig. 4.3).

Dr. Resnick is presently the principal investigator on a grant funded by the National Institute of Aging to test the effectiveness of the Exercise

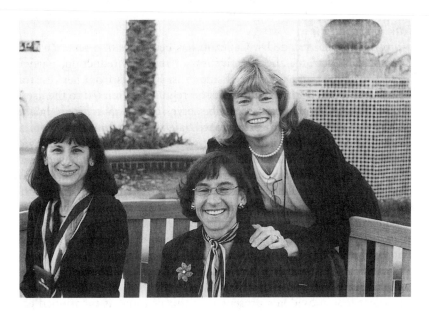

FIGURE 4.3 Elizabeth Capezuti, Barbara Resnick, and Terry Fulmer.

Plus program on older women post-hip fracture. She has also been awarded a grant by AHRQ to test the effectiveness of a restorative care program. Her research studies continue to focus on motivating older adults toward health promoting behaviors (see chapter 8). Currently, Dr. Resnick has over 150 articles published in nursing or medical journals, and numerous chapters in medical and nursing textbooks related to care of the older adult, and has authored a recent book on restorative care nursing (Resnick, 2005). She also has presented on these topics nationally and internationally.

"My ultimate goal is to change the paradigm of care of older adults so that we are no longer simply providing care but are focused on motivating older adults to engage in health behaviors and perform functional activities so that they maintain function and independence for as long as possible. In so doing, I believe that older adults' quality of life will be optimal and there will be a marked decrease in the many age associated problems we presently confront in all health care settings" (Resnick in Ebersole, 2002a, p. 101).

ELIZABETH CAPEZUTI

Elizabeth Capezuti is an associate professor in the Division of Nursing (now the College of Nursing), and also serves as co-director for the John A. Hartford Foundation Institute for Geriatric Nursing at New York University.

Over the last decade Dr. Capezuti has been part of a research team that has demonstrated the effectiveness of restraint reduction, particularly in relation to the use of bed side rails. Findings from her research have been used to draft state and federal regulations related to the use of restraints and nursing home care. She serves on several national boards and is a consultant to the Hospital Bed Safety Workgroup of the United States Food and Drug Administration (FDA) and the Centers for Medicare and Medicaid Services (CMS). Dr. Capezuti has published articles relating to fall prevention, restraint and side rail elimination, elder mistreatment, and legal liability. She is a Fellow of the AAN and GSA, and is one of the energetic young nurses who will impact the future of geriatric nursing care.

CONCLUSION

The select few individuals presented in this chapter, as mentioned earlier, are representative of the numerous geriatric nurses now making outstanding contributions to the care of elders and geriatric nursing education. They and their proteges will carry the momentum forward toward a better climate for aging individuals, and in the process will touch many lives. It follows that these nurses will reap the benefits of their work in their own aging process.

CHAPTER FIVE

Recognition of Geriatric Care as a Specialty Practice

COMPONENTS OF THE GERIATRIC NURSING SPECIALTY

Early in the development of geriatric nursing practice Doreen Norton, of Sussex, England, United Kingdom, provided a model that excited interested nurses in the United States. Her thoughts about geriatric nursing were summarized in a speech given at the Annual Conference of the Student Nurses Association in London, 1956, published by the Student Nurses Association in 1957 and again in *Gerontological Clinics* (1965). It is difficult to extract from her article as everything she said is important. She spoke of nurses, usually focused on "deeds" and the necessity of finding their voice and the importance of her earliest student experiences on a geriatric ward that then became the prime interest of her life.

A half-century ago, she described most nurses as involved in highly technical treatments and saw this as a danger to "unstinted nursing skill." She describes the situation of the aged, who were often cast aside as having "chronic" problems not amenable to treatment. She says, "Man, by his own endeavors, is responsible for the longer life span; he must, therefore, recognize his responsibility towards those he has endowed with it" (Norton, 1956, p. 622).

Doreen has identified the advantages of learning geriatric care in basic nursing education as: (a) learning patience, tolerance, and understanding; (b) learning basic nursing skills; (c) witnessing the terminal stages of disease and the importance of skilled nursing care at that time; (d) preparing for the future, as no matter where one works in nursing the aged will be a great part of the care; (e) recognizing the importance of appropriate rehabilitation, which calls upon all the skill that nurses possess; and (f) being aware of the need to undertake research in geriatric nursing. According to Doreen, the work is hard and exacting but rewarding, as one is able to get to know the person in a way seldom possible when caring for the young. "In conclusion, I can only say that if you elect to nurse old people, and can nurse them successfully, you will be able to nurse anybody, with any condition, anywhere, because, quite simply, you will have learnt how to nurse" (Norton, 1956, p. 624).

In a later publication (1965) Doreen said, of the "two bees in her bonnet" when speaking to students: "One was the firm conviction that no nurse should be launched upon the world as 'qualified' without having had geriatric nursing experience welded into the structure of his or her training." and "The other was the equally firm conviction that the time had come for nurses to acquire the will and skill to critically examine nursing practice—and that the focus for scrutiny must be Geriatric Care—since this is nursing, undiluted and unadorned, and therefore *the sensitive index by which to measure our standards of nursing care.*" She confessed that her appeal to students had been emotional but successful, judging by the responses of the young nurses, "With one accord they expressed an eagerness to share in this work and demanded to know why they were being denied this unique opportunity to learn the nursing art" (Norton, 1965, p. 51).

Doreen has formulated a concept of geriatric nursing in which she diagrams two distinct categories of sick elders: those who have the potential to regain the ability of basic self-care—these are in the rehabilitative category—and those who are beyond "medical reclaim" but will need nursing care for the remainder of their lives. These might be termed irremediable (Fig. 5.1).

Fundamental to this is comprehensive assessment of the individual, including social history as well as social future. The nurse must learn new criteria in the presentation of illness that can be so different in late life. Often the patient lacks energy and initiative toward self-care and the burden falls on the nurse. This requires the highest skill and awareness of just how much care retains the maximum amount of patient independence and affords the greatest opportunity for return to the community. In the "irremediable" category nursing is really all that is available to the patient and involves strengthening whatever remains and maintaining the patient at optimum levels of function for as long as possible. "Patients with a potential to regain independence require *gradual withdrawal of nursing care* and to be surrounded by furniture/equipment which aids independence. Patients beyond medical reclaim need maintenance of their optimum, balanced by *increasing true nursing care* as remaining capabilities decline" (Norton, 1965, p. 59).

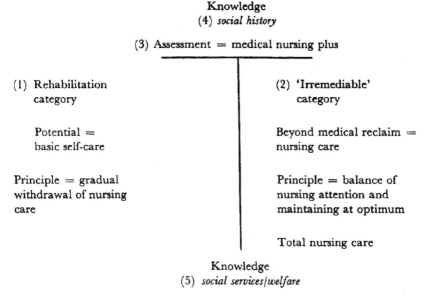

FIGURE 5.1 Norton's concept of geriatric nursing.

In a much later publication Doreen writes of *The Age of Old Age* (1990) and contends that the "ageing population itself will change the climate of the times" (p. 37) and that "this is an era marked by universal public awareness of elderly citizens in its midst." She enumerates the situations that have made this so: the birth of new industries geared to the old; housing and architecture adapted to their needs; promotion of travel and tourism for the aged; and, the elderly have "oiled the wheels of social service" (Norton, 1990, p. 37). Doreen is highly respected worldwide for her cogent and insightful thoughts.

ENDOWED CHAIRS: THE FLORENCE CELLAR GERONTOLOGICAL NURSING CHAIR

Doreen Norton occupied the first endowed chair in gerontological nursing, the Florence Cellar Gerontological Chair at Case Western Reserve University in Cleveland. Doreen writes, "I shall always be indebted to dear Florence and ever conscious of the great honour of having been the first to occupy this first chair in the specialty" (Norton, 1991).

The chair was established May 14, 1982, and has been occupied by Doreen Norton, Beverly Baldwin, Virginia Stone, Joyce Fitzpatrick, Terry

Fulmer, the author, and presently is a permanent chair occupied by May Wykle.

There are presently several gerontologic nursing chairs in the United States; these must be considered significant in elevating the specialty to national recognition. An endowed chair gives distinction to a university and the occupant. Most provide income in perpetuity for a faculty position in a designated area of study, research, and leadership. At Case Western Reserve University one million dollars is required to endow a chair. The earnings from the endowment support a faculty position.

A background in "chairs" is interesting and probably poorly understood in our present era. In the 16th century, a chair with arms, legs, and a back was a rare item of furniture and highly prized. Commoners sat on three-legged stools, gentry used cushions. Only monarchs and high church officials had chairs. When a worthy teacher became a professor and was recognized as outstanding by a king or bishop, a lifetime income was provided and he was given a chair as a symbol of high status in education. Today, an endowed "chair" honors both the donor and the professor (Kohuth, 1983).

Florence Cellar was an obstetrical nurse and administrator at University Hospital, Cleveland, for much of her nursing career. Her decision to endow the chair was based on the excellent nursing care given her parents in their declining years, which clearly shows that nurses never know when their actions will have significant repercussions. Her father was a very successful lumberman and his business thrived. When he was unable to carry on, Florence became president of the company but didn't realize until his death how wealthy he had become. She and her sister, Helen, agreed that they owed a debt to nursing. Later, Florence said, "After all, I'm not getting any younger and when I decide to move into a retirement home, I want to be sure that the best educated and best prepared nurses give me and others of my generation the kind of care we want and should have" (Kohuth, 1983, pp. 241–255).

When I occupied the chair in 1988, I was surprised to be told that Florence wanted to meet me. I had assumed that the donor was long gone. Florence was not only generous of her assets but of herself. She became a treasured friend and shared with me an extensive history of her life. We carried on voluminous correspondence until her death on June 1, 1997.

LICENSURE

Registered nurse (RN) preparation for licensure can be achieved by graduation from 2-year, 4-year, accelerated, alternative (to meet the schedules of working persons), online, or from one of the few remaining diploma programs. The various educational routes toward achieving licensure always have produced contention within nursing and the determination by the American Nurses Association (ANA) to define the truly professional nurse by the type of program from which one graduated. In reality, the quality of programs varies enormously and professional behavior can only be judged by the graduate's actions and level of influence in the profession.

There is one consistent factor in achieving a license to become an RN in every state and from every program. One must pass the NCLEX® examination. The test is developed and controlled by the National Council of State Boards of Nursing. Each nursing program measures some of its success by the percentage of graduates who pass the examination, although most deans and directors disavow that. Various study packages, seminars, and pretests are available for the student after her or his course of study that may enhance one's ability to pass the test. Some are provided by the program from which the person graduated, but most are not and tend to be expensive. An NCLEX examination study package developed in consultation with the National League of Nursing (NLN) is now being marketed. A recent press release from The College Network advertises "Prescription (RX) for NCLEX Success." This package includes a "Diagnostic Readiness Test" and is available for $415, but the advertisement gives no information about content areas covered (April 1, 2005).

What does this have to do with the geriatric nursing specialty? Until very recently there were no test questions specifically focused on caring for the aged. Now, geriatric nurses are encouraged to submit test questions to the national board. It remains to be seen how much actual content will apply to care of older persons.

STANDARDS OF PRACTICE
IN GERIATRIC NURSING

Standards of practice in the various specialties guide nurses in appropriate considerations and are meant to inform nursing programs of goals and directions that should be considered in curriculum development. Nursing was the first of the professions to establish standards of geriatric care. In 1973 ANA defined standards of practice in geriatric care and was the first of the five ANA specialties to do so. Several of the pioneer geriatric nurses were involved in this effort (see chapter 2). In 1976 and 1987 these were updated and revised as the standards of practice of gerontological nursing. In 1995 and in 2001 these were revised again, reflecting the great changes in the knowledge base and growth of the specialty. The 2001 edition was published jointly with the National Gerontological Nursing Association (NGNA) and the National Conference of Gerontological Nurse Practitioners (NCGNP) (Ebersole, Hess, Touhy, & Jett, 2005). The knowledge and skills necessary for the practice of basic gerontological nursing care are listed in Table 5.1.

CERTIFICATION

Certification in a specialty assures the public that an individual has some specialized knowledge in a particular area of practice. Certification informs the public of competency in a given area; increases professional recognition, individually and collectively; and sometimes serves as criteria for an enlarged role in employment and financial reimbursement. It signifies attainment of specific knowledge, skills, and abilities in a specialty field (www.ana.org/ancc, April 14, 2005). Certification programs vary in length, quality, and reliability.

Mezey notes several reasons why one should become certified in gerontological nursing. Geriatric patients are not a subgroup of patients, but the main core of health systems, comprising more than 50% of patients in hospitals. Nevertheless, less than 1% of the RNs are certified in gerontology (www.geronurseonline.org/index.cfm?section_id=8, April 15, 2005).

Gerontological certification can:

- Promote on-the-job success
- Provide high quality care to older adults
- Promote leadership success
- Provide potential increases in pay

The American Nurses Credentialing Center currently offers certification in several specialty areas that strengthen geriatric nursing practice. There is a baccalaureate level examination, the Gerontological Nurse, Registered Nurse, Board Certified (RN, BC, examination #40); and the associate degree/diploma level examination, Gerontological Nurse, Registered Nurse, Certified (RN, C, examination #09). The advanced practice examinations include the Gerontological Nurse Practitioner (Advanced Practice Registered Nurse, Board Certified (APRN, BC, examination #23) and the Clinical Specialist in Gerontological Nursing, Advanced Practice Registered Nurse, Board Certified (APRN, BC, examination #18).

TABLE 5.1 Knowledge and Skills for Basic Gerontological Nursing

- Recognize the right of competent older adults to make their own care decisions and assist them in making informed choices.

- Establish a therapeutic relationship with the older adult to facilitate development of the plan of care, which may include family participation as needed.

- Use current gerontological standards to initiate, develop, and adapt the older adult's plan of care while involving the patient, family, and other providers as needed.

- Recognize age-related changes based on an understanding of physiological, emotional, cultural, social, psychological, economic, and spiritual functioning.

- Collect data to determine health status and functional abilities to plan, implement, and evaluate care.

- Participate and collaborate with members of the interdisciplinary team.

- Participate with older adults, their families if needed, and other health professionals in ethical decision making that is centered on the older adult, empathetic, and humane.

- Serve as an advocate for older adults and their families.

- Teach older adults and families about measures that promote, maintain, and restore health and functional performance; promote comfort; foster independence; and preserve dignity.

- Refer older adults to other professionals or community resources for assistance as necessary.

- Identify common chronic/acute physical and mental health processes and problems that affect older adults.

- Apply the existing body of knowledge in gerontology to nursing practice and intervention.

- Exercise accountability to older adults by protecting their rights and autonomy, recognizing and respecting their decision about advance directives.

- Facilitate palliative care and comfort during the dying process to preserve dignity.

- Support the surviving spouse and family members, providing strength, comfort, and hope.

- Use the standards of gerontological nursing practice and collaborate with other health care professionals to improve the quality of care and quality of life of older adults.

- Engage in professional development through participation in continuing education, involvement in state and national professional organizations, and certification.

From American Nurses Association: *Scope and standards of gerontological nursing practice,* Washington, DC, 2001, ANA, pp. 8–9.

CREDENTIALS

Several specialty credentials are relevant to geriatric nursing and may add to one's professional stature, such as home health nursing and diabetes management, which are offered on the baccalaureate and advanced practice level. Pain management and palliative care are advanced practice certifications. The ANA encourages specialty nurses to obtain dual certification to validate their geriatric competence along with their specialty expertise. This is particularly relevant to those specializing in psychiatric and mental health nursing, family nurse practitioners, wound and ostomy specialists, cardiovascular nurses, and nursing home administrators.

A recent development is a grant encouraging an alliance between specialty nursing associations and the ANA, dubbed the American Nurses Association-Specialty Nursing Association Partners in Geriatrics (ANA-SNAPGs). This project is designed to create a permanent geriatric structure within the primary organization. Some of the expectations of the specialties that become involved include: incorporation of geriatrics into the association scope and standards of practice; incorporating care of older adults in the association mission and strategic plans; developing geriatric competencies, publishing geriatric content in the association journal, newsletters, and e-newsletters; offering geriatric-related preconferences and workshops at annual meetings; and offering a Nurse Competency in Aging Award to members of the association. Eligible applicants receive funds to begin the process. This Nurse Competency in Aging (NCA) project is meant to heighten awareness among specialty nurses of the unique needs of older adults. Information about these grants can be obtained from Karen Horsley, NCA Project Manager.

Many nurses wonder how to display the credentials they have earned. Mary Smolensky posted a discussion in Nursing Spectrum online (http://community.nursingspectrum.com/MagazineArticles/article.cfm? AID=7126, April 15, 2005). Some professionals and consumers find this "alphabet soup" or "Campbell's approach" confusing. To add to the confusion, various states require different designations for advanced practice nurses. Mary insists they must be displayed with pride and that the public has a right to know the nurse has earned distinction in addition to her or his basic RN preparation. However, it is an individual choice. It is the responsibility of the individual to explain the meaning of the credentials in situations where it may be important for professional recognition or advancement. The only credentials that must be used are those required by the state. She reminds us that recently some hospitals did not indicate licensure or credentials on name tags; therefore, patients had no idea of the qualifications of the person attending them. Fortunately, this deceit has almost disappeared.

There are other credentials and certifications available, not specific to nursing but nonetheless providing an additional element of credibility and qualification. These may have no assigned acronyms to follow one's name and generally are only mentioned on vitae or when necessary to establish a level of expertise. Many of the early geriatric nurses completed the gerontological certificate program at Ethel Percy Andrus Gerontology Center at the University of Southern California, Los Angeles, before such certification was available through ANA.

FELLOWSHIPS

Fellow status can be achieved within organizations, usually by application, documentation of outstanding contributions to the organization and profession, sponsorship, and approval of other fellows in the organization. Some that are particularly valued by geriatric/gerontological nurses include Fellow of the American Academy of Nursing (FAAN), Fellow of the National Gerontological Nursing Association (FNGNA), and Fellow of the Gerontological Society of America (FGSA). Many of the nurses cited in this text have multiple fellowships attesting to their contributions to several groups. These have not been noted following their names as sufficient attention has been given to their accomplishments.

Certifications, fellowships, appointments to occupy a dedicated chair, and any special recognition is worthy of notice. These are seldom acquired easily and give evidence of an individual who has gone the extra mile beyond requirements for practice and is expected to continue to achieve. Many of the geriatric nurses featured in this text have attained many credentials that give evidence of their dedication to excellence.

CHAPTER SIX

Geriatric Nursing Organizations and Affiliates

The necessity to organize groups specific to the practice interest in geriatric nursing was recognized near the beginning. Because there are significant differences in education, practice sites, and credentials under the general rubric of geriatric nursing, the geriatric specialty organizations began to form in a response to development of interest in geriatric nursing and the desire for like-minded nurses to gather, form goals, and define their objectives.

Although not a geriatric specialty group, the early "pneumonia nurses" (Wolanin, 1987) emerged from their dedicated interest to the care of the pneumonia patient. They may be some of the progenitors of the infection control nurses of today. This alerts us to the many nurses devoted to geriatric care who have actually defined their work even further. There are now specialty groups of geriatric nurses focused on wound care, incontinence care, pain management, cancer care, rehabilitation, palliative care, and end-of-life care, as well as other very specific specializations. Most major nursing organizations now include special sections for those interested in geriatric nursing. This chapter discusses the origins and expansion of the major geriatric and gerontological nursing organizations and those nursing and interdisciplinary organizations that include a large contingent of geriatric nurses. It is also important to recognize the major philanthropic organizations that have allocated significant funds to the promotion of geriatric nursing research and specialty practice (see chapter 8).

THE NATIONAL GERONTOLOGICAL NURSING ASSOCIATION

The National Gerontological Nursing Association (NGNA) is a nonprofit professional specialty organization founded in 1984 by John McConnell, Martha Baker, Theresa Barrett, and Ana Raley. John was the

185

first president, from 1984 until 1989. He was encouraged and supported to start NGNA by his teacher and mentor, Sr. Rose Therese Bahr of Catholic University. In the beginning it operated out of the home of one of the four founders. The first national conference was held in 1986 in Bethesda, Maryland. Sr. Rose was the chairperson. Mary Opal Wolanin, and Peter Lamy, professor and director of the Center for the Study of Pharmacy and Therapeutics, University of Maryland, were speakers.

Early leaders who were especially influential included first president, John McConnell, followed by Judith Braun in 1990. John was notable for engaging excellent speakers for the annual conferences and in one case, sent a limousine to pick up Mary Opal Wolanin at the airport (Wolanin, 1987). Judith was multitalented and devoted to promoting research interests and strengthening the organization, as well as enhancing the quality of long-term care. Sr. Rose Therese Bahr, ACS, was the annual conference program coordinator for the first 7 years and sought nationally know gerontological nurses as presenters. Sr. Rose, had a natural ebullience that one could not resist. She made each person feel as if his or her involvement was uniquely special.

The NGNA is designed to provide a voice and collective support for RNs, LPNs, CNAs, and associate members involved in the care of the aged. An annual conference featuring educational offerings, presentations from nationally recognized experts, tributes to excellence in geriatric care, and opportunities for interaction with geriatric nurses across the nation was an early goal. NGNA has grown from a small cadre of dedicated nurses to one of more than 1,500 members and at least 25 state chapters. The organization has been under several management groups and is now being dynamically managed by the Puetz Organization in Florida.

The mission of the NGNA is to provide a forum in which gerontological nursing issues are identified and explored; promote the specialty and professional development of nurses whose practice includes older adults; conduct educational programs; disseminate information related to gerontological nursing; engage in programs designed to demonstrate innovative techniques and approaches in gerontological health care to better meet the needs of America's aging population; advocate for legislation that enhances the care of older adults; provide grants to conduct activities which further the goals and purposes of the NGNA; and promote research in gerontological nursing. In 1992, the NGNA Research Committee was established with Mary Ann Anderson, Weber State University, Ogden, Utah, as chair. An advanced practice special interest group also was initiated.

The NGNA board of directors, in conjunction with its committees, task forces, appointed representatives, and NGNA fellows, are dedicated to carrying out the mission and goals of the association. Beginning in 1988, through the efforts of Sr. Rose Therese Bahr and financially supported by Ross Laboratories, annual meetings were held with leaders of the NGNA, the National Conference of Gerontological Nurse Practitioners (NCGNP), the Council of Gerontological Nursing of the American Nursing Association (ANA), and the National Association of Directors of Nursing Administration (NADONA). Later, the National League of Nursing (NLN) was added to the group.

One of the distinctive features that was important in the NGNA's inception was the creation of a forum for the concerns of all nursing personnel providing care to the aged. Thus, registered nurses (RNs), licensed vocational nurses/licensed practical nurses (LVN/LPNs), and certified nurse assistants (CNAs) were included and encouraged to participate. Over the years this multilevel focus is sometimes less apparent but awards are given each year to LPNs and CNAs for outstanding performance. In 2004 Sharon Ruspantine, LPN from the Masonic Home of New Jersey, Burlington, was given the LPN Excellence in Gerontological Nursing Award and Guadalupe Medellin, a CNA at Methodist Hospital in San Antonio, Texas, was the recipient of the CNA Excellence in Gerontological Nursing Award. A reduced membership rate with full benefits is offered to nursing assistants. In the future the commitment to these associate members will continue, although LVN/LPNs and CNAs now have their own organizations and publications.

The NGNA provides a milieu in which members can mature into leaders. Members are encouraged to participate in committees, task force activities, accept positions of leadership on local chapter and national levels, recruit new members to the organization, and are given support while developing their leadership skills. A recent NGNA announcement emphasized this, "One of the benefits of your National Gerontological Nursing Association membership is the opportunity to run for a position of leadership at the national level. All individuals who have been NGNA members at the national level for a minimum of one year are eligible and encouraged to run for office." (March 28, 2005). This may be the first step some geriatric nurses take toward developing professional organizational stature.

An annual *Call for Posters* and presentations at the yearly convention allows members to present their work to the organization. They are also encouraged to submit manuscripts for publication in the NGNA section of *Geriatric Nursing*. Photo contests encourage members to submit their photos that highlight positive aspects of aging.

Winners' photos are posted at the annual convention, and they are awarded complimentary registration at the convention in which their photo is featured.

Benefits of membership include: subscriptions to *Geriatric Nursing;* subscription to a bimonthly newsletter, *Supporting Innovations in Gerontological Nursing* (SIGN); local chapter membership, fellow status availability on application; and an internship and awards program. Online course offerings, certification credits available at conferences, the NGNA core curriculum, books, endowed scholarships, and useful products that are available on order, are other features of NGNA.

In 1994 the NGNA collaborated with the American Nurses Credentialing Center for certification examinations for the Gerontological Nurse; Clinical Specialist in Gerontological Nursing; and Gerontological Nurse practitioner (www.ngna.org). Certification examinations are offered to NGNA membership at discounted rates. The online review course for the generalist gerontological nursing certification is available through the John A Hartford Institute for Geriatric Nursing (www.hartfordign.org).

Recent president, Cindy Shemansky, has markedly contributed to the expansion of the group by her broad background in the field and futuristic awareness of organizational needs. The Cindy Shemansky Travel Scholarship is available to those NGNA members who wish to attend the annual convention and need financial assistance. Each scholarship is a $1,000 cash prize to be used for registration fees, lodging, and other travel costs.

Largely through the inspiration of Virginia Burggraf, the Mary Opal Wolanin Scholarship was established in 1988, to provide two $1,500 scholarships, one to a student in graduate studies and the other to an undergraduate student. The first awards were given in the fall of 1989.

The Judith V. Braun Research Award is given annually in recognition of the scientific contributions of a member or team of nurses who have contributed to advancing the practice of gerontological nursing through research.

The Distinguished Service Award, established in 1999 by the NGNA board of directors, is presented to an NGNA member in recognition of outstanding leadership, participation, and contributions toward achieving NGNA goals.

Recent activities of the NGNA include: chartering of several new NGNA chapters; writing a joint position statement in collaboration with the Canadian Gerontological Nursing Assocation (CGNA); publication of innovations in clinical practice; periodic member needs assessments; revising certification preparation courses; and collaboration with other groups that represent gerontological nurses and the care of the aged (Remsburg & Crogan, 2005).

NATIONAL GERONTOLOGICAL NURSES ASSOCIATION LEADERS

Judy Braun: NGNA President, 1989 to 1994

Judy Braun was one of the most influential of early NGNA leaders. Her early interest in aging was pursued in graduate studies of gerontological nursing at Frances Payne Bolton School of Nursing, Case Western Reserve University, Cleveland. She continued there in doctoral studies and names May Wykle and Mary Adams as some of those who influenced her greatly. While there she served as director of nursing at Margaret Wagner House and co-project director of the Robert Wood Johnson Teaching Nursing Home.

After moving to Virginia, she worked collaboratively with Jiska Cohen-Mansfield at the Hebrew Homes' Research Institute. They chronicled experiences in restraint reduction that resulted in a text, *Toward a Restraint Free Environment* (Braun & Lipson, 1993). After 8 years of progressive positions and professional growth, she achieved the position of president and chief executive officer of the Washington House, Alexandria, Virginia. While there she implemented a community-based program with a state-of-the-art fitness center. Collaborating with Mary Ann Anderson, she copublished another text, *Caring for the Elderly Client* (Anderson & Braun, 1999).

Since 2001, Judy has been the director for affiliate services for the Kendall Corporation, a position in which she is responsible for operations in eight continuing care retirement communities (CCRCs), four residential living communities, and one assisted/skilled nursing facility. She has found that this affords many opportunities for her to support innovation and the blending of research and practice.

One of the highlights of Judy's NGNA presidency was being invited to the White House for lunch with Barbara Bush, and 25 nursing leaders from throughout the nation, in celebration of the May 6, 1990, National Nurses Week. A letter from Mrs. Bush that appeared in the December 10, 1990, *New Horizons,* states: "Our older Americans are a great resource to this country, and it is nurses like you, who are dedicated to their care, who will help provide them with a fuller and more meaningful life. Your fine spirit of professionalism and selfless devotion have on more than one occasion made despair turn to courage, illness abate and better health return."

Shirley Travis, NGNA President 2002 Through 2003

Dr. Shirley Travis, dean of the College of Nursing and Health Science at George Mason University in Fairfax, Virginia, was president of NGNA during the time when the coalition was established with the Canadian Gerontological Nursing Association. Her contributions to the growth of the organization have been noteworthy. Shirley's determination to give research a high priority among NGNA members reflects her own regard for generating clinically significant research. Her research and publications address the patterns of care that dependent older adults and their family caregivers require over time.

Dr. Travis's awards and honors include the 2002 Janssen Eldercare Lifetime Achievement Award for contributions to the health care of older Americans, and the 2000 Springer Geriatric/Gerontological Nursing Research Award for her work on end of life research, among others. Dr. Travis served as a Pope Eminent Scholar of the Rosalynn Carter Institute for Human Development and currently sits on the board of directors of the institute.

Shirley has authored or coauthored more than 100 articles, books, and book chapters on aging and long-term care. She maintains involvement in numerous professional organizations and service activities. In addition to being past president of NGNA she is currently chair of the Clinical Medicine Section of the Gerontological Society of America.

Robin Remsburg, NGNA President Elect 2005

Dr. Robin Remsburg became a member of the NGNA only 10 years ago but in characteristic fashion she immediately became immersed. Her first experience was in submitting a poster abstract that was selected as a finalist for the Judith V. Braun Research Award. This was the beginning of her contributions to the NGNA; in Robin's words, "a remarkable professional association." In addition to serving on the research committee for 2 years, and acting as treasurer for 4 years, she was elected president in 2005. She also served for 2 years as the NGNA representative for the *Geriatric Nursing Journal* and for 3 years as the coeditor of the NGNA section. She attributes her deep involvement in the NGNA to the influence of several "extraordinary gerontological nurses": Karen Armacost, Shirley Travis, Ed Latham, Virginia Burggraf, and Mary Ann Anderson.

The recent alliance with the Canadian Gerontological Association, accomplished through lengthy collaboration and commitment on the part of then current presidents Shirley Travis (NGNA) and Lorna Guse (CGNA), is a significant step in recognizing the importance of shared goals and commitment to the care of the aged on the North American continent.

NATIONAL CONFERENCE OF GERONTOLOGIC NURSE PRACTITIONERS

Geriatric nurse practitioners and gerontological nurse practitioners had their origins in the Primex program. One such program was at Cornell University Medical College, codirected by Doris Schwartz. The Primex design provided a model for the W. K. Kellogg project that focused on recruitment of nursing home nurses and provided support for them to attend geriatric nurse practitioner training programs in one of five universities. The Kellogg project involved nurses from 13 western states and was designed to provide a full-time geriatric nurse practitioner (GNP) in nursing homes with 100 or more beds. From these origins the Western Conference of Geriatric Nurse Practitioners was formed in Oregon in 1981 where nurses' legislative power supported enabling practice laws. The embryonic organization was nourished by Sr. Marilyn Schwab, prioress of the Mount Angel Benedictine Nursing Center in Mt. Angel, Oregon (see chapter 2). In 1984 the organization was incorporated and the name changed to the National Conference of Gerontological Nurse Practitioners. At a small conference in Portland, Oregon, the early leaders formulated the bylaws, mission, and goals of NCGNP. Currently there are more than 3,500 certified GNPs in the nation, many of whom are members of NCGNP.

Dr. Norma Small heads a task force that is completing a historical document of the development of NCGNP. Dr. Small suggests that the NCGNP's history of working with the National Alliance of Nurse Practitioners (NANP), now the American College of Nurse Practitioners (ACNP), is significant because so much of the legislation of the 1980s and 1990s that moved NP (and especially GNP) practice forward came from these cooperative efforts. In 1985, the NCGNP was one of five national nurse practitioner organizations to send a representative, Linda Grissom, to the National Coalition of Nurse Practitioner Organizations Task Force, which became the National Alliance of Nurse Practitioners. The efforts of the task force grew, with NCGNP leadership, to represent more than 13 nurse practitioner organizations. The NANP provided a cohesive force for lobbying for federal and state legislation in the areas of nurse practitioner education and funding, scope of independent practice, reimbursement, and insurance issues. The combined efforts brought about significant changes in Medicare; the result of nurses working together for the common good. The NCGNP continues to collaborate with other nurse practitioner organizations as an affiliate of the ACNP.

The goals of the organization are to advocate quality care for older adults; promote professional development of advanced practice nursing;

provide continuing educational opportunities as well as opportunities for CE credit; promote collaboration and collective strength; support research related to the care of older adults; and be a strong legislative voice of advocacy for the aged. A major part of the legislative effort is to increase practice options and regulatory support for GNPs. There are now almost 100 GNP academic programs. Information about these can be accessed on the NCGNP website (www.ncgnp.org).

Quarterly NCGNP newsletters are sent to members and recent issues are available on the NCGNP website. Conferences are dynamic and provide current information to enhance practice with particular attention to research and pharmacological updates. Annual convention summaries are available on the NCGNP website and some presentations, eligible for CE, are available on Medscape (www.medscape.com/viewprogram/2795). The *Geriatric Nursing Journal* has a dedicated section in NCGNP, and subscription to the journal is a benefit of membership. Barbara Resnick and Ann Luggen are the section editors responsible for organizing the content in the NCGNP section of the journal. Further discussion of their contributions to gerontologic nursing can be found in chapters 4 and 8.

Recently NCGNP was awarded a Technology Assistance Grant from the American Nurses Association. Dr. Barbara Resnick will serve as the clinical coordinator of the project.

In 2005, Barbara Phillips succeeded Barbara Resnick as president of the NCGNP. Barbara was in the first class of students of the blended role (GNP/GCS) Advanced Practice Nurse program in the Christine E. Lynn College of Nursing at Florida Atlantic University (FAU) and recently completed her DNS degree, also at FAU.

NATIONAL ASSOCIATION OF DIRECTORS OF NURSING ADMINISTRATION IN LONG-TERM CARE

The National Association of Directors of Nursing Administration in Long-Term Care (NADONA/LTC) is the only professional nonprofit association specifically serving directors and assistant directors of nursing and RN nurse managers in long-term care and assisted living facilities. It was chartered in 1986 in St. Louis, with 40 founding members. The membership has now increased to more than 6,000 members and 40 state chapters. The phenomenal growth can be attributed to the previous inadequacies of attention in the field to the need, and to compensate for the great dearth of support for providers in long-term care. Joan Warden-Saunders saw the need and envisioned the organization. She has been the force behind this association, the prime mover, and the executive director since its inception.

The organization works vigorously to establish professional relationships with the various disciplines in long-term care, with the constant goal of promoting quality care for long-term care residents and professional recognition for those who serve them. They have established standards of practice and a code of ethics. They endeavor to provide forums for education, as well as a certification system (over 1,400 members are certified through NADONA), communication, and service to members. This commitment has never wavered (www.nadona.org).

The mission of the organization states that the association is to promulgate and foster a network of directors of nursing, assistant directors of nursing, and RN nurse managers in long-term care. Through the NADONA/LTC code of ethics, constitution, and charter, the association supports and promotes quality of care for those individuals receiving long-term care, and concern for those delivering long-term care. The primary goals of the organization are to provide education and support the collegiality, collaboration, and professionalism of its members. The organization has been highly successful and has gained national recognition and cooperation from agencies and organizations devoted to geriatric care. Members enjoy many benefits, including:

- A reference/research library
- A mentoring system available for members
- Educational materials, available through the NADONA Online University (www.nadona.org) or contact Gary Warden.
- A quarterly journal, *The Director* distributed to all members
- Assistance in forming state chapters
- Available professional materials for advancing long-term care
- Scholarships (call 800-222-0539 for particulars)
- National conventions offering CE credits, exhibits, clinical symposia, and entertainment
- Online DON certification (www.nadona.org) with a link to DON Certification Now
- Participation in formulating and promoting appropriate legislation

In 2003, the NADONA/LTC bylaws were amended to include RNs who are in supervisory/administrative positions in long-term care facilities, and certification in long-term care nursing administration is now available.

In 2002 NADONA/LTC became the 13th group to establish an alliance with OSHA and is the first in the long-term care industry to do so. This national affiliation is devoted to workplace safety and health, with a focus on ergonomics, a primary goal of the alliance. In 2003, Mariner Health Care, a provider group of long-term health care in 290 skilled nursing facilities nationwide, joined the NADONA/LTC, providing en bloc membership to all of their directors of nursing (DONs). These and other alliances continue to strengthen the organization and the opportunities for members. Currently, the top 10 long-term care corporations provide complimentary membership to their DONs, a great boon to the morale of any organization. The annual national conventions are truly celebrations of the spirit, expertise, and collegiality of long-term care nurses.

LEADERS OF THE NATIONAL ASSOCIATION OF DIRECTORS OF NURSING ADMINISTRATION/LONG-TERM CARE

Joan Warden Saunders

Joan began her nursing career at age 4, dispensing "pills" from her nurse's kit. By age 16 she was a confirmed seeker and joined the Future Nurses of America (FNA). Although the FNA did not last, Joan's love of nursing did. Joan spent several years attending to a family and working in intensely demanding nursing positions. She always thrived on challenges. As a DON in long-term care she recognized the need for a formalized organization of support and set about establishing one. She invited local DONs to her facility to discuss issues, problems, and careers in long-term care. They began meeting regularly and *McKnight's,* a long-term care publication, ran an article about their meetings. Soon she was deluged with calls from DONs all over the United States. She responded to each individual who expressed an interest in organizing. Soon she was consumed with this mission, left her nursing position, and established a home office. She found that DONs in St. Louis were meeting annually and asked to join them and use their meeting as a nucleus to found a national organization. Joan writes, "The founding meeting in 1986 in St. Louis was one of the most memorable moments of my life. . . . I could not imagine that in years to come the NADONA would have such an impact on the improvement of care for older adults and the education of our staff, and that we would bring the profession of the DON in LTC the recognition it deserves. . . . When people say thanks to me for 'all I have done for NADONA,' I tell them that NADONA has done much more for me" (Warden-Saunders in Ebersole, 2001, p. 157).

Charlotte Eliopoulos

Another important figure in the organization is Charlotte Eliopoulos. She is a specialist in holistic, gerontological and chronic care nursing, and recently was appointed the new director of education of the NADONA/LTC. Eliopoulos has routinely provided a column in the *Director* that provides information about alternative and holistic health care. In her new role she collaborates with the executive director and staff to identify educational needs of the members and develop and implement educational programs to meet those needs. She also evaluates and maintains educational materials for the certification program, conference continuing education programs, website education programs, and scholarship programs.

Charlotte pioneered the role of clinical specialist in gerontological nursing in acute care for the Maryland Department of Health. She has authored several books that emphasize holistic care, alternative therapies, and management of chronic conditions of the aged. She is a past president of the American Holistic Nurses' Association (AHNA) and is sought as a speaker, nationally and internationally.

CANADIAN GERONTOLOGICAL NURSING ASSOCIATION

Canadian gerontological nurses held their first conference in Victoria, British Columbia, in 1983. Over 400 nurses attended from across the country. The excitement was such that the participants spontaneously contributed money to support exploring the founding of a national association and to report the next year at a conference proposed by staff at St. Boniface Hospital, Winnipeg, Manitoba. This conference was chaired by lifetime Canadian Gerontological Nursing Association (CGNA) members, Lynn Mitchell-Pedersen and Lois Abbot. An interim executive committee (Mitchell-Pedersen, Mantle, Abbott, and Jackson) was established in 1984 to develop a constitution and bylaws that would launch a national association. A third historic conference was held in Hamilton, Ontario, in 1985, and was attended by more than 1,100 nurses. At this conference the Canadian Gerontological Association was formally established and Jessie Mantle became the first president.

The mission of the CGNA is to address the health concerns of older Canadians and the nurses who care for them. The organization represents and promotes gerontological nursing across Canada. The association draws its membership from front-line staff nurses working in care programs focused on older citizens, teachers, administrators, and gerontological clinical nurse specialists. In 2003 an alliance was formed with the NGNA to exchange information and share mutual goals and opportunities for the advancement of both groups (Mantle, 2005).

The objectives of the CGNA are to promote high standards of gerontological nursing practice; provide quality educational offerings in gerontological nursing; promote networking opportunities for nurses; disseminate research; and represent the association in government, educational, and professional bodies. In conjunction with those goals, the CGNA became one of the first recognized national interest groups in the Canadian Nurses Association. The first group of Canadian gerontological nurses was certified by the CNA in 1999. Since that time, well over 50% of the members have achieved CNA certification in gerontological nursing. Many nurses take the certification examination even though they are not necessarily members of CGNA. There are 48 gerontological nursing academic programs across Canada and thus opportunities for appropriate education (Springate, 2005).

The CGNA biannual conferences are held in carefully selected sites. The CGNA executive group selects the sites based on proposals submitted by individual groups or provincial associations. Conferences are held across continental Canada, Vancouver Island, Newfoundland, and Nova Scotia, attracting participants from all the Canadian provinces as well as attendees from other parts of the world community. Conferences have been held in such distant places as Corner Brook, Newfoundland, and tourist meccas such as Kelowna, BC, and Vancouver, BC (Mantle, 2005). Further information about CGNA can be obtained on the website (www.cgna.net).

In Canada there have been parallel developments in organizing gerontological nurses in the individual provinces (e.g., Ontario, Alberta, British Columbia). Finding a way to bring these provincial groups into the national association has been the focus of efforts since the beginning of the national association. Recently, satisfactory financial arrangements were effected for those provinces who agreed to opt into the plan (Mantle, 2005).

LEADERS OF THE CANADIAN GERONTOLOGICAL ASSOCIATION

Jessie Mantle

Jessie Mantle was one of the pioneers of the geriatric nursing specialty in Canada. Jessie says, "My interest in aging probably began with my parents. I was the only child of older parents—my mother being 42 when I was born. I grew up being comfortable with older people and was amazed to find that others were uncomfortable around them or considered them 'has beens'" (Mantle, 2005, p. 1).

She followed a rather traditional educational route, initially involving hospital training to achieve her RN, then she attended McGill University for a bachelor of science degree and went on to the University of California, San Francisco for a master's degree. She attended an additional post master's year to become a gerontological nurse specialist. This interest remained her focus until her retirement in 1995. She chose the field because she saw the Canadian population aging but no one seemed to be preparing themselves to meet the challenges of health care for this group.

In 1981 Jessie accepted a joint appointment to teach at the University of Victoria School of Nursing part-time; the other half of her time was spent as a clinical nurse specialist at a long-term care facility, Juan de Fuca Hospital. This government-funded trial project was so successful that it became a permanent position.

From 1991 to 1995 some of her many accomplishments included: founding member of the CGNA and serving as the first official president after the constitution was adopted; pioneering practice innovations; developing and teaching a gerontological nursing course; serving as graduate advisor to master's students; and mentoring nurses interested in clinical geriatrics. She also served on local, provincial, and national boards and committees concerned with the care of older persons; wrote myriad articles; presented workshops; and gave speeches on the subject (Mantle, 2005).

She recently wrote a book entitled *Forgotten Revolution: The Priory Method: A Restorative Care Model for Older Persons* (Mantle & Funke-Furber, 2003), based on the holistic model developed by Vera McIver. McIver recognized the capacity of elders for regaining or maintaining their abilities with appropriate attention. This was a revolutionary idea in the United States and Canada at a time when rehabilitation of the aged was not considered important.

Jessie's consistent devotion to advancing the care of the aged remains important as she actively participates in community gerontological activities and support of quality elder care. She is an honorary life member of the CGNA and the British Columbia Gerontological Nursing Association.

Joyce (Church) Springate, CGNA President 1999 to 2001

Joyce Springate, EdD, RN, speculates that she has always been interested in the care of older adults from her first experiences on the wards as a student in nursing school. Her enjoyment of elders came from a widowed grandfather who lived with her family until he was 86 years old, remarried, and moved 100 miles away.

Dr. Springate has been one of the influential members of the CGNA and served as president from 1999 to 2001. She was the chair of the Conference at Kelowna in 2003. Her dedication and enthusiasm are representative of a cadre of individuals who have contributed to a remarkably effective group of geriatric nurses in Canada. She is energetic, fun-loving, and inspirational. Joyce is an esteemed colleague. Her vivacity and commitment to the progress and recognition of Canadian gerontological nurses has been influential in professional recognition of the CGNA in Canada and the United States. Through her involvement and that of Virginia Burggraf, and the persistence of Lorna Guse (past president of the CGNA) and Shirley Travis (past president of the NGNA) a close and beneficial alliance was fostered between the two groups in 2003.

Joyce has many skills, but her greatest talents seem to be in facilitating change, networking, and developing partnerships. She started the CGNA newsletter and was editor for several years and also developed the CGNA website during her presidency (www.cgna.net).

Joyce has published extensively, is active in a dozen professional organizations related to nursing and gerontology, and has comprehensive experience in long-term care, the community, and education. She is particularly skilled in program development and evaluation, efficient resource use, and customer-focused services. For 10 years (1986–1996) she was the manager of the Education Resource Centre for Continuing Care, which involved coordination and provision of education and resource use in all long-term care facilities and home care in the province of Alberta (Springate, 2004).

She has given many presentations at regional and national conferences, is a prolific writer, and has earned numerous awards. The awards she values most are the Mary Morrison Davis Award of Excellence, Alberta Association on Gerontology, received in 1997 and, most recently the Queen's Golden Jubilee Medal awarded for her work in gerontology.

Presently, Joyce is president of a local organization, the Westside Health Network, that provides health education, and information and referral (I&R) to older adults in the community. Volunteers go to the homes of older adults to program whatever digital appliance they may need. She also teaches two online Masters of Health Sciences courses for Athabasca University. This program reaches students from a small outpost community in Newfoundland to the tip of Vancouver Island.

A very special experience with Joyce occurred after a CGNA conference in Corner Brook, Newfoundland. Her husband Gordon, she, and I traveled together to St. Anthony, the site of Sir Wilfred Grenfell's medical mission work. Gordon found stamps for his collection at remote postal stations. Joyce and I found flowers unique to Newfoundland and in the process welded a lasting friendship.

Others of Historic Significance at the Canadian Gerontological Association

Many nurses have contributed to the development of gerontological nursing in Canada. Some have made huge contributions; some were CGNA presidents and others were significant in other ways. Focusing on particular individuals is bound to neglect others who were equally important. This has been a concern throughout this text, as there are many significant contributors to the geriatric nursing specialty who have simply not been available for input. However, some of particular importance in Canada follow.

Lynn Mitchell-Pederson was the first interim president for the planning executive committee of the CGNA. She is still working in the field, living in Winnipeg and doing pioneering work in sexuality and aging. We have been unable to reach her but are aware that she was pivotal in the development of the CGNA.

Pam Dawson, from Ontario, was the first Gerontological Clinical Nurse Specialist in Canada and the first president of the Ontario Gerontological Nursing Association. This was the first organized group of gerontological nurses in the country. She was honored by Duke University for her contributions and is now retired and living in Toronto.

Mary Gibbon is considered by many to be the "grandmother" of geriatric nursing in Canada. She was the director of the Victorian Order of Nurses in Hamilton, Ontario, and pioneered the first home care program for older people with chronic illness.

Mary Buzzell, an ethicist, works tirelessly on maintaining personhood for individuals in long-term care, developed and currently teaches a family caregiver support group, and participates in national and provincial conferences. She recently received the Queen Elizabeth Medal and was awarded an honorary doctorate from McMaster University for her contribution to gerontology.

Dr. Dorothy Pringle, former dean, Faculty of Nursing, University of Toronto, was one of the first Canadian nurses to obtain her PhD in gerontological nursing. She has played a critical role in conducting nursing-related research projects, mentoring the young nurse researchers and representing gerontological nursing in interdisciplinary and government arenas. She was the cochair of the Third Canadian Gerontological Nursing Conference, which saw the birth of the national association.

GERONTOLOGICAL SOCIETY OF AMERICA

The evolution of the Gerontological Society of America (GSA) began in 1939 when a small group of physicians and scientists formed the Club for Research on Ageing. From this beginning, the Gerontological Society of America was established and incorporated in 1945. The goals and purpose of the GSA are to promote the scientific study of aging, encourage exchanges among researchers and practitioners from various disciplines related to gerontology, foster the use of gerontological research in forming public policy, challenge the myths of aging in order to achieve a more realistic picture of the aged in all their various situations, and revitalize the field by a more balanced view of a healthier and more productive old age. The primary activity envisioned was to start a gerontological publication. In 1946 the first issue of the *Journal of Gerontology* was published. It was the first, and for many years the only, gerontological research journal.

Initially, the large contingent of physician and scientist members led to a concentrated focus on research in aging. Over the years, and markedly under the presidency of Dr. Gene Cohen, it became much broader and more eclectic in activities, giving increased attention to complex quality of life issues, and the position of the arts and humanities in gerontology. Some of this can be attributed to nurses becoming a visible part of the GSA. Shirley Travis, a nurse, active in and a past president of NGNA, is the chair of the Clinical Medicine Section in the GSA. The meeting in Orlando in 2005 celebrated the 58th year of the founding of the GSA. It is fitting that Terry Fulmer was president of the GSA in that memorable year, the first nurse to hold that position.

James Birren's (then director of the Ethel Percy Andrus Gerontology Center at University of Southern California, Los Angeles) interest in developing a cadre of geriatric nurses was influential. He brought Irene Mortenson Burnside to the Center in 1972 and from her courses and others, geriatric nurses formed bonds, obtained gerontological certificates, and began coming together in a group at the annual GSA meetings. Bernita Steffl (see chapter 2) was often the instigator and would simply invite the small cadre of nurses to her room for wine, cheese, and mutual sustenance. The group grew gradually and presently is the largest of the formal interest groups at the GSA, the Nursing Care of Older Adults. Formal status was achieved in 2004. This group disseminates effective nursing interventions for care of older adults, as well as research reports, and advances the study of needs of older adults and their families by encouraging interdisciplinary communication and supporting the development of a scientific basis for nursing care of older adults. The John A. Hartford Foundation has been particularly active in supporting this group in the last few years with the assistance of Donna Algase and Diane Feeney Mahoney.

The GSA is critically important to the augmentation of the geriatric nursing specialty. It forms the backbone of interdisciplinary action that becomes more important each year. Nurses, as noted by Terry Fulmer, must be integrally connected with all the other disciplines, especially as specialties and subspecialties expand and flourish. We are all of one body and must synthesize the functions of each to become whole. The *Journal of Gerontology* and *The Gerontologist* are organs that frequently publish nursing studies. More information about the GSA can be found on the website (www.geron.org).

AMERICAN SOCIETY ON AGING

The American Society on Aging (ASA) was established in 1954 as the Western Gerontological Society. The name change occurred in response to the growing national interest in aging and to meet the needs of a larger group.

The ASA is an association of diverse individuals bound to a common goal: to support the commitment and enhance the knowledge and skills of those who seek to improve the quality of life of older adults and their families. The membership of the ASA is a multidisciplinary group of professionals who are concerned with the physical, emotional, social, economic, and spiritual aspects of aging. The range includes practitioners, educators, administrators, policy makers, business people, researchers, and students. The ASA offers a diverse array of educational programs, outstanding publications, information and training resources, and the largest network of individuals in the field of aging (www.asaging.org/about.cfm).

The goals of the ASA are to infuse a strengths-based model of aging into its publications, conferences, member services, and leadership development activities; provide leadership in integrating research, practice, and policy to address aging issues in an increasingly diverse society; be a leading advocate and partner for information, training, and leadership development in understanding, promoting, and achieving cultural diversity and cultural competence relating to aging; and be a national resource for leadership training, mentorship, networking, and communications to develop and strengthen individual and organizational leaders needed to meet the current and future needs of the diverse older population.

The comprehensive services offered to members include: publications, membership in a constituent group of the member's choice, information, research, career tools, expert advice, online discussion groups, local and national contacts through a membership directory, and leadership mentoring programs. Discounts are given of up to 40% toward the ASA-NCOA (National Council on Aging) annual joint conference, regional Summer Series on Aging, International Care Management Conference and web-enhanced seminars. Web seminars provide CEUs for nurses, nursing home administrators, social workers, case managers, counselors, and other professionals. These are available on demand for a fee and offer such topics as: older driver wellness; comprehensive geriatric assessment; legal and ethical issues of aging; developing caring and competent caregivers; screening for medication related problems; and many others.

Numerous awards are given, including: those for best practice in human resources and aging; graduate and undergraduate students; media; leadership; the ASA hall of fame; Gloria Cavanaugh Award; mental health and aging network award; business and aging awards; and health care and aging awards. Information about these can be obtained from (awards@asaging.org).

The ASA publishes a quarterly journal *Generations*. This topical journal is provided to all members and extra issues are available for sale to any interested professional or individual. Some recent topics include: advocacy; funeral and memorial practices; food and nutrition; silver industries; aging and the senses; getting around in later life; listening to older people's stories; and family caregiving. It has been under the expert guidance of Mary Johnson, editor in chief since its inception. Topics are chosen by a 12-member *Generations* board who also seek appropriate editors for each topical issue.

The bimonthly *Aging Today* is another important publication. This publication, formulated and edited by Paul Kleyman, covers advances in practice, policy, and research nationwide. Other publications include: *ASA Connection; Mind Alert;* and newsletters to members with various specific interests such as *Mental Health and Aging; Business Forum; Forum on Religions and Spirituality; Lesbian and Gay Aging Issues;* and *Network on Multicultural Aging.*

In general the ASA has been concerned with social issues and has a large contingent of members who are in social work, psychology, education, and clinical practice. A great deal of attention of the organization has focused on caregiving. Geriatric nurses are a small but influential group, not specifically identified as a group but integrated into all aspects of the ASA as interdisciplinary participants.

Gloria Cavanaugh, CEO since shortly after the inception of the ASA, has done a remarkable job of expanding and redefining the organization to fit the times and societal trends.

In 2002, the ASA partnered with the NCOA to strengthen both organizations and integrate their mutual goals. The NCOA affiliation brought in additional benefits to members including special mini-conferences on current topics, networking opportunities, and others.

THE AMERICAN GERIATRICS SOCIETY

The American Geriatrics Society (AGS) is dedicated to improving the health and well-being of all older adults. With a membership of over 6,800 health care professionals, the AGS has a long history in the provision of health care for older adults. It has become a pivotal force in shaping attitudes, policies, and practices about the health care of older people. The AGS is a nationwide, not-for-profit association of health care professionals, research scientists, and other individuals concerned with improving health, independence, and quality of life for older people. The roots of the society were planted in 1942 by a group of physicians who were interested in advancing medical care of older adults. At this inaugural meeting, the founding membership decided that any physician with an interest in geriatrics would be eligible to join. In 1994, the society's board of directors decided to expand the AGS to recruit all geriatric health care professionals interested in improving the health care of elders. Membership is comprised of physicians, nurses, researchers, medical educators, pharmacists, physician assistants, social workers, physical therapists, occupational therapists, health care administrators, and others (americangeriatrics.org).

The society welcomes nurses. Terry Fulmer was the first nonphysician board member of the AGS and served from 1998 to 2004. During that time she was the chair of the AGS Geriatric Interdisciplinary Advisory Group that was initiated to engender more interdisciplinary activity in the society. She enjoyed her participation in the organization and encourages others to join, as she has found it very useful. Of particular interest to nurses are the pain management guidelines that she participated in developing.

THE AMERICAN NURSES ASSOCIATION

The American Nurses Association (ANA) is the national organization that represents, advocates, and educates the nearly 2.7 million RNs in the United States through its 54 constituent state and territorial member associations with more than 150,000 members. The ANA advances the nursing profession by fostering high standards of nursing practice, promoting the economic and general welfare of nurses in the workplace, projecting a positive and realistic view of nursing, and lobbying congress and regulatory agencies on health care issues affecting nurses and the public.

Among the priority issues addressed by the ANA are: restructuring of the health care system to deliver primary health care in community-based settings; an expanded role for RNs and advanced practice nurses in the delivery of basic and primary health care; obtaining federal funds for nurse education and training; and helping to change and improve the health care workplace.

The ANA-affiliated organizations include the American Nurses Foundation, the American Academy of Nursing, and the American Nurses Credentialing Center (www.ana.org/about/mission.htm, April 11, 2005). These have all been important in the development and recognition of the geriatric nursing specialty as well as adding to the prestige of individual geriatric and gerontological nurses certified through ANA, or honored by selection as fellows of the AAN.

Barbara Davis has developed a history of the ANA as it pertains to the geriatric nursing specialty; much of that has been included in chapter 1. The Division of Geriatric Nursing Practice was established during the mid-1960s when the attention of the nation was captured by the advent of Medicare. The ANA was identifying the areas of specialization within nursing and eventually came up with five divisions: medical/surgical; psychiatric/mental health; maternal/child health; geriatrics; and community health. Dr. Davis became the first full-time coordinator for the division, then called Geriatric Nursing. In 1973 the ANA first defined the standards of geriatric practice, and the Geriatric Nursing Practice Division was the first within the ANA to establish standards of practice. From 1971 to 1976 Dr. Gunter served on the executive committee of the Division of Geriatric Nursing Practice of the ANA and spent some time during this period working with Barbara Allen Davis to develop certification criteria for geriatric nurses wishing to be credentialed. To the surprise of the committee, more than 100 nurses applied; it kept the committee busy throughout the Thanksgiving vacation reviewing applications. Seventy five nurses completed the process and were credentialed (Ebersole, 1998). Further discussion of Barbara Davis and Laurie Gunter are in chapter 2.

In 2003, the ANA announced the awarding of 12 grants in the *Nursing Competence in Aging* initiative. This initiative is designed to improve quality of care to older adults by enhancing nurse competencies and preparing the nursing workforce for the great increase in elders that will come as baby boomers age. At present only 1% of nurses are certified by the ANCC as gerontological nurses and only 3% are certified as geriatric nurse practitioners and clinical specialists. To address the concern about the shortage of geriatric nurses to meet future needs, the ANA is involved in promoting geriatric structures and activities within nursing specialty associations; facilitating dual certification within these organizations to reflect newly acquired knowledge related to the care of the older adults within the aegis of the specialty; and developing a web-based comprehensive geriatric nursing resource center. Grant assistance is available to help in developing geriatric special interest groups and initiate geriatric educational activities (www.nursingworld.org/pressrel/ 2003/pr0715.htm, April 3, 2005).

THE AMERICAN ASSOCIATION OF COLLEGES OF NURSING

The American Association of Colleges of Nursing (AACN) is the national voice for university and 4-year college education programs in nursing. Representing more than 580 member schools of nursing at public and private institutions nationwide, the AACN's educational, research, governmental advocacy, data collection, publications, and other programs work to establish quality standards for bachelor's and graduate degree nursing education, assist deans and directors to implement those standards, influence the nursing profession to improve health care, and promote public support of baccalaureate and graduate nursing education, research, and practice (aacn.nche.edu, February 20, 2005).

With funding from the John A. Hartford Foundation of New York, grant monies have been provided to the AACN and distributed to 18 schools of nursing to support education for careers in geriatric nursing. Through the Creating Careers in Geriatric Advanced Practice Nursing project, a critical mass of skilled providers will be produced. This project also provides for networking, mentorship, role modeling, and leadership activities. According to Donna Regenstreif, the senior program officer with the John A. Hartford Foundation, this project will not only increase the number of geriatric advanced practice nurses "but it will also enhance the leadership potential of geriatric advanced practice nurses, thus ultimately advancing the Foundation's goal of ensuring quality care for our nation's older adults" (Rosseter, 2005, p. 1).

CONCLUSION

Organizations, both specific to geriatric/gerontological nursing and interdisciplinary, are the seedbeds of new ideas. They provide the venues and vehicles to share accomplishments, receive recognition for contributions, and network with others of similar interests and concerns. The strength of an organization is demonstrated, not necessarily by numbers, but by the realization of continual growth and progress within the specialty. The remarkable progress in the geriatric/gerontological nursing specialty is signaled by the numerous individuals who are serious in their commitment, who have joined organizations of aging and are visible forces for progress.

CHAPTER SEVEN

Educational Programs and Publications for Geriatric and Gerontological Nurses

Because there are so many distinct levels of education among geriatric nurses it is important to recognize the unique contributions of each: the certified nursing assistants, licensed practical/vocational nurses, and all registered nurses. However, this text focuses only on RNs with basic, baccalaureate, graduate, doctoral, and post doctoral preparation. Integral to educational programs are the availability of textbooks and journals that provide current and reliable information. These are also considered in this chapter.

EDUCATION

Hospital Diploma Programs

Many of the nurse pioneers obtained their education through hospital diploma programs. These programs were available to aspiring nurses with little money as, with few exceptions, they worked in the hospital and had "classes," usually given by physicians, sandwiched in between. In most cases these trainees provided an unpaid labor force and were an economic asset for the hospitals. These nurses had extensive experience caring for the aged but no theory in geriatrics.

Burnside (Garand & Buckwalter, 1996) described the experience. Entering nurses training in 1941 at Ancker Hospital School of Nursing in St. Paul, Minnesota, she was in one of the better programs as they were bused to the University of Minnesota to study anatomy, physiology, and other basic subjects. They were on probation (probies) for the first 6 months of the program and, if successful, went through the capping ceremony. Trainees lived in a home, usually adjoining the hospital. Probies lived in the basement and moved to higher floors as they progressed in their training. There were strict house rules, little privacy, and students were dismissed if they married during their training. Students were in charge of entire wards early in their training and often worked split shifts with classes in between. Most were sent to state mental institutions for a few months during their training and there discovered the "back wards" where elders with dementia were incarcerated—neglected and ignored. For many this spurred them into action to change the situation.

The Community College Technical Nursing Programs

Simultaneously with the origins of the Cadet Nurse Corps, discussed in chapter 2, Mildred Montag began a School of Nursing at Adelphi, New York. "The base of the program was at the college and we used the hospitals in the area for clinical experiences for the students. . . . Financing of the program was almost exclusively through the U.S. Cadet Nurse Corps" (Montag in Safier, 1977, p. 220). Her background with the Cadet Nurse Corps formed the foundation of her later thinking. When she was deciding on a doctoral dissertation she began to think about the notion that there were already technical nurses in diploma schools. "I got part of this idea from Louise McManus, who first introduced the notion that you could differentiate the functions of nursing, that nursing had too broad a range of functions to be encompassed in a single individual. . . . Louise McManus enunciated rather specifically the differentiation of function. As a result of many ideas about professional and technical education, my doctoral dissertation was concerned with the introduction of a new worker in nursing, a technician. The dissertation also proposed where these new workers would be prepared (the community college) and a curriculum for their preparation" (Montag in Safier, 1977, p. 220).

The distinction between professional nursing and technical nursing emerged from Dr. Mildred Montag's doctoral thesis, *Education of Nursing Technicians,* in 1951. In 1952 Dr. Montag directed the Cooperative Research Project in Junior and Community College Education for Nursing. A goal of the project was to determine whether functions commonly associated with registered nurses (RNs) could be accomplished in a 2-year academic program. Before the 5-year project was completed the concept mushroomed and programs were developed from coast to coast (Griffin & Griffin, 1965). Guiding principles of these programs included: requirements for appropriate accreditation; the program must have a qualified nurse educator as director and qualified nursing faculty; and the junior college would assume financial responsibility for providing a quality educational program. "The nursing programs became an integral part of the college. That was not true in the fifties in baccalaureate education, and I think that, really, the financing was the most important achievement" (Montag in Safier, 1977, p. 221).

I was a graduate of one such program and in the first RN class at San Mateo Community College, in San Mateo, California. The program was arduous and excellent. Throughout the program we were continually reminded that we were technical nurses and could do all the things RNs should do in hospitals, but not in the community and in public health nursing. This required baccalaureate preparation in the state of California. Fortunately for me, that only fired my intent to obtain a baccalaureate degree. As these programs evolved and proliferated most now include geriatric nursing content. The graduates of these programs provide much of the nursing care in hospitals and the directors of nursing (DONs) in long-term care. The DONs are essential educators of the licensed vocational nurses (LVNs) and certified nursing assistants (CNAs) and are required to provide quality inservice geriatric education.

Baccalaureate Nursing

Nursing education in early baccalaureate degree programs typically required 5 years. The first year (or sometimes two) covered basic college subjects and the second covered science subjects relevant to nursing. The final 3 years were in nursing classes with clinical experiences in hospitals providing medical, surgical, pediatric, and obstetric care. Public health experience was obtained in the senior year and usually in state agencies serving the indigent. Baccalaureate degree nurses were the only ones allowed to work in public health after graduation. Psychiatric care remained in the background and usually was obtained through an off-campus stint in state hospitals. There was little awareness of the deficiency in geriatric knowledge until the advent of Medicare in 1965 when it became glaringly apparent. And, according to Montag, nursing was the stepchild in most colleges and universities; and was not fully integrated.

Mildred Montag (Safier, 1977, pp. 220–230) believed professional nurses should identify the diagnosis that demands nursing intervention, gather the data, put in place an appropriate nursing care plan, and delegate the tasks that can be accomplished by others. She wrote that this is a highly developed skill that the technical nurse does not have and should not attempt. She believed that those who go from an associate degree program to a baccalaureate program are simply technicians with a baccalaureate degree. A professional nurse needs a background, not only in the sciences but also in logic, history, and philosophy. Montag considered all these to be missing in the baccalaureate programs she was aware of when interviewed. One must wonder if geriatric content would be more valued if these were really a part of the expectation of baccalaureate nurses and whether she was right in thinking most baccalaureate nursing education remains technical.

Numerous nurses and faculty have influenced the educational expectations and requirements as they exist today, yet many universities lag and have not yet incorporated solid geriatric content into baccalaureate nursing programs. Most states require at least three credit hours of geriatric content but this is often said to be "integrated," which then is entirely dependent upon the background and knowledge of the faculty. Mezey (2002) found that only one in four baccalaureate nursing schools required a course in the care of the aged.

Terri Brower (see chapter 3) made the valid point that many community colleges (CCs) with 2-year nursing programs have given geriatrics more emphasis than the baccalaureate programs (BSN) simply because BSN programs typically spend the last year on community health and leadership courses that are not the thrust of the CCs. Also, 2-year RNs are more likely working in long-term care settings where geriatric knowledge is essential. However, the differences in nursing programs in CCs and BSN programs are now blurring. In an unpublished study, California community college (CC) and baccalaureate nursing (BSN) educators met several times to define the essential differences in the curricula. Groups were mixed and each member, of course, was wedded to their own type of program. However, it became very difficult to find distinct differences, even in the credit hours given to prerequisites and nursing courses. Some community colleges required more than some baccalaureate programs and some RN requirements in community colleges were not really met in 2 years but required 3 or even 4 years. Some community colleges had invaded the home and community with their educational requirements, although this had been thought to be the distinctive difference in CC and BSN programs!

Defining Geriatric Nurse Competencies

In 1990, a group of 18 leaders in gerontologic nursing practice were invited to a National Invitational Consensus Conference held at Georgetown University School of Nursing, Washington, DC to identify basic nursing competencies.

After a welcome by School of Nursing dean, Alma Woodley, Thelma Wells, PhD, RN, FRCN, FAAN, then professor of nursing at the University of Rochester, New York (and now engaged in research at University of Wisconsin, Madison) reviewed the numerous attempts to identify minimum gerontological nursing competencies in the past, as well as the pitfalls that precluded their implementation.

Small groups then convened to facilitate in-depth discussion of the competencies and identify means of assessment, planning, implementation, and evaluation with an emphasis on realistic expectations of BSN graduates. Nurses involved in these discussions included all of the following: Sarah Greene Burger, National Coalition for Nursing Home Reform; Sr. Rose Therese Bahr, Catholic University of America; Eldonna Shields-Kyle, W.G. Nord Community Mental Health Center; Ella Kick, National HealthCorp, Middle Tennessee State University; Mary Coyne, Manor Health Care Corporation; Marjorie Beyers, Mercy Health Services; Priscilla Ebersole, San Francisco State University; May Wykle, Case Western Reserve University; Judith Braun, Hebrew Home of Greater Washington; Linda Phillips, University of Arizona; Dolores M. Alford, Nursing Associates; Marjorie Jamieson, Block Nurse Program, Inc.; May Futrell, University of Massachusetts, Lowell; Julia Thornbury, University of Wisconsin, Madison; Thelma Wells, University of Rochester; Bernita Steffl, Arizona State University; Toni Sullivan, University of Missouri-Columbia; Joyce Colling, Oregon Health Sciences University (National Invitational Consensus Conference, 1991) (Fig. 7.1).

All of these distinguished nurses, other than Eldonna Shields-Kyle and Bernita Steffl, are from the second generation of geriatric nurse

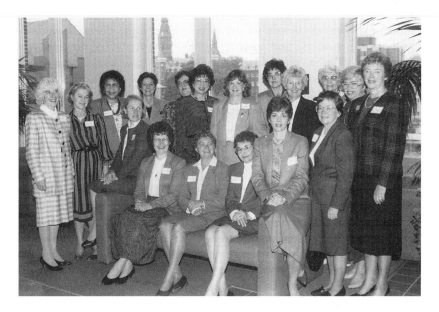

FIGURE 7.1 International Competency Consensus Conference.

leaders, some of whom are discussed in chapter 3. Among the group were educators, researchers, entrepreneurs, administrators, and advocates for the aged. The results of this collaboration of experts were published in 1991 by the Georgetown Press.

Geriatric Curriculum Development

In recent years numerous publications and models of geriatric curricula have been developed, although the first was published by Laurie Gunter and Carmen Estes in 1979 (see chapter 2). Ann Luggen edited a very comprehensive text, *National Gerontological Nursing Association: Core Curriculum for Gerontological Nursing,* with more than 30 contributors. Because of the topical breadth and comprehensive nature of the text, this textbook may be most relevant to graduate programs; however, portions, such as a large section on common health problems, may be used well in undergraduate programs (Luggen, 1996). It considers topics such as professionalism, issues in gerontological nursing including legal and ethical, administrative, reimbursement, regulatory, and environmental issues as well. All are presented in outline form throughout the text. This text remains relevant to curriculum development today.

Fulmer and Matzo compiled several essays to present an overview of means to strengthen geriatric nursing education (1995). These dealt with subjects that remain overriding concerns more than a decade later: integration versus course-specific programs, overcoming ageism, expanding clinical experiences, incorporating geriatrics into the licensure and accreditation processes, and reviving good ideas that have not gone far enough. In addition, the subjects suggested long ago by Montag to develop true professionalism, such as logic, history, and philosophy, must form a bulwark of knowledge and compassion about aging.

Major barriers to the integration of gerontology in nursing curricula were identified: Faculty perceive that there is no room for new content; few faculty are adequately prepared; there are a dearth of well-developed geriatric clinical sites; much of nursing education remains in a medical model; there is a lack of sufficient testing of gerontological content in the NCLEX-RN examination; and the lack of an NLN mandate for inclusion of gerontology in nursing education programs. One can only wonder if any nursing program in the United States has been accredited when lacking a visible maternal/child component. Yet, these form only a small part of actual nursing activities. However, geriatric nursing is flourishing in spite of these obstacles.

The numerous activities of the John A. Hartford Foundation Institute for Geriatric Nursing Practice, within the past 10 years, have provided many options and explicit materials available to incorporate geriatric knowledge into curriculum at all levels of nursing education. In 1997, the Hartford Institute sponsored a 2-day conference at the American Association of Colleges of Nursing (AACN) in Baltimore. At this conference, critical competencies for every entry level professional nurse were defined, including:

1. Assessment of function in the elderly in physical, cognitive, social domains, including activities of daily living
2. Prevention and assessment/management of syndromes common to the elderly (e.g., functional deficits, disturbing behaviors, falls, iatrogenesis, pressure ulcers, dementia and delirium, depression, urinary incontinence, sleep problems, pain)
3. Maximization of independence and maintenance of the elderly in the least restrictive environment
4. Evaluation of the ability to educate nonprofessionals to care for the elderly
5. Collaboration with advanced practice geriatric nurses and other members of the interdisciplinary geriatric team
6. Means to assist the elderly to achieve a peaceful death

Extensive materials are available for faculty development workshops and curriculum lesson plans at www.nyu.edu/education/nursing/hartford.institute/.

A consistent program of awards by the Hartford Institute (hartfordign.org) to programs demonstrating excellence for innovative approaches to teaching geriatric nursing in baccalaureate programs has been in place since 1998. These awards recognize excellence in four categories:

- Geriatric Faculty Member Award
- Infusing Geriatrics into the Nursing Curriculum Award
- Stand-Alone Geriatric Course Award
- Clinical Settings in Geriatric Nursing Award

Technological innovations also reach out to educators. The Consortium of New York Geriatric Education and the Hartford Institute at New York University, under the leadership of Mathy Mezey and Terry Fulmer, using interactive technology, brought teleconferences to 225 nursing educators and staff developers at 10 sites throughout the United States. The goal of these teleconferences was to enhance the skills of nursing faculty and staff developers in order to teach best practice fundamentals in the care of older adults.

The Hartford Institute has raised the consciousness of nursing, other professional providers, and consumers to the needs of older adults in all settings. The Hartford Institute has contributed significantly to the preparation of nurses to care for older adults through a variety of effective mechanisms, such as:

- Widely disseminating geriatric nursing best practices and model geriatric nursing curricula.
- Providing grantsmanship seminars for geriatric nursing faculty.
- Elevating the standard of care of older adults in hospitals through the Nurses to Improve Care of Hospitalized Elders (NICHE) program.

Graduate Nursing Education

Some contend that graduate education is essential to professional nursing and others have even suggested the accelerated baccalaureate programs are in reality just a stepping stone toward professionalism and that the typical baccalaureate programs are really producing mostly technical nurses. Given the lack of a dedicated emphasis on geriatrics in undergraduate programs it is often necessary to progress to graduate education for real professionalism in geriatrics and gerontology.

Advanced Practice Nurses

Advanced practice nurses (APNs) include all those educated as clinical specialists or nurse practitioners. APN is an umbrella term appropriate for a licensed registered nurse prepared at the graduate degree level as either a clinical specialist, nurse anesthetist, nurse-midwife, or nurse practitioner. The broad range of knowledge and skills serve patients in a variety of practice settings. Generally the distinction has been based on practice sites, educational program components, and roles within health care organizations. Nurse practitioners provide direct, primary care to a group of clientele; clinical specialists often have a broader base, seldom a specific group of clients, and function in an advisory, consultative capacity within a health care organization or institution. Some APNs have roles as educators and administrators. All APNs should hold a graduate degree in nursing and be certified. Certification examinations vary for advanced practice nurses, depending on their specialty practice (www.aacn.nche.edu/Publications/positions/cerreg.htm).

A recent press release from Health Orbit states (http://healthorbit.ca. NewsDetail.asp?opt+1&nltid+144250405, April, 29, 2005): "Among urgent-care patients, health outcomes were similar for nurses (primary care nurses) and doctors. Moreover, nurses tended to provide longer consultations, offer more information, recall patients more frequently and receive higher patient-satisfaction ratings." More information is available from Health Behavior News Service (www.hbns.org).

Curriculum development for graduate programs in geriatrics began with the first geriatric nurse specialist graduate program at Duke University, directed by Virginia Stone (chapter 2). Ann Luggen, Shirley Travis, and Sue Meiner have edited a valuable text, *NGNA Core Curriculum for Gerontological Advanced Practice Nurses*, (1998).

A Blended Program

Most graduate programs that educate gerontological professionals are either geared toward a geriatric clinical nurse specialty or to adult/geriatric nurse practitioners. The Christine E. Lynn College of Nursing at Florida Atlantic University has a blended role program of study that prepares graduates for practice as both a gerontological nurse practitioner and a clinical specialist in gerontological nursing. The program, under the leadership of Dr. Ruth Tappen and her colleagues, was funded in 1998 by the Division of Nursing, Bureau of Health Professions, Department of Health and Human Services. Interestingly, the consultants for the grant included some of the notable pioneers and new leaders in gerontological nursing, including Priscilla Ebersole, May Futrell, Christine Kovach, continuing the legacy and mentoring so important to the development of the specialty.

The design of the program as a blending of the roles was congruent with the college's philosophy of nursing, grounded in caring, and was intended to prepare a more marketable graduate who could fill a wide range of roles that were identified as needed by the community served. The faculty was committed to developing a program that prepared advanced practice gerontological nurses who were expert in care of older people as well as in improving gerontological nursing across various settings. As Futrell stated: "Advanced practice nurse preparation should be focusing on the 'person' rather than the place" (2005, p. 23).

A broad survey course entitled Perspectives on Aging provides students with knowledge of gerontology, gerontological nursing, and the social, psychological, and health care needs of older people. Coursework provides content for practice across the continuum of geriatric care and nursing practice experiences are set in primary, acute, and long-term care. All students participate in the development of projects devoted to health promotion in the community and quality improvement in acute and long-term care settings. The graduates of this program are working across the continuum of care to improve the care of older adults in settings ranging from memory disorder clinics, specialized wound care centers, primary care, community-based home care, acute care, and long-term care.

In 2002, the college received continued funding from the Division of Nursing to implement an ethnogeriatric curriculum to better prepare graduates to practice in a culturally diverse society. This program is unique in the country and includes some very innovative content, including an intensive ethnogeriatric interdisciplinary seminar course and projects focusing on cultural disparities and cultural differences. There may be other blended programs in the nation but the Christine E. Lynn College of Nursing, is the first we know of that has developed a specific ethnogeriatric component in the curriculum.

Geriatric Nurse Practitioners

Geriatric and gerontological nurse practitioners combine the best of nursing and primary medical care to holistically assess and manage the common problems of older people and make appropriate decisions about referral to physician specialists and other health care professionals.

The first geriatric nurse practitioners (GNPs) were educated in universities and their programs resulted in certificates rather than master's degrees. In most cases GNPs were developed in response to a crying need for the presence of a nurse able to diagnose, manage primary care on an ongoing basis, and refer to physicians as appropriate. Most were recruited from and for nursing homes or rural areas where, in the 1970s, the need was most pressing. The curricula were quite similar in the universities offering those programs at that time.

In the late 1970s and early 1980s the W. K. Kellogg Foundation funded five such programs to educate and produce GNPs to serve in nursing homes. The universities offering those programs included: University of Arizona, Tucson; University of California, San Francisco; University of Colorado, Denver; State University of New York, Syracuse; and University of Washington, Seattle (see chapter 6). These were modeled after the pattern of the Primex program; one Primex site was at Cornell University, with Doris Schwartz as codirector (see chapter 2).

The programs were 1 year in length and the students spent 4 or 5 months of intensive study at the university with a heavy focus on complex assessment skills, theories of aging, pharmacology, and management of chronic disorders. In the remaining time they were placed in clinics to work alongside a precepting physician. The physician served as their referral source for consultation. In most states they were required to have the facility medical director or physician sign orders, usually after the fact. It was recognized that these nurses were more than physician's assistants and combined the best of nursing and primary medical care. The students returned to the universities weekly for seminars to discuss cases. GNPs were desired as preceptors but there weren't any available at that time. Later, when some geriatric nurse practitioners were obtainable, they were engaged as preceptors. These programs were funded by the W. K. Kellogg Foundation, under the direction of Kellogg officer Barbara Lee.

The program at University of Arizona was based in the College of Medicine. The College of Nursing, with the staff at Prescott Veterans Administration Hospital, prepared adult/geriatric nurse practitioners. Recruitment was nationwide as the need was recognized. In 1982 the Arizona State Board of Nursing approved the curriculum and agreed to certify the graduates. In the 5 years of that program's existence (1982–1987) 78 students were graduated and certified. ANA certification of Adult/Geriatric Nurse Practitioners in that program was achieved in 1984 (DeWalt & Welty, 2004). No such programs currently exist at University of Arizona. University of Colorado had a similar program.

Carole Deitrich, RN, MS, GNP, remains teaching in the GNP program at University of California, San Francisco (UCSF). She provided a brief history of that program. Prior to the GNP program at UCSF, a geriatric specialization was offered through the Core Pathways Program in Adult Primary Care. Carole Deitrich and Gay Kaplan were the first graduates of the primary care geriatric nursing component. In 1981, Barbara Byfield, PhD, RN, secured funding from the Kellogg Foundation to offer a GNP program through the Office of Continuing Education at UCSF, School of Nursing. At that time both the ANA and UCSF School of Nursing, advocated NP preparation at the master's level, but because few nursing home nurses held bachelor degrees, a temporary suspension of the requirement for a BSN was supported because of the critical need for skilled clinicians to work with older adults. The certificate program option at UCSF continued until 1986. Since that time it has been a master's degree program and recruitment to the GNP and GCNS programs has been robust in recent years. Job opportunities for nurses with these qualifications are increasingly available.

In 1975, six nursing schools were funded by the Department of Health, Education and Welfare to develop geriatric nurse practitioner graduate degree programs. These included: University of Massachusetts, Lowell (UML); University of Miami; University of Wisconsin; University of North Carolina; State University of New York, Buffalo; and Rush University. One of these, UML, was the first graduate GNP program in the nation. The others were certificate programs.

Conceptualization, curriculum, and program development for geriatric nurse practitioners leading to a graduate degree initially was accomplished by May Futrell. H. Terri Brower also studied and developed such programs shortly thereafter (see chapter 3). These pioneers led the way and were used, and are still used, as models by many programs across the nation. Now, graduate programs that offer specialization in geriatric/gerontologic advanced practice nursing are readily available.

Geriatric Nursing Excellence

Presently five graduate nursing programs for geriatric nursing practice that lead the nation in educational excellence are sponsored by the John A. Hartford Centers of Geriatric Nursing Excellence (HCGNE). These include University of California, San Francisco, Director Jeanie Kayser-Jones; University of Pennsylvania, Director Neville Strumpf; University of Arkansas, Director Claudia Beverly; Oregon Health Sciences University, Director Patricia Archbold; and University of Iowa, Director Meridean Maas. These Centers are conducted with the guidance of Claire Fagin, program director of the John A. Hartford "Building Academic Capacity Initiative." The goal of these centers is to prepare an exceptional cadre of geriatric nurse scientists who will provide the critically necessary leadership in teaching, research, and clinical practice. Nursing students are enrolled in master's and doctoral programs with a focus on geriatrics and gerontology. In addition, postdoctoral fellowships are available.

The John A. Hartford Foundation awards fellowships annually of $100,000 to 20 promising doctoral and postdoctoral students. At the HCGNE in San Francisco they encourage students from various ethnic groups, and have developed an interdisciplinary program designed to encourage doctoral students and fellows to do research residencies with nonnurse gerontologists (Kayser-Jones, 2004).

Distance Learning and Learning Online

More nursing faculty are offering online courses. Sarah Fishman, PhD, RN, GNP, of Florida Atlantic University, began offering several online gerontology courses in 1996. We believe she is truly the pioneer in online gerontology nursing graduate education. She has found many advantages: The student is more rested when in asynchronous learning; more diverse; more eager to learn; not falling asleep, or leaving early in graduate courses that seem always to be held from 6 to 10 p.m. after the students have already worked a 10- to 12-hour shift.

The courses she has taught include a graduate course, *Perspectives on Aging,* and two undergraduate gerontology certificate courses. The *Social Theories of Aging* does not require the usual clinical work but rather a holistic health interview with a client. Several requirements are built into the courses that enhance interaction with their peers and with her. They develop their philosophy of aging and define the reasons they are taking the course. Their photos, as well as Sarah's, are posted on Doc Sharing (a community bulletin board) and they have periodic chat rooms to clear up questions or problems. Students get instant feedback as Sarah goes to the course website four or five times daily. In addition, Sarah can respond even while "sailing on the high seas" (attested to by her e-mail to me recently while cruising with her husband, Bernie) as well as from her home office. A part of the student assignment is to formulate a question for each other student in the class. In addition, there is a pop quiz each week. Critical-thinking questions and a critique of research articles are required of each student. They do more work than in a traditional class but they receive a great deal more individual attention. Sarah says, "I love it and the students do, too. Evaluations have been very positive. Many students have been recruited into our GNP and Gerontology Certificate programs by taking these courses as electives. It's a wonderful way to spread the love of and knowledge about gerontological nursing" (Fishman, 2005). The main problems are technical; students who think they are computer literate but can't manage downloading, uploading, or doing a PowerPoint presentation.

The online classes that Luggen teaches have students from all over the country, including one who is the director of a graduate GNP program! "The first week, on the discussion board, I ask 'who are we?' and everyone shares a bit about themselves, including me with my picture and info about my parrots, Michael, Ed, and the farm. I have three PowerPoints on lab values for geriatrics, basic geriatric information, and they have book assignments. Each student can choose a case study topic they wish to lead. I push them to choose an area they know little about and want to learn more about. Each week one or two lead a case on the 'discussion board' where each student is graded on their contributions. Tests are online and students have a week to complete them. As we don't have a 2- to 3-hour deadline as there is in class, they can share as each person reads the contributions of the others. My comments are positive and encouraging. If I have a negative reaction, such as they haven't read the material, I e-mail them separately. I think they are pleased by the time they have to prepare, by the positive comments from me and the rest of the class, by the flexibility, and how much they learn" (Luggen, 2005).

Numerous online courses are now available to make geriatric knowledge and geriatric nursing best practices readily available; some are costly, some require membership in various organizations, and some are available at no cost. A description of a course reported by Williams and colleagues is featured in chapter 10 (Williams et al., 2005).

Experiential Learning

Helen Monea, RN, MS, began her teaching career as a child psychiatric nurse specialist (CPNS), and much of the strategy of psychiatric nursing for children, at that time, involved experiential learning. Teaching through experience involved less reliance on verbal abilities and more on feelings that occurred during various exercises. Monea found this worked particularly well in teaching elders as well as gerontology students. Elders were pleased to participate in exercises that did not create test anxiety and allowed them to venture into their own feelings and interpretations of events. Gerontology nursing students in graduate programs usually are immersed in intellectual exercises and often have not had guidance or opportunity in discovering "right brain" activities. They also seem to welcome the opportunity to express their creativity and participate in a different mode of learning. For some it creates anxiety in response to the unusual learning method. This may create resistance in those individuals who are excessively attached to intellectualization, have had little opportunity for innovative learning processes, or expect more teacher intervention.

Monea says, "Experiential learning is an opportunity to be an active learner in which you use your own senses in exploring your beliefs, attitudes, and feelings about aging topics and issues by using a variety of media as a catalyst to develop dialogue within yourself and/or with others. It is a self-journey in the learning process of integrating psychosocial aspects of aging with your intellectual self. It is NOT a sensitivity, nor therapy experience" (Monea, 1978).

Experiential learning is based in Gestalt theory. Gestalt is a German word meaning the whole. The whole is more than the sum of its parts, and forms a particular gestalt that cannot be determined by examining the distinct parts of an experience. Gestalt theorists ascribe to two major goals: self-awareness and self-responsibility. Both require that an individual becomes attuned to their entire being and mobilize their own resources. In its emphasis on awareness, a Gestalt philosophy is a way of life that creates balance, self-discovery and being in tune with one's self, and various modes for expressing feelings (Resnick, 1977).

Monea used experiential exercises in working with elders at the Jewish Home in San Francisco to teach them to counsel their peers. They responded enthusiastically and often wanted to extend the class beyond the allotted time. One particularly fruitful activity was the "clay experience." Clay was used to release unconscious feelings and thoughts as elders were encouraged to poke and squeeze, feel the texture and temperature, and sculpt whatever they felt. One man made a bowl and said, "This bowl is me. I am a happy bowl, deep and round, with a strong base and strong walls" (Monea, 1981, p. 8). There was a great deal of attention throughout the exercise to exploring the sensory impressions. In elders with sensory deficits, the touching exercises were particularly helpful.

In 1971, Helen Monea co-taught with Irene Burnside the class Psychosocial Aspects of Aging at the Ethel Percy Andrus Gerontology Center, University of Southern California, Los Angeles. This was a memorable class for all of us who attended. Again, the "clay experience" produced deep and intense reactions among us. The quality of very personal expression released feelings of which students had been unaware. Students were involved and discovered themselves in new ways.

Given the increasing development and use of online courses to teach nursing we anticipate that an increased use of experiential exercises will be built into courses to provide the personal responsiveness of students that may become lost in distance learning.

PUBLICATIONS

Books

To quote my 17-year-old granddaughter, Ashley Tanti, "Books are transportation for the mind" (Tanti, 2003).

Publications undergird every profession and are the voice of authority, influence, and discovery. As Laurie Gunter noted, the geriatric textbooks in 1959 were often simply mimeographed compilations of articles, mostly written by sociologists and psychologists. One of the first published books devoted to later life was that of Bernice Neugarten, *Middle Age and Aging,* published by the University of Chicago Press in 1968.

Although nurses contributed to several texts and a few articles about geriatric care published in the AJN, those devoted exclusively to geriatric nursing and written by nurses began with Burnside's, *Nursing and the Aged* in 1976 (see chapter 2).

The second round of geriatric nursing textbooks included *Toward Healthy Aging: Human Needs and Nursing Response* (Ebersole & Hess, 1981, now in its 6th edition). That year Mary Opal Wolanin and Linda Phillips wrote the classic text, *Confusion: Prevention and Care.* Both were Mosby publications. Yet, 25 years later, prevention of confusion and promotion of healthy aging are still major concerns among geriatric nurses.

Presently there are dozens of well-written geriatric nursing texts available for all levels of educational programs and as resources for practicing nurses. One might judge, to some extent, the quality of a program or an institution by the selection of texts available to the students and practitioners. I believe, in the present state of knowledge development, there is no one text that can provide sufficient information for the serious pursuit of geriatric nursing knowledge. Therefore, a carefully planned and readily available library of geriatric nursing texts is essential in every nursing program and facility serving the aged. Appropriate selections can be made by considering the qualifications of the authors, the intention of the text as stated in the preface, evidence that the set objectives have been met, and the readability of the text.

Springer Publishing Company: Ursula Springer

Many publishers began responding in the 1980s to the need for geriatric nursing textbooks; prominent among them were Mosby and McGraw-Hill, both since absorbed into larger corporate groups. However, no publishing house devoted as much attention and intense marketing efforts to geriatric nursing textbooks as the Springer Publishing Company. Much of that resulted from the interest and dedication of Dr. Ursula Springer, president and CEO of the company from 1970 until 2005. The publishing program includes a broad array of topics, yet major attention has been given to geriatrics and gerontology, especially to geriatric nursing. In addition to numerous texts, Springer produces the *Springer Series of Geriatric Nursing*. Encyclopedias, such as *The Encyclopedia of Elder Care*, and the *Encyclopedia of Aging*, 3rd ed. form invaluable references for geriatric nurses (www.springerpub.com). The company, established in 1950, has consistently produced high-quality texts addressing basic and current issues and concerns. The first *Encyclopedia of Aging* was published by the Springer Publishing Company in 1987, a landmark volume. Dr. Springer introduced it during the GSA meeting in San Diego at the Springer reception that has become an annual tradition. This was my first introduction to Ursula Springer.

Ursula grew up in Berlin, Germany, an active girl enjoying family support of her varied interests in reading, music, sports, and travel. "Our family in Berlin included, for several years in the 1930s, my grandfather. Interacting with him became my natural introduction to gerontology. I would write letters and articles that he dictated, earning 10 pfennig for each such service. I would buy 'necessities' like chocolate for him, and accompany him occasionally to a movie. I loved to hear his stories—many of the 19th century, about Bismarck, university life, and his work as a director of a Gymnasium (secondary school)" (Springer, March 5, 2005).

Ursula received her PhD in Comparative Education. This led to her professorship at Brooklyn College. She married Bernhard Springer, scion of a German publishing family, who in 1938 had emigrated from Berlin to New York. He established a medical publishing company in 1950 and published the first nursing book related to geriatric care with Doris Schwartz, *Cardiology for Nurses*.

When Bernhard died in 1970, Dr. Springer took over as owner and president and expanded the publishing company program to include nursing, psychology, gerontology, rehabilitation, and social work (Schorr, 2005). As a woman and a pioneering leader of an independent publishing house in this highly competitive business, her success has been phenomenal. In gratitude and recognition of her impact on geriatric nursing she was inducted as a Fellow into the American Academy of Nursing in 2001, and as a Fellow of the Gerontological Society of America in 2004. In addition, Springer gives an annual award in Geriatric Nursing at the Nurses Interest Group of GSA.

Journals

Scholarly journals are meant to keep professionals current on the latest information about their specialties. On average, manuscript publication in journals takes 6 months to a year. Books are less current, as usually 2 years elapse between writing and publishing.

A survey of nursing journal editors done in 2004 (Freda & Kearney, 2005) revealed information never before assessed. Few editors had received any formal education or assistance in learning the role. The vast majority (94%) simply learned on the job, whereas 46% were mentored by an experienced editor. Most noted that it took about 2 years for them to be comfortable with the job.

Numerous geriatric and gerontological journals are available to geriatric nurses in general and journals especially intended for those geriatric nurses in subspecialties. Many of the specialty groups publish their own journals, which are distributed to all members as a benefit of membership.

The first journal devoted to the geriatric nursing specialty, the *Journal of Gerontological Nursing*, was published by Slack in 1974. Edna Stilwell was the first editor. Kathleen (Kitty) Buckwalter is the current editor. Her dynamic contributions to the journal are discussed in chapter 3. The *Geriatric Nursing Journal*, published by *AJN*, was launched in 1980 with Cynthia Kelly as the first editor. In 1991 *Geriatric Nursing* was acquired by Mosby. I then became (and continued to be) the editor through 2005. Barbara Resnick (discussed in chapter 3) assumed the editorship in 2006.

Edna Stilwell: Founding Editor of the Journal of Gerontological Nursing

Edna Stilwell is probably best known as the founding editor of the first geriatric nursing journal, and for almost 25 years continued to edit *The Journal of Gerontological Nursing*. Her remarkable nursing history reveals much more. Edna was involved in many "firsts." In the Maryland area she established the Maryland Geriatric Nurses interest group; the Annapolis Agency on Aging; the Maryland Gerontological Association; and the University of Maryland Master's Program in Gerontological Nursing. On a national level, she served on the ANA first certification committee for geriatric nursing, the Standards of Practice Committee, and the Division of Gerontological Nursing. In addition to her research related to nurse's preferences toward working with older adults, she taught many courses at the undergraduate and graduate level, chaired or served on at least 20 thesis/dissertation committees, and designed and taught continuing education courses. Her innovations as editor, writer, and teacher have increased the knowledge of nurses in the care of elders and her influence continues to compound because of these activities.

Edna's personal history is fascinating. In a recent visit to her home town, Lenoir City, Tennessee, she visited the cemetery to place flowers on her parents' graves and viewed the gravestones of many of her relatives. She reflected on their lives and the positive images of aging they gave her. She lived with her grandparents when they were in their 80s and was greatly influenced by them. The elders of the family seldom complained. They faced their crises, disappointments, and unexpected deaths with fortitude. They had an acceptance of whatever came along and lived in the moment, depending on each other. Loyalty was extremely important to them. The women shared in work and social events, and were supportive and communicative. The social and spiritual life centered around the church. There was much eating and singing but no profanity, smoking, or drinking. Their life style was basic, naturally healthy, and moderate. From this background, Edna grew to value wholesome living and a simple lifestyle.

Her nursing career began in high school when she and her sister, Helen Forgione, were in a work study program and worked in a local hospital. She also served as a reporter for her high school newspaper and thus was introduced to the joys of publishing.

Edna did her undergraduate work at Knoxville General Hospital, the University of Tennessee, and the University of Maryland. She was concerned about the lack of interest in the frail elderly, especially toward rehabilitation potential; therefore, in 1960 she decided to specialize in the care of older adults. During the following decade she sought out nurses in the geriatric field and was especially grateful to Mary Opal Wolanin and Terry Fulmer because they made her realize she was not alone in her zeal to make geriatric nursing a recognized specialty. Colleagues such as Irene Burnside, Priscilla Ebersole, Virginia Stone, Myrtle Irene Brown, Doris Schwartz, Sr. Rose Therese Bahr, Ella Kick, and Dorothy Moses also were inspirational. She followed every lead she could to increase her knowledge and went to the University of Maryland to work on a master's degree. Although they didn't have a specialty program at that time, she was allowed to tailor her courses toward health care of older adults. Now, she notes, there are many experts and resources available and she discovered in 2004 there were 34,000 sites on the Internet for gerontological nursing.

My recollection of Edna goes back to 1981 at an ANA meeting in which I announced the film I would be showing later, *Geriatric Nurse Practitioners: The New Professionals.* In 1981 ANA had some trepidation about these new professionals and only two people came to the showing. Edna was one of them and I will be forever grateful to her!

Cynthia Kelly: Founding Editor of the Geriatric Nursing Journal

Cynthia Kelly has been a hard act to follow. Her journalistic expertise, as shown in the formative years of the *Geriatric Nursing Journal,* is outstanding. There have been excellent editors in the interim but when I began, in 1991, I was a total neophyte to the journalistic trade. I consulted Cynthia frequently and she always provided pertinent comments and guidance. Early on, she wrote, "Your plans for the journal sound ambitious and interesting. My only regret is that you are giving the editorial to others. A strong editorial by the editor in each issue is, I believe, the best means to develop the magazine's character and point of view. Obviously hard work, but worth it. Otherwise, the editorial is apt to become more of a news item. Pat Lewis's editorials in *Nursing Outlook,* Thelma's (Schorr) in *AJN,* and Barb Schutt's in *AJN* are classics" (Kelly, 1994). I took that advice seriously and have since tried to make the editorial carry some sort of significant message.

I became aware of Cynthia Kelly because of Mary Opal Wolanin and their longstanding friendship. Following her retirement from the publishing world, Cynthia joined the Peace Corps and was sent to the island of Chuuk, Federated States of Micronesia. For as long as I have known her, Cynthia has been wiry and sturdy but certainly could not afford to lose weight. I learned that Mary Opal was sending certain high caloric nutritional foods to Cynthia to supplement her island diet. I also sent a package and thus began a fascinating correspondence.

Excerpts from her personal history, handwritten by Cynthia Kelly from Wene, Chuuk, December 12, 1990:

"Living with a great aunt and a grandfather from my birth to their deaths, when I was 8 and 14, respectively, impressed me with their enormous differences. Aunt Lizzie, physically frail but energetic, independent, and a talented seamstress, was vitally interested in everything. Gramp was physically strong but devoid of interests, content to read only the news headlines, look out the window, and exchange comments with a weekly visitor about how the younger generation was surely going to the dogs. These two taught me that old people are not alike."

"A neighbor in her 80s told fascinating tales of her life as a whaling ship captain's wife. Tall, white-haired, and always picture-perfect with a black velvet band around her neck, she seemed happy, serene. Her spinster daughter was neurasthenic, had ulcers, made many doctor visits, and felt 'played out.' Her life, spent caring for her mother, seemed joyless. Another mother–daughter pair impressed me the same way; spunky older woman, 'put upon' daughter. My mother was bitter that she had her father-in-law (Gramp) with her all but 2 years of her married life. The message I got, at 12 or so, was that three generations could not live harmoniously under one roof."

"My first experiences with older adults as a student nurse were more rewarding than clinical experiences with younger adults but I certainly did not plan to specialize in geriatric nursing."

"By the 1970s I knew that old age need not relegate elders to the senseless, sexless, useless category so I was delighted when offered the editorship of *Geriatric Nursing.* This seemed a great opportunity to help change the stereotyping; hence I launched '70+ *and Going Strong.'* Hardly clinical nursing but the best available avenue at my age to contribute to elders and their nurses. . . . My proudest accomplishment in gerontic nursing was persuading Mary Opal Wolanin, Doris Schwartz, Carole Chenitz, and Mary Ann Bartol Yeterian to join *GN's* advisory panel" (Kelly, 1990). Cynthia was a living example of 70+ and going strong.

In her letters she described the people, their customs, and basic existence. Elders were anyone over 45 years old; she was the oldest person on the island of Parem. She was unexpectedly sent home in 1991 because of a dangerous living situation.

In August 1992 an apartment at Foulkeways, a Friends retirement center, became available and Cynthia moved there, where she resided until her death in June, 2005. She had been very active, producing the *Foulkeways Monthly Bulletin,* the *Foulkeways Literary Supplement,* and been involved in many other projects. In addition, she enjoyed singing in the Gwynedd Square Presbyterian Church (Fig. 7.2).

Mentorship in Publishing

Dr. Ann Luggen says, "I feel it is an essential role for those of us who have been professionally involved in geriatrics long enough to be mentors. I have helped many young and older nurses in gerontology to publish, often for the first time. They have proudly seen their work published in

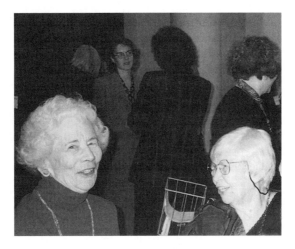

FIGURE 7.2 Cynthia Kelly and Doris Schwartz.

Geriatric Nursing, Advance, and in book chapters. I believe this brings a new level of confidence and professionalism to clinicians who have feared to write and perhaps fail" (Luggen, 2005, p. 1).

CONCLUSION

Making gerontological nursing available through the printed word has been a major accomplishment of gerontological nurses within the last quarter century. Speaking with our own voices, conveying the most current knowledge and the most reliable research, and making available the latest information about best practices, have consumed a major portion of the energies of the nurses featured in this text. The present speed of accessibility and information overload presents a new challenge for geriatric and gerontological nurses. We must thoughtfully consider the knowledge available, wade through the quagmire, and convey only the most reliable.

CHAPTER EIGHT

Nursing Research and Geriatric Care

The greatly increased number of nurses with doctoral preparation and the numerous individuals receiving post doctoral fellowships and research funding for geriatric nursing studies has had a marked influence on the progress of geriatric care and bringing research into practice. The application of best practices has arisen from this research. However, we must credit the earliest geriatric nurse pioneers who seldom had doctoral preparation yet tested their clinical ideas, revised the delivery of care as they saw problems, and progressed in effectiveness, although their studies were neither elegant nor sophisticated. These are the pioneer researchers.

They instinctively began focusing their care on the major geriatric syndromes: instability, immobility, intellectual impairment, and incontinence (Isaacs, 1977). Bernita Steffl has dubbed these "serendipitous researchers" (Steffl, 2005).

Davis (1971) described the goals of geriatric nursing up to the midyears of the last century as quite simple: "(a) keep the aged person fed, keep him safe, keep him quiet, keep him clean, and keep him free from pain (most likely in that order); and (b) follow whatever the doctor prescribes, whenever medical supervision was available to give the orders" (p. 10). When few were interested in or even aware of the unique concerns of elders, the pioneer researchers were challenging the existing paradigm by asking the questions and trying to find the solution, thus providing the foundation for what we accept and study today as best practices in geriatric nursing. Questions such as:

- Why are we tying old people down in our nursing homes and hospitals in the United States? (Schwartz, Strumpf, & Evans)
- What can be done to help little old ladies who wet their pants? (Brink, Colling, & Wells)

- What is this syndrome labeled confusion? (Wolanin)
- How can we provide more humane and dignified care to people with memory problems? (Buckwalter & Wolanin)
- What are the therapeutic benefits of reminiscence and life review? (Burnside, Ebersole, & Haight)
- What are the mental health needs of elders and what are approaches that enhance emotional well-being? (Buckwalter, Harper, & Wykle)
- Could the CNS and NP make a difference in nursing homes and would nursing homes be a site for the education of nursing students to improve practice, teaching, and research? (Lynaugh, Mezey, Wykle, et al.)

Early geriatric nursing research studies focused largely on attitudes toward the elderly. Futrell and Jones's classic study (1977) found that social workers generally had a more positive attitude toward the aged; nurses came in second and physicians third. In 1981 Brower also studied nurses' attitudes toward older people. There were many other similar studies. Whereas gerontologists and psychologists in that era were focused on cognitive decline, nurses were aware that attitudes of professionals significantly affected the care they provided.

Sarah Fishman reports on a student paper that addressed the integration of research and practice as a fundamental need in nurse practitioner programs. Because of the intensity of nurse practitioner programs, the requirement of a scholarly paper or thesis is often omitted from the expectation of students. Forbes (2005) defends and explains the need for such a requirement. In 1996, the NLN noted there is the need for evidence of a scholarly work in all master's degree programs. This is described as an area of inquiry that is important, meaningful, and professionally relevant. This is vital to the evolution of evidence-based practice and significant contributions to the profession.

Published Research Volumes

A notable amount of research into the common conditions of elders has been completed in the last two decades. These have been summarized, categorized, and synthesized in volume 20 of the *Annual Review of Nursing Research* (Fitzpatrick, 2002). Common conditions of elders that are the focus of Part I in the volume include: maintaining and improving physical function; pressure ulcer prevention and management; pain in older adults; and interventions to support persons with irreversible dementia. Part II deals with settings for elder care and of particular significance is Naylor's transitional care investigation. It is noted in Part II that little research has been done on end of life (EOL) care in nursing homes and assisted living facilities. Part III is focused on social, scientific, and political trends that have influenced the development of the geriatric nursing specialty. Research into telehealth interventions is of increasing importance. Part IV emphasizes some neglected areas in geriatric nursing research, specifically hearing impairment and elder mistreatment.

The *Annual Review of Nursing Research,* volumes 18 and 19 (also published by Springer), although not devoted specifically to geriatric research, addressed research into chronic illness and women's health. Both of these topics are closely related to geriatric nursing research. Archbold, Stewart, and Lyons (2002) look back at significant research that has set the stage for future directions in gerontological nursing research. It is suggested by those authors that future gerontological nursing research can be strengthened by larger sample sizes, better conceptualizations, longitudinal research designs, and more attention to testing interventions. Clearly, as has been suggested, the key to valid research findings is based on interdisciplinary approaches.

Doris Schwartz Gerontological Nursing Research Awards

Presently, recognition is given to gerontological nurse researchers at the Gerontological Society of America (GSA) convention during the Nurses' Interest Group annual meeting of the GSA. The Doris Schwartz Gerontological Nursing Research Award recognizes geriatric nurse researchers nationally and internationally. It was established in 1998 to honor Doris Schwartz, a true pioneer in geriatric nursing. Her accomplishments are discussed in chapter 2.

This award, perhaps the most prestigious in geriatric nursing, has been bestowed on the following individuals:

- 1998: Cornelia Beck (chapter 4)
- 1999: Jeanie Kayser-Jones (chapter 3)
- 2000: May Wykle (chapter 3)
- 2001: Lois Evans and Neville Strumpf (chapter 3)
- 2002: Thelma Wells (chapter 3)
- 2003: Ann Whall (chapter 3)
- 2004: Pat Archbold
- 2005: Charlene Harrington

VETERANS ASSOCIATION MEDICAL CENTERS

Much of the earliest geriatric research can be traced back to the Veterans Administration Medical Centers (VAMCs). The captive subjects, the great preponderance being males with some disabilities or chronic health problems, provided readily accessible research participants. Those who were institutionalized found that their involvement in research studies added variety to their daily existence. In addition, most VAMCs were affiliated with universities; therefore, they became training grounds for clinicians and clinical research investigators. We credit the VAMCs with a great deal of the early research in aging.

Vernice Ferguson

Vernice Ferguson, RN, MA, FAAN, FRCN, served for 12 years as the Assistant Chief Medical Director for Nursing Programs in the Department of Veterans Affairs. From 1993 to 1996 she was the Senior Fellow at the University of Pennsylvania School of Nursing (Penn Nursing). She currently serves as a member of the University of Pennsylvania School of Nursing Board of Overseers, and held the Fagin Family Chair in Cultural Diversity at Penn Nursing from 1993 to 1997.

Ms. Ferguson is the recipient of eight honorary doctorates and two fellowships, one in physics and the other in alcohol studies. She is an Honorary Fellow in the Royal College of Nursing of the United Kingdom, the second American nurse so honored, following the late Virginia Henderson. In 2002, Vernice was selected as a "Living Legend" by the American Academy of Nursing, and in 2004, was honored by the National Academies of Science, Engineering, and Medicine (http//nursing.cua.edu/news/ferguson2.cfm, April 20, 2005).

Her interest in and support of nursing research has been consistent throughout her career.

A recent experience at the San Francisco VAMC, Ft. Miley, was an eye opener. Research is not only conducted by affiliated universities in the area but the clinical staff conduct numerous research studies with the guidance and encouragement of Martha Buffum, DNSc, APRN, BC, CS, director of Nursing Research. These are presented annually to the staff and others in the community who are interested. The current 10th Annual Nursing Research Day included topics such as: preoperative teaching for deep brain stimulation surgery; symptom trajectory and quality of life after brachytherapy for prostate cancer; music intervention to reduce anxiety before vascular angiography procedures; comparison of two pain assessment tools for the cognitively impaired; factors associated with resource use after discharge from psychiatric intensive care; retention of experienced staff nurses; complementary/holistic care survey; aromatherapy for the treatment of postoperative nausea and vomiting, intervention to reduce staff nurse stress; and many others. Clearly, this is an example of VAMC nursing research that provides a unique opportunity for nurses in practice to conduct research that directly influences patient care (San Francisco VAMC, 2005).

NATIONAL INSTITUTE FOR NURSING RESEARCH

The National Institute for Nursing Research (NINR), a division of the Department of Health and Human Services (DHHS), was established as the National Center for Nursing Research (NCNR) in 1986. The impetus for establishing the NCNR came from studies by the Institute of Medicine (IOM) and the National Institutes of Health (NIH) recommending that nursing research be included in the mainstream of biomedical and behavioral science. In 1993 the NCNR was elevated to the status of an NIH Institute and established as the NINR (http://.nih.gov/ninr/about/history.html).

The mission of the NINR is to promote and support clinical and basic research on the care of individuals across the life span, including the underserved, minorities, and families within community-based settings. The NINR work group, headed by Dr. Patricia A. Grady, Director of NINR since 1995 and chair of the National Advisory Council for Nursing Research, provides updates on nursing research and disseminates information through mailings, press conferences and on the website. Nurses from all disciplines regard the NINR Strategic Plan as a road map for future nursing research (http.ninr.nih.gov/ninr/research, March 17, 2005).

The influence of the NINR on geriatric research has been particularly notable in studies of sleep, restraints, infection, confusion, urinary incontinence, hospice and most recently EOL care.

Patricia Archbold, DNSc, RN, FAAN, has been a key participant in formulating plans for the future goals of the NINR. Dr. Archbold is the Elnora E. Thomson Distinguished Professor of Nursing at the Oregon Health Sciences University, director of the Hartford Center of Geriatric Nursing Excellence, and an adjunct investigator at the Center for Health Research at Kaiser Permanente Medical Centers in Portland, Oregon. Her research on family caregiving for frail older people has been funded by the NINR and is directed toward developing and evaluating home health interventions for this population. She has served as a member of two Institute of Medicine Committees and is a member of the National Advisory Council for Nursing Research, which advises the NINR. She is a Fellow of the Gerontological Society of America and the American Academy of Nursing. Among her honors are the Helen Nahm Award from the School of Nursing, University of California, San Francisco; the Distinguished Research Lectureship of the Western Society for Research in Nursing; Outstanding Alumni Award, Columbia University School of Nursing; Charles Dolen Hatfield Award, Alzheimer's Association; Gerontological Nursing Research Award, Western Institute of Nursing; and the Doris Schwartz Gerontological Nursing Research Award as mentioned earlier. She has served as advisor to the World Health Organization (WHO) on the subject of nursing research in primary care (http://ninr.nih.gov/ninr/research/vol3/Biosketch.html, March 17, 2005).

Another person of influence in the NINR is Nancy Bergstrom, PhD, RN, FAAN, of University of Nebraska Medical Center in Omaha. She is actively involved in research related to nutrition and the etiology of pressure sores, and has been instrumental in the testing and further development of the Braden Scale for Predicting Pressure Sore Risk. She has received research grants from the NCNR, NIH, and the Division of Nursing at the Health Resources and Services Administration (HRSA). She has many publications and awards to her credit; most notably the Jessie M. Scott Award of the American Nurses Association for demonstrating the interdependence of nursing education, nursing practice, and nursing research.

THE NATIONAL INSTITUTE ON AGING

In 1974, the National Institute on Aging (NIA) was established in the National Institutes of Health (NIH). Robert Butler, MD, was appointed the first director. The agency was poorly funded and in 1975 Dr. Butler found that in the whole NIH only 12 grants were funded to study the aging brain. He decided that the study of Alzheimer's disease and related dementias (ADRD) must be among the major national research priorities. Dr. Robert Katzman, in 1976, described Alzheimer's disease (AD) as a major public health problem. By 1984, T. Franklin Williams, MD, the second director of the NIA, established the Office of Alzheimer's Research at the NIA and Alzheimer's disease research was declared the highest research priority. Large clinical trials of cholinesterase inhibitors soon were being conducted as well as other studies (Alzheimer's Disease Education and Referral Center, 2004 to 2005). However, it was nurses who began investigating ways to care for those who were afflicted.

RESEARCH CONTRIBUTIONS OF NATIONAL SIGNIFICANCE BY GERIATRIC NURSES

Kathleen (Kitty) Buckwalter, PhD, RN, FAAN, is discussed in chapter 4, but should be mentioned here as a member of the National Advisory Council on Aging, which advises the National Institute on Aging (NIA), a component of the National Institutes of Health. She, Joanne Rader, Ann Whall, and many other nurse researchers have added to the knowledge needed to provide more humanistic, patient-centered care for Alzheimer's patients.

Freida Butler, PhD, RN, FAAN, formerly of Howard University School of Nursing, has served as consultant to numerous organizations, including the American Public Health Association, the Senate Special Committee on Aging, and the National Center on Black Aging. Her research interests have included behavioral problems of nursing home residents, and the effects of neuroleptic medications on these behaviors. Dr. Butler was founder of a nurse-managed wellness center for minority elderly.

Margaret F. Dimond, PhD, RN, FAAN, has investigated the effects of the various transitions commonly experienced by older adults, including residential relocation, bereavement, environmental factors, and the quality of care in nursing homes. She is a member of the Human Development and Aging Study Section in the Division of Research Grants at the National Institutes of Health.

Marquis (Mark) Foreman has focused his research for more than 20 years on the prevention, recognition, and management of delirium in elders. His first investigation of the literature was on how to prevent or treat acute confusion (Foreman, 1984).

An early and key accomplishment was the result of working with Christine K. Cassel and Peter Pompei on a project funded by the John A. Hartford Foundation in the late 1980s to examine early identification and management of delirium in older hospitalized patients. Dr. Foreman was on one of six projects funded and was one of three with a nurse co-principal investigator: Yale with Terry Fulmer; the University Hospitals of Cleveland with Denise Kresevic; and the University of Chicago with Mark Foreman. This was the first John A. Hartford Foundation grant to include nurse co-investigators. This initiative was followed by the NICHE initiatives (I and II), and the numerous other contemporary nursing initiatives supported by the Hartford Foundation. Research conducted by Mark, and that collaborating with other researchers, such as Sharon Inouye, Donna Fick, and Koen Milisen, is contributing to a better understanding of who is at risk for delirium, how to prevent it from occurring, and how to better manage it when it does occur. Mark continues to champion prevention of delirium and improved hospital care for older patients. Those that did not include a nurse co-investigator were: St. Mary's Hospital affiliated with University of Wisconsin-Madison; Palo Alto Veterans Affairs Medical Center; and Cedars of Sinai Medical Center.

Charlene Harrington, PhD, RN, FAAN, has focused her research primarily on public policies in long-term care at the state and federal level. In a prior position as Deputy Director of Licensing and Certification at the California State Department of Health in Sacramento, she served as principal investigator on several large research projects addressing state long-term care policies, supply, access, use, and social health maintenance organizations. Her work resulted in a data base that is in great demand nationally.

Dr. Ann Horgas, University of Florida, Gainesville, has focused much of her research on pain assessment in nursing home residents, especially those with dementia. She is a Fellow of the Gerontological Society of America. Dr. Horgas has earned several awards, among them the Southern Nursing Research Society Hartford Institute Geriatric Nursing Award, the Springer Award for Geriatric/Gerontological Nursing, and the Nightingale Award for Excellence in Nursing Research.

Diane K. Kjervik, JD, RN, FAAN, has been a member of the National Advisory Council for Nursing Research that advises the National Center for Nursing Research (NCNR). Her chief interest is in mental health nursing and the law. Her research projects have addressed informed consent, inequality in service delivery, and incompetency assessment for older persons. She has been a member of panels to set research priorities on medical malpractice for the Agency for Health Care Policy and Research (AHCPR) and ethics for the NCNR.

May L. Wykle, PhD, RN, FAAN, is discussed in chapter 4. Her research focuses on care of the aging, self-care, care in psychiatric settings, and caregiving of African-American and white families. She was a member of the Institute of Medicine Committee to study nursing home regulations; the National Institutes of Health Consensus Panel on Geriatric Assessment; and a research review committee of the National Institute on Aging.

PRIVATE NONPROFIT FOUNDATIONS

One must credit the support of nonprofit foundations for a great deal of the geriatric nursing research that has substantially affected geriatric and gerontologic nursing practice.

The W. K. Kellogg Foundation

The W. K. Kellogg Foundation, located in Battle Creek, Michigan, was established in 1930 by Will Keith Kellogg, the cereal entrepreneur. Their slogan is "to help people help themselves." In 1996 it was ranked the second largest private foundation in the United States.

Two Projects of National Significance

The W. K. Kellogg Foundation, through the advocacy of Barbara Lee, Nursing Project Officer, granted funds to the Mountain States Health Corporation (MSHC), Boise, Idaho, to recruit nurses from sponsoring nursing homes and to return them to GNP positions in the sponsoring facilities. The impact of this program was investigated by Robert Kane, then of the Rand Corporation and now at University of Minnesota. It was found that the GNPs remained in long-term positions that implemented the model for a median of 4½ years, demonstrating the success of the MSHC program in introducing and retaining GNPs in nursing homes.

The W. K. Kellogg Foundation also supported the Community College-Nursing Home Partnership model that began in Florida and has spread across the United States. Verle Waters, MA, RN, Dean Emerita, Ohlone College, Fremont, California, was the project consultant. Essential factors in these programs were to influence the redirection of associate degree nursing education to include active participation in long-term care settings and develop nursing potential in long-term care settings. The active participation of nursing home staff with community college faculty was assiduously cultivated. Factors that created this partnership included: collaborative planning, pragmatic goal setting, clear communication, and mutual respect (Mengel, Simson, Sherman, & Waters, 1990).

In 1986, six associate degree in nursing programs were funded to initiate the project. The initial programs were at Community College of Philadelphia; Ohlone College, Fremont, California; Shoreline Community College, Seattle, Washington; Triton College, River Grove, Illinois; Valencia Community College, Orlando, Florida; and Weber State University School of Allied Sciences, Ogden, Utah. Ms. Carignan surveyed the program participants in 1989. Results showed improved leadership and management skills, improved assessment skills, improved documentation, and improved attitudes (Carignan, 1992).

The Robert Wood Johnson Foundation

The Robert Wood Johnson Foundation, located in Princeton, New Jersey, was established in 1972 and is the largest philanthropy devoted exclusively to health and health care in the United States. The founder's, Robert Wood Johnson, life work lives on with the foundation that bears his name (www.rwjf.org/about/index.jhtml, January 24, 2005). Linda Aiken has been an advocate for nursing studies funded by the Robert Wood Johnson Foundation.

The Robert Wood Johnson Foundation concentrates its grant making in four goal areas: access to quality health care at reasonable cost; quality care and support for people with chronic health conditions; promotion of healthy communities and life styles; and reducing the personal, social, and economic harm of substance abuse (www.rwjf.org, January 10, 2005).

The Teaching Nursing Home Project

The Robert Wood Johnson Foundation Teaching Nursing Home Program was designed by Dr. Linda Aiken. The idea evolved from her American Academy of Nursing presidential address in 1980 (as did the idea for the Magnet Recognition Program) (Aiken, 1981). Problems in nursing homes, public hospitals, and VAMC hospitals had been ameliorated successfully by affiliation with medical schools. Linda thought a similar strategy of affiliation with nursing schools would have a similar beneficial effect on the quality of nursing home care. She proposed a 5-year multisite national initiative that was funded by the Robert Wood Johnson Foundation. Mathy Mezey and Joan Lynaugh at the University of Pennsylvania School of Nursing, Philadelphia, were appointed to administer the national program. A key feature of the program was the introduction of geriatric nurse practitioners. Ultimately the evaluation of the Teaching Nursing Home Program showed that the program improved the quality of life and functional status for nursing home residents and reduced hospitalizations (Aiken, 2005).

The National Hospice Study

In the early 1980s Dr. Aiken was instrumental in creating a public/private partnership between the Robert Wood Johnson Foundation and the Health Care Financing Administration (now the CMA) to commission a national hospice study. The findings showed better symptom control and patient satisfaction of those under hospice care and resulted in approval by Medicare of a hospice benefit (Aiken, 1986).

The John A. Hartford Foundation

The John A. Hartford Foundation, Inc., of New York, is a private philanthropy established in 1929 by John A. Hartford. Mr. Hartford and his brother, George L. Hartford, both former chief executives of the Great Atlantic and Pacific Tea Company, left the bulk of their estates to the foundation on their deaths in the 1950s. Prior to 1979, the foundation primarily supported clinically oriented biomedical research projects. Subsequently, it focused its support on improving the quality and financing of health care and enhancing the capacity of the health care system to accommodate the nation's growing elderly population. Since 1995 the foundation has focused extensively on enhancing the nation's capacity to provide effective and affordable care to its growing older adult population through grant making related to enhancing geriatric research and training of physicians, nurses, and social workers, and integrating and improving health services for older adults (www.hgni.org, February 20, 2005). The John A. Hartford Foundation commitment of 35 million dollars to supporting the development of geriatric nursing has had immense influence throughout the nation.

The Atlantic Philanthropies (USA) Inc.

The Atlantic Philanthropies (USA) Inc. project involves partnering with ANA through the American Nurses Foundation (ANF), the American Nurses Credentialing Center (ANCC), and the John A. Hartford Foundation Institute for Geriatric Nursing, New York University, with an investment of $5 million, to promote the Nurse Competency in Aging Program's (the ANA-SNAPG), alliances. The Steinhard School of Education and the School of Nursing are working with specialty nursing associations to incorporate a geriatric presence and enhance member competencies in aging (www.GeroNurseOnline.org). The *AJN* series on aging, edited by Diana Mason, is a part of the project that brings information to nurses who will then gain exposure to current aspects of geriatric care.

Additional Foundations

The Henry J. Kaiser Family Foundation funded studies related to efficacy of geriatric case managers, and medication usage among elders, and has a large body of current health statistics (www.kff.org).

The William R. Hearst Foundation has set up endowments for several scholarships for master's students in geriatric nursing in several schools of nursing.

The Retirement Research Foundation was established by John D. McArthur and endowed in 1978. The foundation invests approximately $9 million each year to support efforts that enable elders to maintain independent living, improve the quality of care in nursing homes, use the wisdom and experience of older adults to promote community involvement, and increase understanding of the aging process and age-association diseases (www.rrf.org/overview).

Many other foundations have funded projects important to progress in gerontological nursing research. Further information about nonprofit foundations interested in geriatric nursing can be found at the Foundation Center (fconline.fdncenter.org) and the Foundation Directory (fdncenter.org/funders).

CURRENT RESEARCH IN GERIATRIC NURSING

Dr. Barbara Resnick

Dr. Barbara Resnick is currently one of the very prolific geriatric nurse clinical researchers. Her research interests focus on care of the older adult and include health promotion and disease prevention; outcomes after rehabilitation, functional performance, a special focus on motivation related to functional activities and exercise behavior, testing outcomes of restorative care nursing programs, and other innovative long-term care projects. Currently Dr. Resnick has an RO1 from the National Institute of Aging to test the effectiveness of the Exercise Plus Program in older adults post hip fracture, and a second RO1 from AHRQ to test the effectiveness of a restorative care nursing program in long-term care. She is also principal investigator on a behavior change consortium challenge grant exploring measurement of physical activity among older adults, and principal investigator and co-investigator on numerous other projects related to health promotion, particularly physical activity and exercise in older adults (Resnick, 2005). Resnick reports the launching of a Center for Research Excellence—the Center for Occupational and Environmental Health and Justice at the University of Maryland. The goal is to compile research directed at preventing occupational and environmental causes of illness and injury, which is of great concern to nurses.

Dr. Cornelia Beck

Dr. Beck is conducting both clinical and health services research in older adults with cognitive impairment (CI). In her clinical research, she is concentrating on three conditions: disruptive behaviors, sleep disturbance, and pain. Currently, elders who suffer from these conditions are more likely to become institutionalized and receive pharmacologic treatments, which often have detrimental side effects. Her long-term goal is to develop and test nonpharmacologic treatments to delay or prevent institutionalization and minimize the need for pharmacologic treatments. In her health services research, Dr. Beck is studying caregiving issues in institutions and in the home care of the 3 million older adults who have CI and live in the community. Dr. Beck also has focused on availability and accessibility of services to diagnose and treat memory-related disorders, particularly in African American and rural older adults, two underserved populations that are prevalent in Arkansas.

At the National Conference of Gerontological Nurse Practitioners (NCGNP) in 2002, Dr. Beck presented an intriguing correlation of the continuous cycle of nursing research and nursing practice by using the Mobius strip to illustrate the interdependence. The Mobius strip was co-discovered by German mathematicians, August Ferdinand Mobius and Johann Benedict. Unlike Euclidean geometry, in which objects have one surface, the Mobius strip has a continuously twisting surface. It has served as the basis of continuous-loop recording tapes and the universal recycling symbol created by Gary Anderson (Jones & Powell, 1999) (Figs. 8.1, 8.2, and 8.3).

FIGURE 8.1 Recycling symbol.

Dr. Beck created a Mobius strip (see Fig. 8.2) showing that geriatric nursing practice and research represent a continuous process in which the geriatric nurse practitioner has a pivotal role. For instance, Crowther, Maroulis, Shafer-Winter, and Hader (2002) reported that a Heart Failure Center directed by physicians and run be an advanced practice nurse with a broad cardiology background better served patients with heart failure and reduced the high rate of hospital admission, readmissions, and the high cost of care. Space was allocated for the outpatient

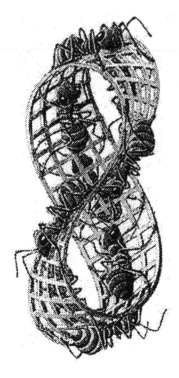

FIGURE 8.2 Mobius strip.

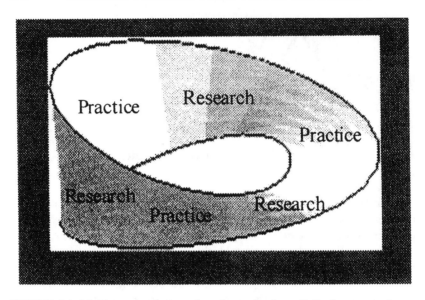

FIGURE 8.3 Mobius strip of research and practice from C. Beck presentation.

center, which included an office, an examination room, and a treatment room, at Jersey Shore Medical Center. The advanced practice nurse performed physical assessments and provided treatment based on research findings from the literature, and made follow-up telephone calls. In the first 6 months, lengths of stay decreased from 8.4 to 6.5 days for a cost savings of more than $360,000. The first full year of operation led to continued decreases in lengths of stay and savings of $250,000 more. Other findings showed that recidivism dropped from 33% to 20% or less and out patients indicated a 33% improvement in functional status and physical endurance, and a 25% improvement in quality of life. Other studies have reported similar findings for geriatric nurse practitioner/physician teams. The integration of research and practice demonstrates the Mobius strip in action.

Graham McDougall

Graham McDougall, PhD, RN, FAAN, has devoted much of his research to the study of CI, age-associated memory impairment (AAMI) and the study of memory enhancement techniques. Cognitive decline is a major concern of elders, the middle-aged, and clinicians. Graham's research is designed to abate older adult's memory loss and shift the perception that it is inevitable as one ages. The timing, depth, and breadth of his research has had great influence. Evidence of the impact of his work began with publication in the *Nurse Practitioner Journal* in 1990 and *Applied Nursing Research* in 1993. Since that time he has contributed numerous articles, book chapters, and presentations focused on cognition and mental health of the aged; and has been given extensive media coverage, awards, and accolades. Presently, he has a 5-year grant from the National Institutes of Aging, Mental Health and Nursing Research to test the Cognitive-Behavioral Model of Everyday Memory (CBMEM) with healthy older adults to determine the efficacy of mentally stimulating activities in preventing cognitive decline. This includes the effects of physical, emotional, and control beliefs as they affect subjective and objective memory performance in community dwelling elders. The studies were designed to moderate adults' memory loss complaints and evaluate the intervention on everyday function. The self-efficacy paradigm frames the interrelationship between subjective and objective memory function in a health promotion model rather than inevitable decrement and loss. We expect these studies will have important ramifications on the future understanding of cognitive function.

Mary Naylor

With the support of the Alzheimer's Association, the Marian S. Ware Alzheimer Program, and the National Institutes of Aging, Dr. Mary Naylor and her team currently are investigating interventions of varying intensities, nurse staffing, and skill set requirements to improve the care management and coordination of cognitively impaired elders and their caregivers during the challenging transition from hospital to home. In January 2005, Mary assumed the leadership role in the University of Pennsylvania's Center for Interdisciplinary Geriatric Health Care Research. This is one of only five such centers in the U.S. funded by RAND and the John A. Hartford Foundation with the primary goals of advancing the science in geriatric intervention research by bringing together scholars from nursing, medicine, social work, and other disciplines. They also provide mentorship and interdisciplinary research opportunities for students and junior faculty.

RESEARCH NEEDED

Dr. Beck has suggested four vital enhancements to strengthen research in older adults with cognitive impairment (CI). One, researchers must begin to examine the resource use, cost, organizational facilitators and barriers of enacting interventions. If clinicians are to adopt efficacious interventions, more health services studies are needed. Two, the effect of genotype on the type of behavioral symptoms that persons display and their response to treatment require further exploration. Three, researchers must start conducting trials that involve both behavioral and pharmacologic treatments to answer such questions as, "Does an enhanced environment potentiate the effect of acetylcholinesterase inhibitors (AChEIs)?" Four, the biological basis for the efficacy of interventions requires measurement. For instance, researchers have discovered that enriched environments and training lead to increased cholinergic neural activity and neural synapses.

Gender differences are emerging in many research studies and there is much more that needs attention, particularly for very old men and women. Much of the attention has been given to how treatment for men and women varies. There is no question that some of this relates to how male and female providers relate to the recipient of care. Other factors of significance include the levels of hormone fluctuation that predominate much of a female's life, males' readiness for certain interventions and numerous other factors that have been given insufficient consideration.

Biorhythms and their effect on medication utilization, particularly in relation to time of medication dosage, sleep patterns, learning patterns, cognition, and cardiac rhythms, are being explored. As mentioned earlier, it will be up to nurses to shift the institutional patterns to accommodate individuals rather than common routines. Nurses that are interested may want to review some of the more than 5000 studies cited on PubMed under circadian rhythms. A good resource for chronobiology is found on www.circadian.com.

Allen, Francis, and O'Connor (2004) emphasize the need for research into the special aspects of rural nursing care and the merit of making the appropriate research into rural nursing care delivery more readily available to professionals. They suggest such research be integrated into nursing specialist programs in order to produce evidence of best practices generated through empirical research. While they do not focus specifically on rural geriatric care it is well known that this has been neglected and holds potential for much improvement if sufficient emphasis is placed on this growing problem. Worldwide it is a problem to identify specific modes of care delivery suitable to those "aging in place" when that is a rural, relatively inaccessible population; the elders left behind as the younger generation leaves home to "seek their fortunes."

Whall feels that research to be reliable and implemented in practice requires the following: "Availability, feasibility, and evaluation of such research depends upon the range of contexts in which gerontological nursing occurs, the clarity in which the research is presented in order to translate into practice initiatives, and of a cooperative chain of colleagues. The ability to participate as a trusted member is absolutely essential, and almost guarantees success" (Whall, 2004, p. 6). Citing a comment by

Angela McBride, Archbold (2005) says "good research takes a village" (p. 5). We would add that many of the geriatric nurse researchers cite the importance of interdisciplinary team work, and the inestimable value of the contributions of graduate and doctoral students working with them. Clarity of evaluation is necessary to provide evidence of patient-centered outcomes in gerontological nursing practice (Conway & FitzGerald, 2004).

CONCLUSION

Of continuing concern is the dearth of nursing students entering gerontological master's and doctoral programs. Whall (2004) suggested that "we need to act now to capture the hearts and minds of these wonderful students" and need to provide more opportunities for funding for doctoral and post doctoral students (p. 6).

To end this chapter, we would like to share some of the reflections of Dr. Ruth Tappen and Dr. May Wykle, gerontological nursing research leaders. At a recent conference on culture and aging sponsored by the Christine E. Lynn College of Nursing at Florida Atlantic University, they were asked to informally share their thoughts on the past, present, and future of gerontological nursing research for this book.

Dr. Tappen and Dr. Wykle discussed what they perceived as milestones in the development of research in the specialty. These included the influence of the development of master's programs in gerontological nursing that moved research forward by producing experts and increasing recognition that nurses need to study old people. In reflecting back on the development of master's programs in the late 1970s and 1980s, they commented that the master's preparation in the specialty really got ahead of the baccalaureate preparation. This area needs considerable attention now to prepare nurses competent in care of the elderly and to recruit bright young nurses into the specialty.

Grant and research funding availability were cited as other factors that spurred the growth of research. Foundations such as Robert Wood Johnson and the Hartford Foundation, and others cited in this chapter, as well as federal grant funding, are absolutely critical to the development of gerontological nursing knowledge. The awarding of the first geropsychiatric post doctoral fellowships for nurses from the National Institute of Mental Health that were given to Wykle, Kitty Buckwalter, and Ann Whall were considered another milestone, recognizing the need to study the mental health of older people.

Another milestone mentioned by Dr. Tappen and Dr. Wykle included the Teaching Nursing Home project funded by the Robert Wood Johnson Foundation. The Teaching Nursing Homes (TNH) demonstrated that advanced practice nurses made a difference in outcomes in this setting and that we could educate students by bringing them into nursing homes. Research on delirium, mental health, pressure ulcers, and urinary incontinence during the TNH project laid the foundation for best practice nursing in these areas.

Other milestones included the landmark research of Strumpf and Evans on restraints (spurred by Doris Schwartz), Beverly Baldwin's seminal research in nursing homes, the inclusion of nursing in the establishment of the GRECs, the beginning inquiry into confusion, dementia, and delirium by Mary Opal Wolanin, the Institute of Medicine Study leading to OBRA, caregiver studies, the effect of interventions from NICHE projects, and the discharge studies conducted by Brooten and Naylor demonstrating the effectiveness of follow-up post hospitalization of elders by advanced practice nurses. Charlene Harrington's research on staffing and professional nursing in nursing homes was another milestone and Wykle suggested that Harrington's work is to gerontological nursing what Linda Aiken's work is and has been to the rest of nursing.

Dr. Tappen noted that gerontological nursing research is naturally interdisciplinary and that the study of care concerns and development of scientific knowledge across disciplines is important. The contribution of gerontological nursing research is widely recognized across disciplines and compared to other health-related fields, Wykle and Tappen feel we have been the leader in contributions toward improvement of care outcomes.

Looking to the future, these two researchers identified the following as areas most in need of gerontological nursing research:

- Staffing patterns and the most appropriate mix to improve care outcomes in long-term care settings
- The influence of culture, diversity, ethnicity on aging
- Health disparities and health literacy
- Factors contributing to successful aging, health promotion, and wellness with the upcoming Baby Boomer generation
- Retirement decisions of Baby Boomers, how they are made and how they are changing from our current knowledge level
- Dementia as a chronic illness and staying well with the disease
- Caregiving, particularly intergenerational
- Values and attitudes of the current generation toward aging and their expectations
- Interventions to assist with the increasing prevalence of drug and alcohol abuse and other mental health problems of the current and future generation of people who are aging
- Integration of current best practice protocols into settings across the continuum in cost-effective and care-efficient models

- Models of acute care designed to prevent negative outcomes in elders
- Strategies to increase preparation in gerontological nursing at all levels of nursing education and increased recruitment of the brightest and best into gerontological nursing
- Models of interdisciplinary practice
- Health promotion and illness management interventions in the assisted living setting; role of professional nurses and advanced practice nurses in this setting; aging-in-place
- Development of models for end-of-life care in home and nursing home

Gerontological nursing research is poised to continue its significant contribution to the future of health care for older people. Standing on the shoulders of those who have come before, we are hopeful for our future and agree with Brink and Wells (2003) when they say "a wonderful thing about looking forward is the certainty that gerontological nursing will thrive" (p. 5).

CHAPTER NINE

Elements of Attracting Nurses to the Field

There was a time when care of the old was the least attractive choice one could make in nursing. Young nurses headed for the excitement of surgery, obstetrics, intensive care, or other foci that stimulated the adrenal rush. This, we like to think, has changed as nurses see the many opportunities on the horizon in the care of the old. As individuals in acute care are shuttled through in supermarket style, those nurses seeking gratification from actual nursing practice find it possible in the extended exposure to the older person in various long-term care situations.

MENTORSHIP

One of the most important aspects of attracting nurses to the field is mentorship. Dr. Dolores Alford speaks of many mentors during her early life and professional career. From her numerous learning experiences with her mentors, she has developed a clear sense of the process.

"The role of mentoring is a natural outgrowth of the desire to help others. What I have chosen as the definition, concept, and practice of mentoring are the following:

- Mentoring is being there for the mentees to encourage them, to give them ideas for decision making, to be a sounding board, to be a confirmer, and to be a challenger.
- Mentoring is primarily a person to person encounter that may involve talk, hugs, touch, kind words, and realistic comments that the mentee might not want to hear.

- The process of mentoring includes allowing mentees to express their ideas, problems, worries, and the desired results they wish to achieve. The mentor listens and makes suggestions. The mentor may communicate ideas, resources, and kind words via email, telephone, fax, or even an appropriate greeting card.
- Let mentoring happen. You do not need to tap someone on the shoulder and say, I'm going to mentor you.
- Listen to what people say to you. Suggest ideas and direction without saying, You have to do . . . In other words, do not control the mentee's life. Just give the mentee ideas and options for his/her own decision making.
- Do not let the mentee control your life. Yes, the mentee can contact you when needed, but discourage dependency.
- Make the relationship professional, but warm and comfortable."
- I would add that mentors must learn to let go at the appropriate time and even allow the mentee to exceed them professionally. Dr. Alford says this beautifully, "Now, you younger nurses will be the ones who must open the next door, put the light on, and let your ideas and visions illuminate nursing for the future. My spirit will be applauding you if any of your visions come to pass. My spirit will haunt you if you do not ensure that gerontic nursing remains the wonderful specialty it is" (Alford, 2004, pp. 22–23).

Ann Schmidt Luggen (chapter 4) writes about mentorship in publishing and the importance of the "old girls' network" (Luggen, 1994). Those older, wiser in some respects, and willing to take the fledgling into the circle of contacts have the ingredients for mentoring. Age is not a criterion of mentorship, but some studies indicate the mentor is usually 8 to 15 years older than the mentee. The critical element in publishing mentorship is the ability to cultivate the unique voice of the neophyte. One must refrain from attempting to clone oneself. Luggen says that enthusiasm, energy, and drive are the essentials in mentorship for the protege and the mentor. It is also important for both to listen, question, and analyze and for the mentee to be grateful. In reading the experiences of nurses included in this text they all express gratitude for the mentor relationship.

May Futrell notes she has had a 27-year relationship as mentor to Karen Melillo, watching her growth and participating in it at several points. They have coauthored several publications and worked as a team on proposals and projects. May writes, "Mentorship can be a lifelong process. In the case of Dr. Melillo, that has come to fruition. Continued opportunities for mentoring in the educator, administrator, clinician, and scholar role abound. Together we continue to conduct research, publish, think, dialogue, and grow. Offering a mentoring relationship to an interested, enthusiastic, hardworking colleague is one facet of a true pioneer and leader. I am proud so say I have had that opportunity with Dr. Melillo" (Futrell, 2004, p. 2).

Virginia Burggraf has found a unique way to mentor as she hosts an annual "mentoring luncheon" at the Gerontological Society of America (GSA) annual convention. After 5 years, this has become a tradition, although initially she had simply brought 6 or 7 of her graduate students to GSA to meet some of the geriatric nurse leaders in an informal luncheon, rather hastily cobbled together. The students talked a lot about their problems working, going to school and, for several, maintaining a home and raising children as well. One was getting little help from her husband as he resented her efforts to advance herself professionally. We, the potential mentors who attended, autographed textbooks and spoke with some individually after the luncheon. Presently, her graduate students, those potential scholars funded by the John A. Hartford Foundation, lunch with gerontological nurse leaders and discuss their current research and projects. This expands their horizons to begin seeing themselves as prospective leaders. Many of the current geriatric nurse leaders have taken part in these mentoring events. Virginia is the *metamentor*. From these group meetings, we expect great things to emanate, thanks to Virginia's "out of the box" thinking. She says she is mainly a futurist and facilitator.

THE IMPORTANCE OF FACULTY

All of the leaders in the geriatric nursing specialty have identified individuals who were important in their decision to enter the field. Often grandparents or other significant persons from their childhood made a deep impression and instilled a love for the aged. However, we know that for the initial seed to grow and flourish it must be fed, tended, watered, and encouraged. The importance of nursing faculty cannot be neglected or overestimated. Eldonna Shields-Kyle noted how significant Virginia Stone was in her development. Barbara Davis and Laurie Gunter found no geriatric nursing faculty available and had to seek inspired faculty outside nursing.

There is now no excuse for a lack of well-informed and enthusiastic geriatric specialty faculty. Knowledge of geriatric care abounds, but what are the factors that kill enthusiasm? Joanne Hall cites some of the problems in keeping faculty enthused about students and teaching: exhaustion with nonteaching activities and the burden of academic expectations that have very little to do with teaching (e.g., the expectation of obtaining funded grants, scholarly endeavors, university and clinical service, and community service). Enthusiasm and optimism are squelched by unrealistic requirements. How do some rise above these exhausting expectations? Dr. Hall believes that identifying our strengths, celebrating our differences, and persistent communication of our needs and those of students form the basis for excitement and enjoyment of teaching and learning (Hall, 2004). One nurse faculty, I shall not name, said to be selective and focus on the things you do well and neglect the things you do poorly. Soon, you will not be asked to do those things that do not fit your special attributes.

A FIELD OF DREAMS

Nursing is perhaps the only profession that gives one a wide open field of opportunity. A nurse can be anything he or she wants to be. Two outstanding examples give this message most clearly.

Director of Probate Court: Mary Quinn

The first example is Mary Joy Quinn, RN, MA, and director of the Probate Court of San Francisco Superior Court since 1989. This court was named by the U.S. General Accounting Offices in 2004 as one of four exemplary probate courts in the United States. Ms. Quinn is a member of the California Judicial Council Probate and Mental Health Advisory Committee and a commissioner with the American Bar Association Commission on Law and Aging. She is also a board member of the National Committee for the Prevention of Elder Abuse.

Ms. Quinn, early on, thought she wanted to be a physician but says, "If I had become a physician, I would have missed the joys and pleasure of being a nurse, which have given such deep meaning and purpose to my life. Nursing is multidisciplinary, holistic, and disciplined. The general public trusts nurses and recognizes that they are helpers in time of deep need. Those professional realities provide nurses with untold opportunities. They provide a platform for intellectual adventure, service, and challenge. But, opportunities must be sought out or recognized when they present themselves" (Quinn, 2005, p. 1).

Quinn credits her many opportunities to curiosity, an innate trust in herself, a willingness to take risks as well as leave situations she found unrewarding, and to those important people who were there for her at critical times—teachers, fellow nurses, family, friends, supervisors, and employers who liked her spunk and were willing to give her a chance.

Her early nursing education in an excellent diploma nursing program in North Dakota grounded her in nursing. After that she went to the University of Oregon School of Nursing and graduated with a bachelor of science degree in 1964. Her clinical work was varied, including: a summer emergency nursing in Yellowstone Park; teaching operating room nursing; working as a public health nurse in an urban area; acting as visiting nurse with a geriatric mental health team; and becoming the director of a geriatric psychiatric day treatment center. She then sought more specific education, which included a master's degree in psychology specializing in gerontology. After graduation she began casting around for new challenges that would benefit her monetarily as well as stimulate her intellectually.

"A personal friend who was a judge, told me about new legislation that created a new position in Probate Court. The position was called court investigator and entailed going into homes and facilities of adults who were alleged to need a guardian to handle their personal and financial affairs. It also involved explaining what their legal rights were and arranging for an attorney to represent them. Most were frail elders, the population I had worked with for many years. It was clear the position had advocacy and protective elements because no other person in the proceeding could give the elder's perspective to the judge or provide a neutral viewpoint.

I was intrigued by the possibilities, applied, and was accepted. I was a court investigator for 12 years and then became the director of the Probate Court, a position I have held since 1989. During that time, I realized that many of the cases involved elder abuse and neglect. From the experience of dealing with these problems I, together with a medical social worker I met at a conference, wrote one of the first books on elder abuse and neglect. It is now in its second edition and will go into a third. I also was aware that what I had learned in probate court about adult guardianships was not known by health and social service practitioners. In fact, there was precious little information on guardianships. So, I wrote another book (Quinn, 2005), which was just published. Writing also has brought deep satisfaction" (Quinn, 2005, p. 2).

"If it hadn't been for my maternal grandfather, I would never have known the joie de vivre, wisdom, and amusement that can come with old age. Old age became and remains intriguing to me. Obituaries are fascinating and educational. Wisdom or the lack of it in old age, curiosity, and seeking provide guidance for my own life. The pioneering spirit that I have found as a nurse came from my parents, who were in many ways themselves pioneers in their small midwestern town. My parents also imparted a no-nonsense mandate: Work is good and plenty of it is better. Work brings meaning to life, keeps you out of trouble, and gives you opportunities for financial independence. I will never be able to truly retire. I imagine I will continue to seek out work that will provide 'food' for the restless and energetic mind I was given" (Quinn, 2005, p. 3).

The United States Surgeon General: Richard H. Carmona

Richard H. Carmona, RN, MD, MPH, FACS, began as an army medic, then a paramedic, then a registered nurse, a surgeon, and now United States Surgeon General. Carmona holds the rank of vice admiral in the U.S. Public Health Service and oversees 6,000 members of the Corps, articulates health policy analysis, and advises the president and the secretary of Health and Human Services. An interview in Sigma Theta Tau's, *Reflections on Nursing Leadership* (2005) related the path he has followed. Joining the army when he was 17 years old, his advanced medical training in the army while in Vietnam allowed him, upon discharge, to sit for the nursing examination, which he passed. He moved to California, was licensed as an RN, and practiced in intensive care, critical care, and the emergency room while pursuing a bachelor of science degree at the University of California, San Francisco. Dr. Carmona continued to work as a nurse during the years before 1979, when he graduated from the University of California, San Francisco School of Medicine. At that time he no longer maintained his RN licensure but says, "I really feel, once a nurse, always a nurse, because if you have come up in that culture . . . there is a certain way you see patients and you see care and you see life. To me it very much complements who I became as a physician, and certainly I draw upon those skills every day as U.S. Surgeon General. . . . Nursing is the true caring profession. That doesn't mean that doctors don't care, but doctors have multiple, rapid, episodic care throughout the day with their patients. . . . It's the nurses who provide that continuity, the holistic approach. . . . I have often said that if there was no restraint on time or money, the ideal situation would be that all physicians should pass through nursing, because it gives you a different dimension. It really makes a much broader defined, wholesome person" (Carmona in Mattson, 2005, p. 15).

This truly amazing nurse, surgeon, and U.S. surgeon general says, "One of my primary goals is to increase health literacy in the United States. We are largely a health-illiterate society. Because nurses play a critical role in enhancing health literacy, cultural competence is important" (Carmona in Mattson, 2005, p. 15). Carmona is the second Hispanic surgeon general. The first, Antonio C. Novello, served from 1990 to 1993 during the first Bush administration.

While there is no evidence that Carmona has a special interest in geriatric care, his example emphasizes the unusual possibilities open to nurses.

Mid-Course Career Move: Robin Remsburg

Dr. Robin Remsburg entered the geriatric nursing field late. She is the prime example of mid-course career correction. It is classic to find people evaluating and reassessing their goals, turning to new interests, and making important shifts in priorities at mid-life. It is not surprising that awareness of growing older influences these decisions. Some of the factors that influenced Robin's career shift were a growing awareness of the aging population, and the ethical, social, political, economic, and technologic factors that must be addressed if the last half of life is to be fulfilling rather than simply a test of endurance. These require dedicated efforts to become immersed in specialized knowledge. Of interest to geriatric nurses will be a new journal launched online, *The Online Journal of Health Ethics,* edited by Sheila Davis. It can be accessed at (http://ethicsjournal.umc.edu/ojs, April 3, 2005).

Robin emphasizes again, as has Terry Fulmer, that interdisciplinary involvement is essential. Nurses must be cognizant of team work and their special place on the team. Their focus on the whole person integrates all of the various approaches to care. As she states, "Each specialist brings something unique to the team but, isolated, these can be cold, lonely, and painful. The glitzy technology dulls and the longing for time to connect with the aging individual becomes uppermost" (Remsburg, 2005, p. 4).

She has the following suggestions for recruiting students and established nurses in the field of geriatrics:

- Those who are geriatric nurses need to applaud what they do and spread the word. An excellent example of this was a gathering of geriatric nurses from across the nation at the Waldorf-Astoria in March 2005, to honor and celebrate the accomplishments of Mathy Mezey, Mark Beers, and others that, through the generous support of the John A. Hartford Foundation, have brought geriatric nursing out of the shadowland and into the sunlight.
- The image of geriatric nurses must be promoted through an inclusive view of the numerous activities and possibilities afforded within the specialty. Most of the geriatric nurses featured in this text have commented on the myriad opportunities that have been available to them within the specialty.
- Education about the realistic and positive aspects of aging should begin in kindergarten. Some futuristic teachers have brought elders into the classroom to interact with children in various ways. And it is noteworthy that with few exceptions the geriatric nursing leaders mention the significance of grandparents in their decision to work with the aged. In some places there have been "adopt a grandparent" programs that

connect school children with some lonely elder in a nursing home or elsewhere.

• Religious and community organizations have an important role to play in connecting elders and youth in various activities. Children singing at a senior center or church-sponsored alliances between the young and old are already occurring in some places.

• Changing the societal focus on the image of youth as the ideal state of being needs to be shifted to a realistic appreciation of the activities and appearance of the old. Marketing admonitions are largely responsible for the youth focus, while the main targets for elders are pharmaceuticals. Reaching the business world with the realization that the aged as a whole have more discretionary funds available than any other segment of the population is important. Generally, reports of the poor, neglected, abandoned, and the sensational, receive the attention of the public. The American Society on Aging (ASA), the National Council on the Aging (NCOA), and the American Association of Retired Persons (AARP) are three organizations that have made concerted efforts to shift marketing attention to the older consumer. The vast majority of elders are quite comfortable and interested in aging well and looking the part.

• Active recruitment of mid-career nurses should be a high priority. All dedicated geriatric nurses should in some way show others the rewards and satisfactions of working with the aged.

CONCLUSION

A recent news release from the ANA online noted that in a survey of 76,000 nurses the elements of job satisfaction included interactions with other RNs, their professional status, and the professional development opportunities (www.nursingworld.org/pressrel/2005/pr0401.htm, April 7, 2002). This then alerts us to elements of the position that must be enhanced if we wish to attract nurses to the geriatric specialty.

CHAPTER TEN

Nursing and the Future Care of the Aged: Possibilities and Opportunities

OLDER AMERICANS' WELL-BEING

A 2004 report from the National Center for Health Statistics gives some idea of trends for the future health of elders (Federal Interagency Forum on Age Related Statistics, 2004).

A major function of geriatric nurses in the future will be the dissemination of current knowledge in a manner understandable and acceptable to a diverse population of elders. Many elders will be managing their own care to the best of their ability and the geriatric nurse will in a sense act as an information gatekeeper. Awareness of directions in health care and health behaviors will be essential as individuals seek more control of their health outcomes.

Directions at present are uncertain, although we are well aware that the very old are increasing dramatically and the majority of these are women, often frail and living alone. Approximately 7 million elders have chronic disabilities. The increase in obesity among all ages is alarming. The percentage of individuals 65 to 74 years old who are overweight rose from 57% to 73% between 1976 and 2002. Drug costs and usage among elders has gone up exponentially; the average annual cost in 2000 for elders was $1,340 and the average number of prescriptions filled rose from 18 to 30 (Federal Interagency Forum on Aging-Related Statistics, 2004).

The greatest challenge to the society and geriatric nurses at present is the impending impact of the baby boomers upon health care in the

United States. Another equally important trend is the emigration of a growing stream of families to the United States. Often, the younger immigrant brings not only the nuclear family but the extended family and numerous "aunties." The HHS Agency for Healthcare Research and Quality (AHRQ, 2005) reports significant disparities remain within health care delivery related to race, ethnicity, and socioeconomic status in the American health care delivery system. These now require focused efforts to produce gains needed in the future of this rapidly growing segments of the aging population. Some improvements are evident as best practices have been and are being identified, but we expect much greater attention will be given to these strategies. The most notable recent changes, foretelling some of the future trends, are better management of pain in nursing home residents, more appropriate care of the dying, and decreases in the percentage of elderly patients who are given inappropriate medications.

Now, we must also consider such things as stem cell research, growing and harvesting organs, cloning, the prolongevity and antiaging movements, the outer limits of inner space, and how and from whom will ethical decisions be made. There are as many opinions about future care of the aged as there are pundits willing to speculate about it. The Boomers will likely have a major influence on health systems and policy, but our interest and commitment must be to the very old who most need nursing. Rather than the esoteric, we focus this chapter on the projections of gerontological nurses presently most active in the field and concerned with *nursing* care of the aged, and the emergent geriatric nursing roles.

Kathleen Buckwalter says, "I am personally very optimistic about the future of geriatric nursing. As my colleague, Meridean Maas, and I noted some years ago, nurses must work to create the professional and political will to avoid a crisis in long-term care. We must work to create models of care that are appropriate for the elderly and their families; pursue adequate funding and reimbursement for programming and services; support the preparation and retention of adequate numbers of qualified nursing providers; increase our research to assess the effectiveness of care strategies; increase our emphasis on health promotion, community based services, and continuity of care; and strengthen the gerontological and professional ethics content of our curricula. If we in the nursing community can focus our concerted efforts on these most critical areas, gerontological nursing will be well prepared to thrive in the 21st century" (Maas & Buckwalter, 1996, p. 247). "I am confident . . . that geriatric nursing will not only survive but thrive in the years to come. It's truly an exciting time to be a geriatric nurse, and I feel so lucky to have gotten in on the 'ground floor' of geropsychiatric nursing almost 20 years ago" (Buckwalter in Ebersole, 2001, p. 93).

Jessie Mantle (discussed in chapter 6), a Canadian gerontological clinical specialist, projects into the immediate future of geriatric nursing in Canada, "I see a specialty being caught in the economic crunch and again downgraded in status, decreased staffing, and a disinterest in fostering innovation in the field. I believe this will change quickly as the baby boomers retire and already we are seeing their impact as their parents require help" (Mantle, 2005, p. 3).

In the long haul she expects that nurse practitioners will gain wide acceptance in both community and institutional settings; more nurses will have graduate training in the specialty and they will exert pressure for positive change; Canadian gerontological nurses will develop politically and wield significant influence on national drug committees, policy initiatives, and research directions. Jessie also expects nurses in acute care and in the community will become more knowledgeable about the specialized aspects of long-term institutional care (Mantle, 2005).

Terry Fulmer believes that nursing will evolve toward more interdisciplinary support, coordination, and requirements in action and education. The patient's needs and desires will be at the center of service and nurses will be central to the cohesion of the team (Fulmer, 2005).

HEALTH AND WELLNESS

Futrell and Alford have focused on the visible movement of the population toward goals of health promotion and wellness with a shift from the common perception that being an older adult inevitably means poor health, sickness, and dependency (Futrell & Alford, 1996).

The World Health Organization (WHO), in 1948, defined health as a state of complete physical, mental, and social well-being, and not merely the absence of disease or infirmity. Clearly, this definition must be examined in terms of age, gender, ethnicity, and circumstantial variations. Wellness may exist in the presence of disease and infirmity. The present emphasis of health promotion has been to promote physical fitness, exercise, smoking cessation, and dietary modifications. These are only the material aspects of health. Dignity, self-esteem, personal regard, and commitment to someone or some idea are some of the more elusive elements of wellness.

More than a decade ago (1992), Alford and Futrell proposed the development of gerontic nursing institutes, housed in colleges of nursing, to be regional health resource centers and health education libraries, and to provide continuing education in gerontological nursing. The institutes would also provide clinical practice settings for nursing students, emphasizing wellness concepts for elders whether they were sick or well. These institutes would generate aging and gerontological nursing research, advocate for elders, and seek social policy change to better meet the needs of elders (Alford & Futrell, 1992). "The institutes would be a 'one-stop' resource for older adults, their families, and caregivers. Older persons would be used as cherished advisors on programs, curricula, grants, and health policy proposals" (Futrell & Alford, 1996, p. 99). This is now being done in a less comprehensive manner in several sites, but certainly is a feasible idea that could be facilitated in the future.

Serious health promotion is a relatively new and evolving area but one we expect will become a much greater part of health care. The biggest barrier at present is the lack of professionals prepared to provide wellness/health promotion services rather than the illness services that have characterized the *health* professions (Futrell & Alford, 1996).

Gene Cohen, a respected gerontologist, is greatly interested in creativity and soul-feeding programs for elders and the amazing capacities of the brain. His exciting synthesis of the phases of post-midlife human development is partially based on emerging neurological research into the aging brain. He writes, "Brain tissue is creatively restless tissue. The tissue *wants* to express the human potential it holds, and there are developmental mechanisms at work that allow this potential to be expressed . . . throughout the whole life cycle" (Cohen, 2004, p. 1). As we refocus our lens, we see that the medicalization of old age has resulted in a materialistic concept of aging. We don't discount the importance of adequate health care and attention to basic needs, but do know elders who rise above these to attain a meaningful old age in spite of pain, loneliness, physical deprivation, and chronic disorders. We are just beginning to understand that there are developmental issues that shift and change after midlife. Dr. Cohen speculates there are four phases of later life: *midlife reevaluation;* the *liberation phase* that follows, including a desire to experiment and innovate; the *summing-up* phase that we see so frequently, including periods of life review, conflict resolution, and legacy identification; and the final *encore* phase. The *encore* phase at first glance seems like the last bow before leaving the stage. Dr. Cohen sees it as increased interest in the young, the ones coming on stage, and species survival. Celebrations, reunions, and generational continuity become increasingly important. With new exploration of the brain and its capacities for rejuvenation, we expect the tasks and abilities of later life will become increasingly apparent. Geriatric nursing activities will incorporate new expectations of elders.

Dr. Edna Stilwell, the founding editor of the *Gerontological Nursing Journal,* served as editor for 25 years. She has seen and been a real contributor in many aspects to the growth of the geriatric nursing specialty. Edna says, "One characteristic of leaders in a specialty area is to view the future and be prepared. I feel that the thousands of nurses that I have influenced either directly or indirectly are ready to do this. This current age of biotechnology is completely changing the way we view aging. I used to ask my students, 'What does it mean to be old?' 'What is the difference between an older person and a younger person?' Answers used to be, 'You are closer to the end of your life than the beginning.' 'You are more likely to have certain diseases.' 'You are the oldest living member of your family.' 'Many of your age group have died.'

"These answers are changing. Landmark events such as completion of the genome project, high-tech diagnostic tools, tissue engineering, gene therapy, brain/machine interface, and drugs tailored to genetics are dramatically changing the way we must view health and aging. It is an exciting time to be an older person" (Stilwell, 2005, p. 3).

ONLINE EDUCATION

It seems clear that future progress in geriatric nursing proficiency will be largely dependent upon technology; remote and Internet sources. A recent online course was developed in Florida to meet mandated state legislation to provide dementia training for long-term care staff. Florida House Bill 1971 charged the American Health Care Administration (AHCA) with the establishment of a program to better meet the needs of Florida's increasing population of frail elders. An advisory committee composed of representatives from the major elder health care organizations met to formulate appropriate plans. The advisory committee realized that LPNs were the largest group of licensed caregivers in long-term care and decided to tailor the course toward them. This led to the development of dementia care competencies that would guide a competency-based curriculum to meet the training demand; LVNs were the target group. The competencies for dementia care and the curriculum based on those competencies are currently available through the Teaching Nursing Home online educational site, (www.GeriU.org). From there the learner is directed to a link in Florida's Teaching Nursing Home Program. Any health care provider can use the dementia education learning modules without cost (Williams et al., 2005). Obviously, more available training for the vast number of paraprofessionals will be reflected in improved long-term care. Such online courses are a wave of the future that will greatly enhance the availability of geriatric nursing education.

EMERGING GERIATRIC NURSING ROLES

One of the certainties is that more and more geriatric care will be delivered in the home and through community clinics and agencies. Those informal caregivers providing the majority of this care seldom have adequate assistance or preparation. Spousal caregivers presently provide twice the hours of care of other family members. This has been gradually increasing in the past decade with the growing number of frail elders and their caregivers. There will be a greater need for assistance through the complex maze of multiproblem management. We expect a cadre of primary care advanced practice nurses will develop in each community, perhaps dispatched from senior centers and nurse managed clinics to guide and counsel caregivers. The model was developed long ago by Dolores Alford (as discussed in chapter 3), and many other advanced practice nurses with an entrepreneurial bent undoubtedly will follow.

Curb service, as occasionally practiced by GNP staff at the Louise and Anne Green Memory and Wellness Center developed by Martha Anderson at the Carillion Health Center, Healthy Aging Service in Roanoke, Virginia, has the potential for development as well. In this model, an appraisal of a particular problem, such as a medication reaction, may be done from an auto without the necessity of a well-known frail client entering a clinic and waiting. Also, geriatric telemedicine and telenursing will grow and flourish in response to the increasing use of computers by elders and the difficulties in transportation that often occur among the very old. Mobile health units with advanced technologic equipment are increasing, delivering services to the door of high-risk elders. The New York Visiting Nurse Service has a long and outstanding record of care to elders. Doris Schwartz (discussed in chapter 2) was one of the geriatric nurse pioneers who foresaw the great need for expansion of these services.

A role that will become more accessible and important for geriatric nurses is that of the certified legal nurse consultant. More attention is being given to the quality of geriatric care in all settings and litigation about questionable practices is on the increase. Meiner (2005) names several roles that are rapidly being developed by geriatric nurses throughout the nation: legal nurse consultant, medical records reviewer, legal assistant, forensic nurse, and expert witness. Currently, certification is not essential but is available for nurses in these roles.

Roles of Gerontological Nurse Practitioners

In the 35 years since the first geriatric/gerontologic nurse practitioners (GNPs) began practicing, their role has become much more independent and clearly that of the primary care provider, particularly in nursing homes and managed care settings where the majority of GNPs are employed. The medical aspects of the role have become more integrated into their total function and GNP activities are less often seen as that of physician-extender. During the 1990s substantial pharmacologic courses, emphasis on social and health policy issues, more research, and a health promotion/wellness focus that includes the use of alternative and complementary therapies has strengthened the role (Futrell & Melillo, 2002). The blending of clinical nurse specialist (CNS) and nurse practitioner (NP) education into advanced practice nursing (APN) has created further changes in the role. Futrell and Melillo point out that this conjunction moved the erroneous idea about different practice arenas for CNSs and GNPs to one of a focus on the person rather than the place of care delivery. The Florida Atlantic University Nursing Program is one of the first to formalize this blend into an educational program (see chapter 7).

Futrell and Melillo (2005) predict that GNPs and APNs will be instrumental in improving availability and effectiveness of care delivery in acute care, home care, community, hospice, and institutional long-term care. Further discussion of APNs can be found in chapter 7.

End of Life Care

Long before nursing curricula were giving much attention to geriatric care, death, and dying courses appeared on campuses as electives, often within the schools of nursing. Dr. Patricia Hess developed such a course in 1972 and it was always oversubscribed. Students became very aware of their own grief experiences as well as aspects of attending their dying patients. Pat became deeply interested in geriatrics and gerontology through her interest in the dying. After that early course, she began seeking more education in the specialty and earned certificates in gerontology from the Ethel Percy Andrus Gerontology Center, University of Southern California, Los Angeles and Holy Names College in Oakland, California.

Pat's baccalaureate education was at Frances Payne Bolton School of Nursing, Case Western Reserve University. She earned a nursing master's degree at the University of Colorado, Boulder, and a doctorate from Walden University in Naples, Florida. In 1986 she completed the geriatric nurse practitioner program at the University of California, San Francisco, School of Nursing. She is a board certified GNP, a member of the National Academies of Practice, and has been a professor in the School of Nursing, San Francisco State University since 1971. She also has held appointments in the Applied Gerontology Certificate Program at San Francisco State University as well as being an instructor in the continuing education death and dying course (by correspondence) at University of California, Berkeley. She served on the board of directors during the inception of the Hospice of Marin in Marin County, California. She also visited St. Christopher's Hospice, Sydenham, England, during that time.

She has been involved in gerontological nursing for over 40 years and has conducted workshops and seminars on aging nationally and internationally. Her expertise is in the areas of health promotion, wellness, death and dying, and education of students and staff to the specific needs of the aged in acute care settings. She has coauthored eight textbooks focused on healthy aging (Ebersole & Hess, 1981, 1985, 1990, 1994, 1998, 2001; Ebersole, Hess, & Luggen, 2005; Ebersole, Hess, Touhy, & Jett, 2005).

A great deal has changed about death and dying since the first courses, particularly within the last decade. Families are relying on hospice for support and assistance that allows individuals to die at home when they wish. Jeanie Kayser-Jones reports on a model long-term care hospice unit in a large metropolitan county hospital (Kayser-Jones, Chan, & Kris, 2005). There is a great need for the blending of long-term and hospice care. The program developed by Kayser-Jones provides a model for the proliferation of such agenda.

Palliative care in hospitals is becoming more acceptable. Advance directives, in the best circumstances, protect individuals from treatments they do not wish, and end of life (EOL) care has become more humanistic and less mechanical (Matzo & Sherman, 2004). The End-of-Life Nursing Education Consortium (ELNEC), a national initiative to improve EOL care, shows widespread acceptance. Over 19,000 nursing students from 460 institutions have received ELNEC training (Rosseter, 2005). We look for these trends to gain significant strength. The ELNEC courses were funded by a major grant from the Robert Wood Johnson Foundation and administered jointly by the City of Hope National Medical Center and the American Association of Colleges of Nursing. Betty Ferrell, PhD, RN, FAAN, the principal investigator of the ELNEC Project, says, "Over the next few years, we estimate that ELNEC-trained educators will touch the lives of 6 million patients and their families facing the end of life" (Brown, 2005).

The Second Global Summit for Hospice and Palliative Care Associations was held in Seoul, Korea, March 18, 2005. Seventy delegated attendees from 35 countries drafted an international declaration on care for the dying. The progress on this declaration will be assessed and made public in 2 years. Dr. Cynthia Goh, from the Asia Pacific Hospice and Palliative Care Network, stated, "We accept the need to support people at the start of life but we are failing to give equal importance to the inevitable end. Death and dying are natural journeys that we must take, but we need strong support on that journey, particularly if we or someone we love is in pain. It's a shocking indictment of our global society that we don't do more to support hospice and palliative care, an issue which literally affects every one of us" (HELP THE HOSPICES Press Release, March 18, 2005).

A publication of *Generations* (Spring 1999) was entirely devoted to EOL care. Topics considered included pain, palliative care for the demented, cultural considerations, assisting caregiving families, legalities, anticipatory coping, training of advance practice palliative care nurses, and palliative care in the nursing home. There is definitely an international groundswell of concern about the care of the dying that we expect to continue to spread.

We expect that the parish nurse movement may link with hospice care and both fields gain strength. Elders will be involved in ways meaningful to them; biologic and spiritual needs will be seen as equally important in achieving wellness and a good death.

Evidence-Based Nursing Practice

Nursing practice has gone along fairly comfortably for a few decades, making clinical and policy decisions based on the usual, ritualistic, and unsystematic forms of clinical practice. In geriatric care this has been particularly prevalent as it has been generally accepted until recently (and still is by some) that caring for the old entailed no special considerations. There is presently a strong and growing movement toward establishing evidence-based nursing practice (EBNP) in which research and practice outcomes are evaluated to produce sound interventions that will result in the best possible care available (Udod & Care, 2004). This intertwining is discussed in chapter 8 as Cornelia Beck explains the Mobius strip concept. The outcomes of the union of research and practice will be increasingly available to the public and professionals, effecting changes in standards of practice in geriatric/gerontologic nursing and more precise outcomes and expectations. There will no longer be passive acceptance of the status quo. An informed public will seek the best and most effective care and attentive geriatric nurses will instill their research and knowledge toward evidence-based practice. Melnyk, Fineout-Overholt, and Feinstein (2004) surveyed 160 nurses attending EBNP conferences as to their awareness of, participation in educational opportunities for, and belief in the value of evidenced-based practice. Most believed in the value but felt their knowledge was weak. Fewer than half (46%) say their practice is based on clinical research evidence. Some key leaders in the movement, such as Dr. Melnyk, will further the melding of research and practice. Almost half of the nurses (44%) indicated they had access to faculty or clinical nurse specialists who helped them to integrate research evidence into practice. With the rapid growth of knowledge and increased communication, it appears the future will be greatly influenced by EBNP.

Continence Clinic Managers

Urinary incontinence is one of the issues receiving a great deal of attention as strategies are being developed for optimal continence management. A large group of concerned nurse leaders gathered at a conference in 2003, sponsored by the University of North Carolina and the University of Pennsylvania, to explore methods to address this sensitive topic more openly and effectively. This will continue to generate interest and ultimately greatly affect the dignity and quality of life of older persons (http://todaysseniornetwork.com/bladder_problems.htm, April 24, 2005). Nurses are in the best position to banish the stigma by education of the public to the availability of effective solutions.

I know one of those involved in the conference, Joyce Colling, a professor emerita from Oregon Health Sciences University, Portland, quite well. Her studies, which cover a span of over 20 years, as well as her proactive approach to urinary incontinence, have been beacons to others. Continence specialists, such as Dr. Colling, have tested the effectiveness of various management strategies. Dr. Colling has contributed greatly to the research on incontinence in the frail elderly in the community and particularly in long-term care settings, with emphasis on staff education to improve continence care, and has published numerous research articles on incontinence in the elderly.

Dr. Colling and her colleague, Dr. Rondorf-Klym, examined the physical and psychological factors that affect the quality of life of men after radical prostatectomy. Their studies concurred with previous ones indicating that sexual and urinary function are adversely affected by prostate surgery but concluded that age, self-esteem, locus of control, and social support affected the outcome (Rondorf-Klym & Colling, 2003).

Joyce provides continence services to clinic patients and consultation to numerous groups. She is a Fellow of the AAN and GSA and serves on two international panels on urinary incontinence. Chapter 2 presents early work in incontinence by Ella Kick, and chapter 3 by Thelma Wells.

Progress in this field has enormous future implications as many of the very old frequently experience urinary incontinence and have hidden it from public knowledge because it seemed nothing could be done. In the future we expect the concentrated attention that these disorders are now receiving will result in accessible information and a more forthright approach among professionals and afflicted individuals.

CELEBRATING PROGRESS

In January 2005 a gala celebration was held in New York City at the Waldorf-Astoria to honor Mathy Mezey and Mark Beers, and to express gratitude to the John A. Hartford Foundation for their massive support of geriatrics and gerontological initiatives. Outstanding geriatric nurses from across the United States were there to give recognition and laud the progress in geriatric nursing so influenced by their efforts. We see this as a signal event that launches geriatric nursing into the limelight and portends increasing efforts in the future.

FUTURISTIC THOUGHTS

Thirty years ago Mary Ellen Ianni, in a progressive school, designed and taught a class to fourth and fifth graders asking them as a final project to video interview an elder with whom they had worked in class. The children enjoyed the creative project and the elders. Why should we not be using our elders in such a meaningful manner? The children need more attention than they are getting in this hurly burly world of blended families, working parents, and overburdened teachers. Geriatric nurses have a place in generating interest of aging among the young, particularly in schools. Virginia Burggraf's (see chapter 4) dedication to thinking "out of the box" can be done.

Nurses can play a vital part in designing and participating in programs to link well children and well elders. This is proactive nursing at its best. Elders, children, and adolescents share some of the same needs: managing appropriate levels of independence, finding a way to make valued contributions to the society, and expressing their creativity. Elders can teach history and children can excite enthusiasm. These are not new ideas but have seldom been embellished to their fullest potential. Let us think about youth as we plan for the future of all.

The ANA centennial celebration brought out "voices from the past and visions of the future." A voice from Janet Holt, assistant director of nursing at Maple Knoll Village, Cincinnati, Ohio, said, "There is such a need for gerontological nurses. It is a fast growing field. . . . I've found a lot of fulfillment in caring for the elderly. There are so many needs there to be met" (*The American Nurse*, April 1989, p. 9; reported in www.nursingworld.org/centenn/cent1980.htm, April 3, 2005). Nurses nationwide are discovering the opportunities and satisfactions of working with the elderly. A search of recent gerontological articles posted on *Nursing World* reflects the increasing interest in care of the frail elderly, ethical issues, specialty certification, and pain management. These, to some extent, portend directions of the future (http://nursingworld.org/search/vfp_search.cfm, April 2, 2005).

Preparation for the Future

Significant progress in geriatric nursing has occurred because of advanced nursing practice that has allowed nurses to develop primary care practices in many situations. The additional education and expertise of NPs,

CNMs, CNSs, and CRNAs has garnered status and respect among the various health professionals. In the future it appears they will be shouldering more of the burden of geriatric care.

The American Association of Colleges of Nursing (AACN) in an October 2004 position statement recommends that APNs be prepared at the doctoral level in "practice doctorates" (www.aacn.nche.edu/DNP/pdf/DNP.pdf). However, the American Nurse Credentialing Center (ANCC) recommends that in the future the doctor of nursing practice (DNP) will be a requirement for eligibility to sit for the advanced practice exams (www.ana.org/ancc, April 14, 2005).

Frances Payne Bolton School of Nursing at CWRU launched the first ND (Nursing Doctorate) in 1979, the inspiration of Roselle Schlotfeld. Several programs currently offer a nursing doctorate, but the AACN recommends more consistency and that future programs consider conferring a DNP (Doctor of Nursing Practice). It is felt that the complexity of the health care delivery system requires ever more knowledge and sophistication to keep pace with the needs of the population and be considered "equal players in the health care arena." Some specific benefits of a practice-focused doctorate include: additional educational preparation for those not desiring a strong research focus; preparation for increasingly complex clinical, faculty, and leadership roles; parity with other health professionals; enhanced ability to attract individuals to nursing from nonnursing backgrounds; increased supply of faculty; and improved image of nursing.

Ann Whall (2005) discusses the move toward more DNPs. Whall suggests there is a less metaphysical focus in the DNP and a view that nursing practice be approached as a stand-alone phenomenon, based in science and specific domains of practice. The DNP has the potential for moving nursing forward into greater awareness of the foundations of present practice and to define the nature and possibilities of future practice. Whall says, "As nursing discusses ways to develop the DNP, it is important to keep in mind the philosophic views of the science that have negatively affected nursing practice and research in the past. *Practice is not a 'stand alone' phenomenon;* rather, it is a direct outcome of philosophic beliefs. DNP graduates will lead nursing practice forward and they need a clear grounding in philosophy of science (or metatheoretical) issues that define the nature of nursing practice and research. . . . nursing has the tendency to approach current issues as not having a 'past' and of repudiating our disciplinary past experience. Hopefully this will not be forgotten in current discussions of the DNP" (Whall, 2005, p. 1).

Others have suggested another possible route to the nursing doctorate; that of bypassing the master's degree and going directly from the

BSN to the doctorate. If this develops as a feasible option it must be thoughtfully considered. It will be important in the future to the success of DNPs because they influence best practices through research and clinical innovation. These individuals are in the best position to activate the Mobius strip that Cornelia Beck suggests (see chapter 8).

Future trends include increasing numbers of doctoral programs for nurses interested in aging. The Duke University School of Nursing provides one example of this trend. Their new PhD program, admitting students in fall 2006, targets chronic disease. They are dedicated to interdisciplinary collaboration. Program codirectors are Professor Elizabeth Clipp, who holds a dual appointment in the Schools of Nursing and Medicine, and Ruth Anderson, an associate professor of nursing (Duke University School of Nursing, 2005). Although this program is not specific to the aged or a nursing doctorate, the focus on chronic care will be attractive to geriatric nurses who may be seeking doctorates.

Advancing the Professional Through Expanding Awareness

Future possibilities in the profession depend upon being heard; books, speeches, publications, and workshops are the vehicles. Numerous excellent ideas never come to general attention in geriatric nursing simply because individuals are too busy to share them, or are held back by personal or professional constraints. Teamwork may be the solution for some, or connecting with a mentor who knows the ropes. Often, one may be the idea person and the other proficient at conveying those ideas in pleasing forms. More importantly, we now have a vast number of electronic means to convey ideas and information as more and more journals go online.

Alternative Health Care

In the near future it appears that the flight to self-care, when traditional care is exorbitantly expensive or simply not available, will attract more and more elders. In reality, medical care as it is today is not "traditional" but simply the prevailing method of providing care. Many of the "alternative" methods are rooted in centuries of tradition.

Wellness programs and alternative/complementary medicine are being sought to a larger extent than ever before. Interestingly, a recent selective summary from the Gerontological Society of America (GSA), provided weekly by Doody for subscribers, listed seven articles related to advanced practice, and 24 related to alternative therapies (April 1, 2005). A study from Ohio State University posted on Health Orbit (http://healthorbit.ca/NewsDetail, April 24, 2005) found that 70% of older adults use some kind of alternative medicine and noted many types have not been tested for safety and effectiveness. It was noted that there is a serious need for consumer education.

As is evident, increasing numbers of aging individuals are managing their own health through alternative and complementary medicine and Internet information. Many of these strategies prove effective and particularly for the chronic disorders that may accompany aging. This is likely to increase markedly as people become more and more disenchanted with rocketing costs of drugs and medical care, and patent medications are withdrawn from the market because of adverse effects. There are cautions in self-care: fraudulent claims for various alternative care methods, over-the-counter remedies, and neglect of serious disorders. The consumer must become sophisticated in assessing traditional and nontraditional medicine. It seems there is a vital role to be developed by geriatric nurses who may form a cadre of Internet health managers, gatekeepers of accurate information that consumers may access with confidence.

Evolution of an Ordinary Nurse

Grypma (2005) writes of the use of biographic methods in nursing history and suggests that the ordinary nurse is a worthy but often neglected subject. Beyond the "heroic" figures, what do the commonplace nurses tell us about the development of a specialty such as geriatric nursing? Contemplating this, I began to see a pattern that holds great expectations for the future. A nurse I have known very well for over 50 years provides an example. In 1950 she entered a typical hospital school of nursing, neither the best nor the worst. She, young at the time, was enchanted by obstetrical and maternity care in which she continued for most of her working life, usually working nights as there was more freedom; fewer staff and professionals complicating the situations. Becoming disenchanted with OB nursing, what became of the initial appeal of obstetric/maternity nursing? How had the milieu changed?

However, in 1985, long-term care positions were readily available and she was welcomed into a supervisory position in a facility in another state. She found that she loved working with the elders as she got to know them and their various idiosyncrasies. She found the work gratifying and her unique sense of humor made even the difficult situations tolerable. She had found her niche and completed her working years in a state rehabilitation unit serving the aged. Was she an ordinary nurse, who evolved into a geriatric nurse through circumstance, or had hospital "nursing" changed so much over the years that staff nursing was no longer gratifying? It appears that "real nursing" is seldom possible currently except in the situations where the individual nurse and patient/resident become respected in all their uniqueness. This is simply not possible in many situations. I look for more and more nurses to find satisfaction in long-term care and discover their niche. Fortunately, the difficulties confronting nurses in acute care are being addressed by the Hartford Institute of Geriatric Nursing. Several models of providing expert, humanistic care have been developed and are available on their website (www.hartfordign.org).

Transitional Care

The futuristic geriatric nurse must look carefully at changing practices of nursing in acute and intensive care situations. Increasing the connections, monitoring availability to elders of carefully coordinated care as they move from one health care venue to another, and readily available information must all lead the way in the future. Rapid discharges from acute care situations have made this of the highest priority.

Dr. Mary Naylor, Marian S. Ware Professor in Gerontology, University of Pennsylvania, Philadelphia, has developed such a model. Dr. Naylor and her multidisciplinary research team have conducted clinical trials focused on discharge planning and home follow-up of high-risk elders by advanced practice nurses (APNs). For over two decades she and her colleagues have been building models of transitional care, designed to improve outcomes and reduce costs of care for vulnerable community-based elders, testing care management interventions that improve health outcomes and reduce hospitalizations. However, this research-based approach to care has not been integrated into clinical practice yet. In response to this challenge and with the support of the Commonwealth Fund and the Jacob and Valeria Langeloth Foundation, Mary and her team formed a partnership with Aetna Corporation to promote rapid adoption of the APN care model in a manner that enables widespread adoption by major health care insurance corporations, and health policy changes that support reimbursement for this approach to care (Naylor, 2005).

As health care becomes more and more specialized, individuals will need a selected geriatric nurse case manager/advocate who follows each person through the entirety of their wellness/illness trajectory. This will require a dedicated interdisciplinary effort so envisioned by Terry Fulmer and Mary Naylor.

A Vision and a Legacy: Nursing Home Reform

Joanne Rader has a plan, a vision, and is developing a legacy. Her early professional years were spent as an army nurse caring for neurologically impaired Vietnam veterans. She learned that rehabilitation nursing was a good fit for her; meeting physical and psychological needs and getting to know the person over time rather than in brief interactions. Later, working in a "rehab" hospital among indigents in Washington, D.C., she met a 70-year-old African American woman who had suffered a stroke, and lost two sons simultaneously to street violence, "yet emanated a sense of self, calm and knowing that I had not observed before. She had the wisdom that can only come from lived experience. She had chosen to become wise, rather than broken. She had triumphed over adversity and become a loving, connected, caring crone. I wanted what she had and decided the best path was to work with elders" (Rader, 2005, p. 2).

Joanne wanted to know how to be a better long-term care nurse and entered the graduate program in mental health nursing at the Oregon Health and Science University in Portland, Oregon. Her clinical work took her to the Benedictine Nursing Center (BNC) in Mt. Angel, Oregon. After finishing her graduate program she was employed by Sr. Marilyn Schwab as a mental health nurse clinical specialist at BNC. This was a model nursing home with a longstanding reputation for innovation and quality. She began her focus on improving the care of persons with dementia.

Joanne began programs, with the blessing of Sr. Marilyn and Sr. Lucia Gamroth, administrators at BNC, to remove restraints, question the way reality orientation had been used, study the motives in wandering behaviors, and design bathing situations for resident satisfaction rather than the "industrial" model of care. Pairing with notable researchers and scholars such as Joyce Colling, Joyce Semradek, Beverly Hoeffer, Philip Sloane, Darlene McKenzie, and Barbara Stewart, she was able to establish demonstration projects on agenda behaviors, wandering, restraint-free care, individualized wheelchair seating, and pleasant bathing experiences. She was most proud of her work on bathing and with others created a video and interactive CD-ROM illustrating how to create person-directed, pleasant bathing. In addition she and several others published a book, *Bathing Without a Battle,* that was given a 2004 AJN Book of the Year Award (Barrick et al, 2002).

In 1996, Joanne participated in a panel convened at the National Citizen's Coalition for Nursing Home Reform (NCCNHR). The panel members recognized the need to totally revolutionize the long-term care system and began working to create a new, positive vision for elder care. As others became interested in the work they formed a Pioneer Network (PN) to address needed changes by linking all stakeholders who shared the common goal of improving care and services for elders. The many individuals and facilities linked with PN include Bill Thomas, through the Eden Alternative and the Greenhouse Project; Charlene Boyd from Providence Mt. St. Vincent in Seattle; Theresian House in Albany, New York; Steve Shields from Meadowlark in Kansas; Wellspring; La Vrene Norton's, Action Pact; the Paraprofessional Health Institute (PHI); NCCNHR; and the disability movement.

Joanne says, "After 30 years in LTC, I am now old enough and wise enough to spend time only on efforts I feel will make a difference. I know the preciousness of time. That is why as a founding member, board member and volunteer for the PN, I choose to push for the evolution, revolution, and transformation of our long-term care system. . . . In addition, I want to remind nurses that we should not let the *business* of health care define the art and practice of nursing" (Rader, 2005, p. 5).

Virginia Burggraf was a contributing author to Stanley, Blair, and Beare's (2005) *Gerontological Nursing: Promoting Successful Aging With Older Adults.* In her chapter, The Future of Gerontological Nursing, she has developed a model giving specific expectations and means to achieve them in the areas of policy, research, education, and clinical practice. Figure 10.1 provides very specific goals that could be used as guides to the future of gerontological nursing.

Progression of Gerontological Nursing

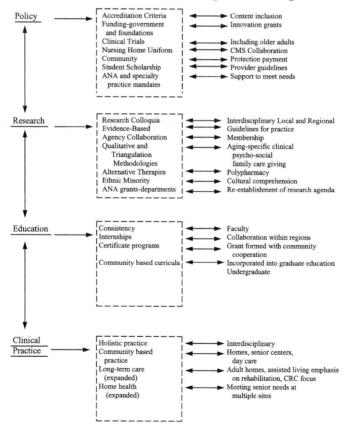

FIGURE 10.1 The future of gerontological nursing.

CONCLUSION

Most of the outstanding nurses featured in this text developed their interest in aging early in their careers. It would be an interesting research study to interview a number of nurses who took on geriatric care late in their professional lives. These then could be mentored and given opportunities to fully develop their special talents. Nurses are never too old to become geriatric nurses!

There is much to be done in the future; however, reading of the heroic efforts among earlier geriatric nurses, and the amazing energies displayed by the current ones, there is no question that geriatric nursing holds a bright and stimulating future.

Web Sites of Interest to Geriatric Nurses

American Geriatrics Society
http: www.americangeriatrics.org

American Nurses Credentialing Center
http://www.nursingworld.org/ancc/

American Society on Aging
http://www.asaging.org/

Creating Careers in Geriatric Advance Practice Nursing
http://www.aacn.nche.edu/Education/Hartford/creating.htm

Faculty Development in Geriatric Nursing—Mather Lifeways
http://www.matherlifeways.com/Re_facultydevelopment.asp

Geriatric Nursing journal/books
http://www3.us.elsevierhealth.com/gerinurs/

geronurseonline.org

Gerontological Society of America
http://www.geron.org

Hartford Institute for Geriatric Nursing
http://www.hartfordign.org

John A. Hartford Centers of Geriatric Nursing Excellence:
University of California San Francisco:
Nurseweb.ucsf.edu/www/hcgne.htm

University of Arkansas for Medical Sciences:
http://hartfordcenter.uams.edu

Oregon Health Science Center:
http://www.ohsu.edu/hartfordcgne/

University of Pennsylvania:
http://www.nursing.upenn.edu/centers/hcgne/

University of Iowa:
http://www.nursing.uiowa.edu/hartford/

Nurse Competence in Aging
http://www.ana.org/anf/nca.htm

National Conference of Gerontological Nurse Practitioners
http://www.ncgnp.org

National Gerontological Nursing Association
http://www.ngna.org

National Association of Directors of Nursing Administration
     in Long-Term Care
http://www.nadona.org

Springer Publishing Series on Geriatric Nursing
http://www.springerpub.com/store/SSGN/html

References

Abdellah, F. G. (2003a, December). *Curriculum vitae: Dr. Faye Glenn Abdellah.*

Abdellah, F. G. (2003b, December 15). Personal communication.

Abdellah, F. G. (2000). Faye Glenn Abdellah, 1919–. In V. L. Bullough & L. Sentz (Eds.), *American nursing: A biographical dictionary* (vol. 3). New York: Springer Publishing.

Abdellah, F. G. (1991a, February 5). Personal communication.

Abdellah, F. G. (1991b, February). *Curriculum vitae: Dr. Faye Glenn Abdellah.*

Abdellah, F. G. (1961). *Patient centered approaches to nursing.* New York: Macmillan.

Achterberg, J. (1991). *Woman as healer.* Boston: Shambhala.

Aiken, L. H. (2005, April 24). Personal correspondence.

Aiken, L. H. (1986). Evaluation research and public policy: Lessons from the the national hospice study. *Journal of Chronic Diseases, 39*(1), 1–4.

Aiken, L. H. (1981). Nursing priorities for the 1980s: Hospitals and nursing homes. *AJN, 81*(2), 324–330.

Alford, D. M. (2004). *Dolores Marsh Alford, PhD, RN, FAAN: An autobiography.*

Alford, D. M., & Futrell, M. (1992). Wellness and health promotion of the elderly. *Nursing Outlook, 40,* 221–226.

Allen, S., Francis, K., & O'Connor, M. (2004). Research an exciting journey and a career statement: A means to an end, putting rurality on the nursing research agenda. *Australian Journal of Rural Health, 12*(6), 279–280.

Alzheimer's Disease Education and Referral Center (ADEAR). (2004–2005). Alzheimer's disease centers program celebrates 20th anniversary. *Connections* (ADEAR newsletter), *12*(3–4), 1–2.

American Nurse. (1989). Career parallels history of gerontology. *The American Nurse, 21*(4), 6.

American Nurses Credentialing Center. (2003). *Annual Report.*

American Nurses Foundation. (1996). Virginia Stone RN Award. Flyer from the American Nurses Foundation. Awards funded to a maximum or $10,000. Awards given annually. Information and applications available <anf@ana.org (Specify subject: NRG97)>

Anderson, M. A., & Braun, J. V. (Eds.). (1999). *Caring for the elderly client* (2nd ed.). Philadelphia: F. A. Davis.

Archbold, P. (2005). Research takes a village. *Journal of Gerontological Nursing, 31*(3), 5–8.

Archbold, P. G. (2005, March 6). Personal communication.

Archbold, P. G., Stewart, B. J., & Lyons, K. S. (2002). In J. J. Fitpatrick (Ed.), *Annual review of nursing research.* New York: Springer Publishing.

Bahr, R. T., Sr. (1998). Biographical information.

Bahr, R. T., Sr. (1992). *Curriculum vitae.*

Bahr, R. T., Sr. (1990, November 17). Videotaped interview. Boston.

Barrick, A. L., Rader, J., Hoeffer, B., & Sloane, P. (Eds.). (2002). *Bathing without a battle: Personal care for individuals with dementia.* New York: Springer Publishing.

Basson, P. (1967). The gerontological nursing literature search: Study and results. *Journal of Gerontological Nursing, 6,* 527–532.

Beck, C. K. (2005). *Curriculum vitae.*

Beck, C. K. (2002, September). *The Mobius strip of outcomes and research: Geriatric nurse practitioners as nonEuclidian change agents.* Presented at the National Conference of Gerontological Nurse Practitioners.

Beck, C. K. (1999). Doris Schwartz: An exemplar of personal, social, and creative courage. *Journal of Gerontological Nursing, 25*(11), 7–9.

Benedictine Sisters. (1986). In Sr. M. Schwab (1984). A gift freely given: The personal journal of Sister Marilyn Schwab, OSB. Benedictine Sisters, Mt. Angel, Oregon.

Berman, A., Mezey, M., Kobayashi, M., Fulmer, T., Stanley, J., Thornlow, D., & Rosenfeld, P. (2005). Gerontological nursing content in baccalaureate programs: Comparison of findings from 1997 and 2003. *Journal of Professional Nursing, 21*(5), 268–275.

Berman, A., & Thornlow, D. (2005). Your bright future in geriatric nursing. *NSNA Imprint,* 24–26.

Braun, J., & Lipson, S. (Eds.). (1993). *Toward a restraint free environment: Reducing the use of physical and chemical restraints in long-term and acute care settings.* Baltimore: Health Professions Press.

Breeze, J. (1909). *The care of the aged.* New York: McGraw-Hill.

Brimmer, P. (1979). The past, present and future in gerontological nursing research. *Journal of Gerontological Nursing, 5*(1), 27–34.

Brink, C., & Wells, T. (2003). Spotlight. Looking back, looking forward. 2002 Doris Schwartz Award Presentation. *Journal of Gerontological Nursing, 29*(2), 4–5.

Brower, H. T. (2005, January 9). Personal correspondence. Auburn, AL.

Brower, H. T. (1991a, May 7). Personal correspondence. Auburn, AL.

Brower, H. T. (1991b). Biographical data information.

Brower, H. T. (1991c). *Curriculum vitae.*

Brower, H. T. (1990, October 6). Videotaped interview. Washington, DC.

Brower, H. T. (1981). The social organization of nurses' attitudes toward older persons. *Journal of Gerontological Nursing, 7*(5), 293–298.

Brower, H. T., & Christ, M. A. (1982). A Delphi study of research priorities for long term care nursing. Supported by grants from the Beta Tau Chapter of

Sigma Theta Tau and Department of Health and Human Services (DHHS) Division of Nursing, Nurse Practitioner Section DHHA, BHM, HRA, 1 D24, NU 00157.

Brown, N. (2005, February 28). ELNEC press release regarding strengthening nursing care. American Association of Colleges of Nursing <www.aacm.nche.edu>

Buckwalter, K. C. (2005, February 20). Personal correspondence.

Buckwalter, K. C. (2003). *Curriculum vitae.*

Buckwalter, K. C. (2002, May 15). Personal correspondence.

Buckwalter, K. C. (2000). *Curriculum vitae.*

Buckwalter, K., Ebersole, P., Fulmer, T., McDowell, J., Whall, A., & Wykle, M. (1997). Nursing. In S. Klein (Ed.), *A national agenda for geriatric education.* New York: Springer Publishing.

Buckwalter, K. C., Gerdner, L. A., Hall, G. R., Kelly, A. Kohout, F., Richards, B., et al. (1999). Effects of family caregiver home training based on the progressively lowered stress threshold model. In S. H. Gueldner & L. W. Poon (Eds.), *Gerontological nursing issues for the 21st century.* Indianapolis, IN: Sigma Theta Tau International Publication Center Nursing Press.

Buckwalter, K. C., Smith, M., Zevenbergen, P., & Russell, D. (1991). Mental health services of the rural elderly outreach program. *The Gerontologist, 31*(3), 408–412.

Buckwalter, K. C. in Ebersole, P. R. (2001). Kathleen Coen Buckwalter, PhD, RN, FAAN. *Geriatric Nursing, 22*(2), 92–94.

Buckwalter, K. C., Smith, M., Zevenbergen, P., & Russell, D. (1991). Mental health services of the rural elderly outreach program. *The Gerontologist, 31*(3), 408–412

Bullough, V. L., & Sentz, L. (2002). Irene Mortenson Burnside. *American nursing: A biographical dictionary* (vol. 3). New York: Springer Publishing.

Bullough, V. L., & Sentz, L. (2002). Laurie Martin Gunter. *American nursing: A biographical dictionary* (vol. 3). New York: Springer Publishing.

Burggraf, V. (2005). The future of gerontological nursing. In M. Stanley, K. A. Blair, & P. G. Beare (Eds.), *Gerontological nursing: Promoting successful aging with older adults* (3rd ed.). Philadelphia: F. A. Davis.

Burggraf, V. (1997). Memories of Mary Opal Wolanin: Geriatric nurse, mentor, friend. *Geriatric Nursing, 18*(5), 234.

Burnside, I. M. (1988). *Nursing and the aged* (2nd ed.). New York: McGraw-Hill.

Burnside, I. M. (1985). Gerontological nursing research: 1975–1984. In *Overcoming the bias of ageism in long-term care.* New York: National League for Nursing, Pub # 20-1975.

Burnside, I. M. (Ed.). (1983). *Working with the elderly: Group process and techniques* (2nd ed.). North Scituate, MA: Duxbury Press.

Burnside, I. M. (1980). Why work with the aged? *Geriatric Nursing, 1*(1), 33.

Burnside, I. M. (Ed.). (1978). *Working with the elderly: Group process and techniques* (1st ed.). Boston, New York: McGraw-Hill.

Burnside, I. M. (Ed) (1976). *Nursing and the aged.* New York: McGraw-Hill.

Burnside, I. M. (1975). Listen to the aged. *American Journal of Nursing, 75*(1), 1801–1803.

Burnside, I. M. (1973). *Psychosocial nursing care of the aged.* New York: McGraw-Hill.

Burnside, I. M. (1971). Gerontion: A case study. *Perspectives in Psychiatric Care, 9*(3), 103–108.

Burnside, I. M. (1969). Group work among the aged. *Nursing Outlook, 17*(6), 68–72.

Burnside, I. M., & Schmidt, M. G. (Eds.). (1994). *Working with the elderly: Group process and techniques* (3rd ed.). Sudbury, MA: Jones and Bartlett Publishers.

Butler, R. (1975). *Why survive? Growing old in America.* New York: Harper & Row.

Butler, R., & Lewis, M. (1982). *Aging and mental health.* St. Louis: C. V. Mosby.

Capezuti, E., Talerico, K., Strumpf, N. E., & Evans, L. (1998). Individualized assessment and interventions in bilateral siderail use. *Geriatric Nursing, 19*(6), 322–330.

Carignan, A. M. (1992). Community college-nursing home partnership: Impact on nursing. *Geriatric Nursing, 13*(3), 139–141.

Carson, M. (1947). Improving standards in nursing homes. *Public Health Nursing, 39*(3), 312–314.

Chow, R. K. (2004a, December 16). *Synopsis of the history of Carville Leprosarium.* Personal correspondence.

Chow, R. K. (2004b). *Rita K. Chow: A tailor's daughter.* Unpublished manuscript prepared for Priscilla Ebersole.

Chow, R. K. (2002). Initiating a long-term care nursing service for aging inmates. *Geriatric Nursing, 23*(1), 24–27.

Chow, R. K. (1975). *Cardiosurgical nursing care: Understandings, concepts, and principles for practice.* New York: Springer Publishing.

Chow, R. K. (1972). Research + PRIMEX=improved health services. *International Nursing Review, 19*(4), 319–327.

Chow, R. K. (1969). Postoperative cardiac nursing research: A method for identifying and categorizing nursing action. *Nursing Research, 18*(1), 4–13.

Cohen, G. D. (2004). *Uniting the heart and mind: Human development in the second half of life. Special lecture by Gene Cohen.* Mind alert: A Joint program of the American Society on Aging and MetLife Foundation. San Francisco, CA: American Society on Aging.

Conway, J., & FitzGerald, M. (2004). Processes, outcomes and evaluation: Challenges to practice development in gerontological nursing. *Journal of Clinical Nursing, 13*(6B), 121–127.

Cora, V., & Lapierre, E. (1986). ANA speaks out (current research and ANA's statement on the scope of gerontological nursing practice). *Journal of Gerontological Nursing, 12*(6), 21–26.

Crane, C. (1907). Almshouse nursing: The human need. *American Journal of Nursing, 7,* 872–881.

Crowther, M., Maroulis, A., Shafer-Winter, N., & Hader, R. (2002, March 5). Clinical column. Evidence-based development of a hospital-based heart failure center. *Online Journal of Knowledge Synthesis.* Nursing clinical Column, Document N 5C.

Cumming, E., & Henry, W. E. (1961). *Growing old: The process of disengagement*. New York: Basic Books.

Davis, B. H. (2004). Personal communication.

Davis, B. H. (1991, February 1). Excerpts from taped interview. Los Angeles, California.

Davis, B. H. (1984). Nursing care of the aged—Historical evolution. Conference proceedings Historical Basis of Clinical Nursing Practice in the United States. Edited by S. Fondmiller, New Orleans, LA, 6/26/84. American Association for the History of Nursing, Chicago, Illinois, 42–53.

Davis, B. H. (1982). *History of nursing care of the aged: The last hundred years*. Research prospectus personal papers shared by author.

Davis, B. H. (1980). Nursing care of the aged: Past, present, future. *Imprint, 38*(65), 72–73.

Davis, B. H. (1971). Geriatric nursing through the looking glass. *Journal of the NYS Nurses' Association, 2*(3), 7–12.

Davis, B. H. (1968a). ANA and the geriatric nurse. *Nursing Clinics of North America, 3*(4), 741–748.

Davis, B. H. (1968b). Coming of age: A challenge for geriatric nursing. *Journal of the American Geriatrics Society, 16*(10), 1100–1106.

De Walt, E., & Welty, M. J. (2004, December 5). Personal communication.

Dimond, M., Infield, D., Kethley, A., & Pfeiffer, E. (1997). Long term care. In S. Klein (Ed.), *A national agenda for nursing education*. New York: Springer Publishing.

Dock, L. (1912). *A history of nursing* (vol. 3). New York: Putman.

Dock, L. (1908). The crusade for almshouse nursing. *American Journal of Nursing, 8*, 520–523.

Dock, L. (1906). Rural nursing. *American Journal of Nursing, 7*(4), 181–182.

Donahue, M. P. (1985). *Nursing: The finest art. An illustrated history*. St. Louis: C. V. Mosby.

Dowling-Castronova, A. (2000). Gerontological nursing—Advanced practice. In J. Fitzpatrick & M. Wallace (Eds.), *Geriatric nursing research digest*. New York: Springer Publishing.

Drill, H. (1999, August 28). Doris Schwartz, nurse and author. *Philadelphia Inquirer*.

Duke University School of Nursing. (2005, February 16). *Good news from the Duke school of nursing*. Brochure from the Office of Development and Alumni Affairs, Duke University Medical Center, Durham, NC.

Ebersole, P. R. (2004). *Recollections of Sr. Marilyn Schwab 1981–1984*. San Bruno, CA.

Ebersole, P. R. (2003a). Irene Mortenson Burnside: Her light shines on. *Geriatric Nursing, 24*(4), 232–233.

Ebersole, P. R. (2003b). The dynamic partnership of Lois K. Evans and Neville E. Strumpf. GN Leaders. *Geriatric Nursing, 24*(2), 110–112.

Ebersole, P. R. (2002a). Researchers who have made a difference: Beverly Baldwin, PhD, RN, FAAN, FGSA, and Barbara Resnick, PhD, CRNP, FAAN, FAANP. *Geriatric Nursing, 23*(2), 99–101.

Ebersole, P. R. (2002b). Rita K. Chow, EdD, RNC, HNC, FAAN: A life in the light. *Geriatric Nursing, 23*(1), 43–44.

Ebersole, P. R. (2001). Kathleen Coen Buckwalter, PhD, RN, FAAN. *Geriatric Nursing, 22*(2), 92–94.

Ebersole, P. R. (1999a). Ann Schmidt Luggen, PhD, RN, CS, CNNA, A force to reckon with. Leaders in Geriatric Nursing. *Geriatric Nursing, 20*(4), 217, 222.

Ebersole, P. R. (1999b). May L. Wykle, Phd, RN, FAAN. Leaders in Geriatric Nursing. *Geriatric Nursing, 20*(1), 50–51.

Ebersole, P. R. (1999c). The dynamic duo: Mathy Mezey, EdD, RN, FAAN, FGSA, and Terry Fulmer, RN, PhD, FAAN, FGSA. *Geriatric Nursing, 20*(2), 106–107.

Ebersole, P. R. (1998). Looking for a few good nurses. *Geriatric Nursing, 19*(1), 49.

Ebersole, P. R. (1998). Continence care pioneers: Thelma Wells, RN, PhD, FAAN, FRCN, and Joyce Colling, RN, PhD, FAAN. *Geriatric Nursing, (2)*, 103–105.

Ebersole, P. R. (1997a). Interview with Sister Rose Therese Bahr, pioneer in NGNA. *Geriatric Nursing, 18*(1), 29–32.

Ebersole, P. R. (1997b). Doris Schwartz: A Living Legend. *Geriatric Nursing, 18*(6), 277.

Ebersole, P. R. (1997c). Memories of Mary Opal Wolanin: Geriatric nurse, mentor, friend. *Geriatric Nursing, 18*(5), 232.

Ebersole, P. R. (1997d). Mary Starke Harper: Nurse/politician extraordinaire. *Geriatric Nursing, 18*(4), 175.

Ebersole, P. R., & Hess, P. A. (2001). *Geriatric nursing & healthy aging.* St Louis: C. V. Mosby.

Ebersole, P. R., & Hess, P. A. (1981, 1985, 1990, 1994, 1998). *Toward healthy aging: Human needs and nursing response* (5 editions). St Louis: C. V. Mosby.

Ebersole, P. R., & Hess, P. A. (1990). A personal view of gerontic nursing. Perspectives of gerontic nurse pioneers. In *Toward healthy aging; Human needs and nursing response* (3rd ed.). St Louis: C. V. Mosby.

Ebersole, P. R., Hess, P. A., & Luggen, A. S. (2005). *Toward healthy aging: Human needs and nursing response* (6th ed.). St Louis: C. V. Mosby.

Ebersole, P. R., Hess, P. A., Touhy, T. A., & Jett, K. (2005). *Geriatric Nursing & Healthy Aging* (2nd ed.). St Louis: C. V. Mosby.

Editorial. (1906). A neglected field in nursing: The county almshouse. *American Journal of Nursing, 6*, 493–494.

Evans, L. K. (2003a). The dynamic partnership of Lois K. Evans and Neville E. Strumpf. In P. R. Ebersole, GN Leaders. *Geriatric Nursing, 24*(2), 110–112.

Evans, L. K. (1987). Sundown syndrome in institutionalized elderly. *Journal of the American Geriatrics Society, 36*(2), 101–108.

Evans, L. K., & Strumpf, N. E. (1989). Tying down the elderly: A review of the literature on physical restraint. *Journal of the American Geriatrics Society, 37*(1), 65–74.

Evans, L. K., Strumpf, N. E., Allen-Taylor, L., Capezuti, E., Maislin, G., & Jacobsen, B. (1997). A clinical trail to reduce restraints in nursing homes. *Journal of the American Geriatrics Society, 45*(6), 675–681.

Ezekiel 3:15.

Federal Interagency Forum on Age Related Statistics. (2004, November). *Older Americans 2004: Key indicators of well being.* Federal Interagency Forum on Age Related Statistics. Washington, DC: US Government Printing Office.

Fishman, S. (2005, March 20). Personal correspondence.

Fishman, S. (2003). In Ebersole, P. R. (2003). Irene Mortenson Burnside: Her light shines on. *Geriatric Nursing, 24*(4), 232–233.

Fitzpatrick, J. J. (Ed.). (2002). Geriatric nursing research (vol. 20). *Annual review of nursing research.* New York: Springer Publishing.

Fitzpatrick, J. J., Fulmer, T., Wallace, M., & Flaherty, E. (Eds.). (2000). *Geriatric nursing research digest.* New York: Springer Publishing.

Forbes, N. (2005, April 4). *Promoting scholarship in nurse practitioner programs.* Student paper submitted to Sarah Fishman, faculty in master's program, Florida Atlantic University. Boca Raton, FL.

Foreman, M. D. (2005, March 29). Personal communication.

Foreman, M. D. (1984). Acute confusional states in the elderly: An algorithm. *Dimensions of Critical Care Nursing, 3,* 207–215.

Frances Payne Bolton School of Nursing. (2004, Summer/Fall). *FPB Nursing,* A Publication of Frances Payne Bolton School of Nursing. <http.//fpb.case.edu/>

Freda, M. C., & Kearney, M. (2005). An international survey of nurse editors' roles and practices. *Journal of Nursing Scholarship, 371,* 87–93.

Freeman, J. (1961). Nascher: Excerpts from his life, letters and works. *The Gerontologist, 1,* 17–26.

Fulmer, T. T. (2005, March, 5). Personal correspondence.

Fulmer, T. T. (1999). *Curriculum vitae, Terry T. Fulmer.* New York.

Fulmer, T. T., & Matzo, M. (1995). *Strengthening geriatric nursing education.* New York: Springer Publishing.

Futrell, M. H. (2005). Gerontological nurse practitioners: Implications for the future. *Journal of Gerontological Nursing, 31*(4), 19–24.

Futrell, M. H. (2004, February 4). Karen Devereaux Melillo biography prepared by May Futrell.

Futrell, M. H. (2002). Written comments to add to videotaped interview done previously. Lowell, MA.

Futrell, M. H. (1991). *Curriculum vitae, May Holmes DiPietro Futrell, PhD, RN, FAAN.* Lowell, MA.

Futrell, M. H. (1990, November 17). *Videotaped interview.* Boston, MA.

Futrell, M. H., & Alford, D. M. (1996). Health promotion: Its role in enhancing the health of the elderly. In E. A. Swanson & T. Tripp-Reimer (Eds.), *Advances in gerontological nursing, volume 1, issues for the 21st Century.* New York: Springer Publishing.

Futrell, M. H., Brovender, S., Mullett, E., & Brower, H. (1980). *Primary health care of the older adult.* North Scituate: Duxbury Press.

Futrell, M. H., & Jones, W. (1977). Attitudes of physicians, nurses and social workers toward the elderly and health maintenance services for the aged: Implications for health manpower policy. *Journal of Gerontological Nursing, 3*(3), 42–46.

Futrell, M. H., & Melillo, K. D. (2002). Evidence-based protocol: Wandering. *Journal of Gerontological Nursing, 28*(11), 14–22.

Gamroth, L. (1998). Marilyn Schwab: A vision shared. *Geriatric Nursing, 18*(3), 160–162.

Garand, L. J., & Buckwalter, K. C. (1996). The psychosocial care of older persons: The pioneering work of Dr. Irene Burnside. In E. A. Swanson & T. Tripp-Reimer (Eds.), *Advances in gerontological nursing: Issues for the 21st century* (vol. 1). New York: Springer Publishing.

Gelbach, S. (1945). Nursing care of the aged. *American Journal of Nursing, 43*(12), 113–114.

Generations (1999). Care at the end of life: Restoring a balance. *Generations, 23*(1).

Georgetown News. (1990, October 26). Conference at Georgetown University identifies gerontological nurse competencies. Washington, DC.

Gerdner, L. A., Hall, G. R., & Buckwalter, K. C. (1996). Caregiver training for people with Alzheimer's disease based on a stress threshold model. *Image: Journal of Nursing Scholarship, 28*(3), 241–246.

Gress, L. (1979). Governance and gerontological nursing in schools of nursing. *Journal of Gerontological Nursing, 8*(10), 576–580.

Griffin, G. J., & Griffin, H. J. (1965). *Jensen's history and trends in professional nursing.* St. Louis: C. V. Mosby.

Grypma, S. J. (2005). Critical issues in the use of biographic methods in nursing history. *Nursing History Review, 13,* 171–187.

Gubersky, B., & Burke, V. (1941). A modern home for the aged. *Public Health Nursing, 41.*

Gunter, L. M. (2005, January 3). Personal communication.

Gunter, L. M. (1990, September 10). Videotaped interview. Seattle, WA.

Gunter, L. M., & Estes, C. A. (1979). *Education for gerontic nursing.* New York: Springer Publishing.

Gunter, L. M., & Miller, J. (1977). Toward a nursing gerontology. *Nursing Research, 26,* 208–221.

Haight, B., & Gibson, F. (2005). *Working with older adults: Group process and techniques* (4th ed.). Sudbury, MA: Jones and Bartlett.

Hall, J. M. (2004). Dispelling desperation in nursing education. *Nursing Outlook, 52,* 147–154.

Hall, G. R., & Buckwalter, K. C. (1990). From almshouse to dedicated unit: Care of the institutionalized elderly with behavioral problems. *Archives of Psychiatric Nursing, 4*(1), 4.

Hall, G. R., & Buckwalter, K. C. (1987). Progressively lowered stress threshold: A conceptual model for care of adults with Alzheimer's disease. *Archives of Psychiatric Nursing, 1,* 399–406.

Hannefin, Sr. D. (1981, May 29). *The Daughters of Charity at Carville: 1896–1981.* Manuscript submitted to Vicentian Studies, St. Louis, MO.

Harper, M. S. (2005, March 15). Personal correspondence.

Harper, M. S. (1996). Condensed Resume for Mary S. Harper, PhD, DSc, LLD, RN, FAAN. Provided by Mary Harper in personal communication.

Harper, M. S. (1992). Videotaped interview. Washington, DC: Home at Geranium St. October 6, 1990.

Harper, M. S. (1991). *Management and care of the elderly: Psychosocial perspectives.* Newbury Park, CA: Sage.

Harper, M. S., & Liebowitz, B. (Eds.). (1986). *Mental illness in the nursing home: An agenda for research*. Washington, DC: The National Institute of Mental Health.

Harrington, C., Kovner, C., Mezey, M., Kayser-Jones, J., Mohler, M., Burke, R., et al. (2000). Experts recommend minimum staffing standards for nursing facilities in the United States. *The Gerontologist, 40*(1), 5–16.

John A. Hartford Foundation Institute for Geriatric Nursing & American Association of Colleges of Nursing. (2003). Awards for baccalaureate education in geriatric nursing. New York, New York. <www.nyu.edu/education/nursing/hartford.institute/>

John A. Hartford Foundation Institute for Geriatric Nursing. (2000, November 14). Hartford Institute/AACN award honors nursing schools for innovative gerontology education. *NYU News*. New York <www.nyu.edu/education/nursing/hartford.institute/>

John A. Hartford Foundation Institute for the Advancement of Geriatric Nursing Practice. (1997, February 5–7). Baltimore. Paper Prepared for the American Association of Colleges of Nursing Invitational Round Table.

John A. Hartford Foundation Institute for Geriatric Nursing. (undated). Baccalaureate nursing program: Partner for dissemination of best practices in care of older adults. New York <www.nyu.edu/education/nursing/hartford.institute/>

John A. Hartford Foundation Institute for Geriatric Nursing. (undated). Incorporating geriatric content into undergraduate education and staff development. *NYU News*. New York <www.nyu.edu/education/nursing/hartford.institute/>

HELP THE HOSPICES. (2005, March 18). Hospice and palliative care is a human right: Global summit in Korea demands governments do more to meet the needs of the dying. Press Release. Drafted by HELP THE HOSPICES, 34–44 Britannia St., London WC1X 9LG, UK. Registered charity no 1014851 <www.helpthe hospices.org.uk>

Houde, S. (2002). Methodological issues in male caregiver research: An integrative review of the literature. *Journal of Advanced Nursing, 40*(6), 1–14.

Houde, S. (2001). Age-related vision loss in the older adult: The role of the nurse practitioner in prevention and early detection. *Clinical Excellence for Nurse Practitioners, 5*(4), 185–195.

Houde, S. (1998). Predictors of elders' and family caregivers' use of formal home services. *Research in Nursing and Health, 21*, 533–543.

Houde, S. (1996). *Predictors of the utilization of formal home services by family caregiver/care recipient dyads*. Doctoral dissertation, Brandeis University. Dissertation Abstracts International.

Houde, S., & Huff, M. (2003). Age-related vision loss in the older adult: A challenge for the gerontological nurse. *Journal of Gerontological Nursing, 29*(4), 25–33.

Houde, S., & Melillo, K. D. (2000). Physical activity and exercise counseling in primary care. *The Nurse Practitioner: The Journal of Primary Health Care, 25*(8), 8–37.

Ianni, M. A. (2005, February 9). Personal communication.

Isaacs, B. (1977). Five years experience of a stroke unit. *Health Bulletin, 35,* 94–98. In J. E. Morley, (2004). A brief history of geriatrics. *Journal of Gerontology: Medical Sciences, 59A*(11), 1132–1152.

Jones, P., & Powell, J. (1999). Gary Anderson has been found. *Resource Recycling, 18*(5), 25.

Kalisch, P., & Kalisch, B. (1978). *The advance of American nursing.* Boston: Little Brown.

Kane, R., et al. (1980). *Geriatrics in the United States: Manpower projections and training.* Santa Monica, CA: Rand Corporation.

Kayser-Jones, J. S. (2004, July 12). Personal correspondence.

Kayser-Jones, J. S. (1977). Gerontological nursing research revisited. *Journal of Gerontological Nursing, 7,* 217–223.

Kayser-Jones, J. S. (1990). *Old, alone and neglected: Care of the aged in the United States and Scotland.* Paperback edition with new epilogue. Berkeley, CA: University of California Press.

Kayser-Jones, J. S. (1981). *Old, alone and neglected: Care of the aged in the United States and Scotland.* Berkeley, CA: University of California Press.

Kayser-Jones, J. S., Bird, W. F., Paul, S. M., Long, L., & Schell, E. S. (1995). An instrument to assess the oral health status of nursing home residents. *Gerontologist, 35*(6), 814–824.

Kayser-Jones, J. S., Chan, J., & Kris, A. (2005). A model long-term care hospice unit: Care, community, and compassion. *Geriatric Nursing, 26*(1), 16–20.

Kayser-Jones, J. S., & Minnigerode, F. A. (1975). Increasing nursing students' interest in working with aged patients. *Nursing Research, 24*(1), 23–26.

Kelley, L. S., Buckwalter, K. C., & Maas, M. (1999). Access to health care resources for family caregivers of elderly persons with dementia. *Nursing Outlook, 47*(1), 8–14.

Kelly, C. (1994, March 7). Personal communication.

Kelly, C. (1992, August 17). Personal communication.

Kelly, C. (1991, March 5). Personal communication.

Kelly, C. (1990, December 12). Personal communication.

Kelly, C. (1987). 70+ and going strong. Dorothy Moses: Gerontologist and professional volunteer. *Geriatric Nursing, 8*(5), 277–278.

Kelly, C. (1984). 70+ and going strong. Mary Opal Wolanin, a nurse for all reasons. *Geriatric Nursing, 5*(6), 339.

Kick, E. (2004, November 18). Personal correspondence.

Kick, E. (2003, May 31). Health care and the aging population: What are today's challenges. *Online Journal of Issues in Nursing, 8*(2). <www.nursing world.org/ojin/topic21/tpc21ntr.htm>

Kick, E. (1990a, October 8). Videotaped interview. Murfreesboro, TN, home.

Kick, E. (1990b). *Curriculum vitae.*

Kick, E. (1990c). Gerontic nursing: A personal experience. In P. R. Ebersole & P. A. Hess, (1990). A personal view of gerontic nursing. Perspectives of gerontic nurse pioneers. In *Toward healthy aging; Human needs and nursing response* (3rd ed.). St Louis: C. V. Mosby.

Klein, S. (Ed.). (1997). *A national agenda for geriatric education.* New York: Springer Publishing.

Knollmueller, R.N. (1998). In her own words: The story of Doris R Schwartz, RN, MS, FAAN, public health nurse. *Public Health Nursing, 15*(2), 67–73.

Kohuth, B. J. (1983). A national first: The endowment of a professorship in gerontological nursing makes history. *Journal of Gerontological Nursing, 9*(4), 237–241, 255.

Kovner, C., Mezey, M., & Harrington, C. (2000). Research priorities for staffing, case mix, and quality of care in U.S. Nursing Homes. *Journal of Nursing Scholarship, 32*(1), 77–80.

Lacey, D. (1999). The evolution of care: A 100 year history of institutionalization of people with Alzheimer's disease. *Journal of Gerontological Social Work, 31*(3/4), 101–131.

Lambertson, E. (1975). Preface. In T. Christy. The methodology of historical research: A brief introduction. *Nursing Research, 24,* vii.

Luggen, A. S. (2005, April 4). Personal communication.

Luggen, A. S. (1998a). Comfort and pain control. In M. A. Rosswurm (Ed.), *Health care for older adults: A guide for families and other caregivers.* New York: Springer Publishing.

Luggen, A. S. (1998b). Comfort and pain control module. In M. A. Rosswurm (Ed.), *Health care for older adults: Instructor's manual.* New York: Springer Publishing.

Luggen, A. S. (1998c). Healthy people 2000: Chronic pain in older adults, a quality of life issue. *Journal of Gerontological Nursing, 24*(2), 48–54.

Luggen, A. S. (Ed.). (1996). *National Gerontological Association: Core curriculum for gerontological nursing.* St. Louis: C. V. Mosby.

Luggen. A. S. (1994). The old girls' network: Mentorship in publishing (guest editorial). *Geriatric Nursing, 15*(6), 291.

Luggen, A. S., & Meiner, S. (2000). *Handbook for care of the older adult with cancer.* Pittsburg: Oncology Nursing Press.

Luggen, A. S., Travis, S., & Meiner, S. (Eds.). (1998). *NGNA Core curriculum for gerontological advanced practice nurses.* Thousand Oaks, CA: Sage.

Lund, M. (2004, May 5). *Autobiography.* Personal correspondence. Brookfield, WI.

Lund, M., & Wei, F. F. (1990). Speaking out on ethics. *Geriatric Nursing, 11*(5), 223–227.

Maas, M. L., & Buckwalter, K. C. (1996). Epilogue—Gazing through the crystal ball: Gerontological nursing issues and challenges for the 21st century. In E. A. Swanson & T. Tripp-Reimer (Eds.), *Advances in gerontological nursing: Issues for the 21st century* (vol. 1). New York: Springer Publishing.

Mack, M. (1952). Personal adjustment of chronically ill old people under home care. *Nursing Research,* 9–30.

Mahoney, D. F. (2003). Biography prepared for the University of Massachusetts, Lowell, Alumni Annual Award for Health Professions.

Malone, L. K., Fletcher, K. R., & Plank, L. M. (2004). *Management guidelines for nurse practitioners working with older adults* (2nd ed.). Philadelphia: F. A. Davis.

Mantle, J. H. (2005, March 2). Personal correspondence.

Mantle, J. H. (2005). Biographical notes.

Mantle, J. H., & Funke-Furber, J. (2003). *Forgotten revolution: The priory method. A restorative care model for older persons.* Victoria, BC: Trafford Press.

Marsh, E. (1941). The care of the chronically ill at the Cuyahoga County nursing home. *American Journal of Nursing, 7,* 161–166.

Mattson, J. E. (2005). Been there, done that. *Reflections on Nursing Leadership, 31*(1), 10–15.

Matzo, M. L. (2004). Personal communication and professional vitae.

Matzo, M. L., & Sherman, D. (Eds.). (2004). *Gerontological palliative care nursing.* St. Louis: C. V. Mosby.

Matzo, M. L., & Sherman, D. (Eds.). (2001). *Palliative care nursing education: Toward quality care at the end of life.* New York: Springer Publishing.

McAllister, M., DiMarco, M., Houde, S. C., & Miller, K. (2000). Module III: Preceptor guidelines. In M. A. S. Dumas (Ed.), *Partners in NP education: A preceptor manual for NP programs, faculty, preceptors and students* (pp. III-1–III-28). Washington, DC: National Organization of Nurse Practitioner Faculties.

McDougall, G. J. (2000). Graham McDougall, Jr., PhD, RN, CS: Academic, leader, and researcher. In P. Ebersole, Leaders in Geriatric Nursing. *Geriatric Nursing, 21*(5), 2000.

McDougall, G. J. (1993). Older adult's metamemory: Coping, depression, and self efficacy. *Applied Nursing Research, 6*(1), 28–30.

McDougall, G. J. (1990). A review of screening instruments for assessing cognition and mental status in older adults. *The Nurse Practitioner, 15*(11), 18–20, 22–24, 26–28.

McNeil, P. (1998). In Gamroth, L. Marilyn Schwab: A vision shared. *Geriatric Nursing, 18*(3), 160–162.

Meiner, S. E. (2005). Legal nurse consultant. *Geriatric Nursing, 26*(1), 34–36.

Melillo, K. D. (2004, February 4). *Biography of Karen Devereaux Melillo.*

Melillo, K. D., & Futrell, M. (1998). Wandering and technology devices: Helping caregivers ensure the safety of confused older adults. *Journal of Gerontological Nursing, 24*(8), 32–38.

Melillo, K. D., & Houde, S. (Eds.). (2005). *Geropsychiatric and mental health nursing.* Sudbury, MA: Jones and Bartlett Publishers.

Melillo, K. D., Williamson E., Houde, S., Futrell, M., Read, C.Y., & Campasano, M. (2001). Perceptions of older Latinos regarding physical fitness, physical activity, and exercise. *Journal of Gerontological Nursing, 27*(9), 38–46.

Melnyk, B., Fineout-Overholt, E., & Feinstein, N. F. (2004). *Worldviews on Evidence-Based Nursing, 1*(3), 185–193.

Mendelson, M. A. (1974). *Tender loving greed.* New York: Vintage Books.

Mengel, A., Simson, S., Sherman, S., & Waters, V. (1990). Essential factors in a community college-nursing home partnership. *Journal of Gerontological Nursing, 16*(11), 26–31.

Mezey, M. (2005, January 5). Personal communication.

Mezey, M. (2002). Excellence in advanced practice nursing: Kathleen Ryan Fletcher, RN, APRN, BC, GNP. Leaders in Geriatric Nursing. *Geriatric Nursing, 23*(3), 164–165.

Mezey, M., & Fulmer, T. (2003). In Ebersole, P. R. Irene Mortenson Burnside: Her light shines on. *Geriatric Nursing, 24*(4), 232–233.

Mezey, M., & Fulmer, T. (2002). The future history of gerontological nursing. *Journal of Gerontology: Medical Sciences, 57A*(7), M438–441.

Mezey, M., & Fulmer, T. (1999). Shaping the quality of health care for the elderly. *Nursing and Health Care Perspectives, 20*(3), 118–120.

Mezey, M., Harrington, C., & Kluger, M. (2005). Nursing expertise in caring for older adults. *American Journal of Nursing, 104*(9), 72.

Mezey, M., & Lynaugh, J. (1989). The teaching nursing home program. *Nursing Clinics of North America, 24*(3), 769–780.

Military Medicine: International Journal of AMSUS. (2004, November). Interview with Rear Admiral Faye Glenn Abdellah. *Military Medicine, 169*(11), ix.

Miller, M., Keller, D., Liebel, E., & Metrowitz, I. (1966). Nursing in a skilled nursing home. *American Journal of Nursing, 66*(9), 321–325.

Monea, H. E. (2003). In Ebersole, P. R. Irene Mortenson Burnside: Her light shines on. *Geriatric Nursing, 24*(4), 232–233.

Monea, H. E. (1981). *Peer counseling: Training elders to counsel their peers.* San Francisco, CA: Jewish Home for the Aged. Unpublished manuscript.

Monea, H. E. (1978). Experiential teaching/learning: Integrating psycho-social aspects of aging. Educational Curriculum and Instruction Course # 582K. San Francisco, CA: University of California, San Francisco, unpublished syllabus.

Monea, H. E. (1976). Instructor's manual to accompany I. M. Burnside. *Nursing and the aged.* New York: McGraw-Hill.

Morley, J. E. (2004). A brief history of geriatrics. *Journal of Gerontology: Medical Sciences, 59A*(11), 1132–1152.

Moses, D. V. (1990a). Gerontic nursing. A personal view of gerontic nursing. Perspectives of gerontic nurse pioneers. In P. R. Ebersole & P. A. Hess (Eds.), *Toward healthy aging; Human needs and nursing response* (3rd ed.). St Louis: C. V. Mosby.

Moses, D. V. (1990b, September 14). Videotaped interview. San Diego, Wesley Palms Retirement Center.

Moses, D. V. (1988). *Short vita form.* San Diego, CA.

Moses, D. V. (1979). The nurses role as advocate with the elderly. In A. Reinhardt & M. Quinn (Eds.), *Current practice in gerontological nursing.* St. Louis: C. V. Mosby.

Munson, H. (1930). The care of the sick in almshouses. *American Journal of Nursing, 30*(10), 1226–30.

National Invitational Consensus Conference. (1991). Georgetown University Press.

Nascher, I. (1914). *Geriatrics.* Philadelphia: P. Blakiston's Son & Co.

Nascher, I. (1909). Geriatrics. *New York Medical Journal, 90,* 358–359.

Naylor, M. (2005, April 25). Personal correspondence.

Neugarten, B. L. (Ed.). (1968). *Middle age and aging*. Chicago: University of Chicago Press.

Newton, K., & Anderson, H. (1966). *Geriatric nursing*. St. Louis: C. V. Mosby.

Norman, E. M. (1999). *We band of angels: The untold story of American nurses trapped on Bataan by the Japanese*. New York: Random House.

Norton, D. (1991, April 15). Personal correspondence.

Norton, D. (1990). *The age of old age: The story of care provision for the elderly over the centuries*. London: Scutari Press.

Norton, D. (1965). Nursing in geriatrics. *Gerontological Clinics, 7*, 51–60.

Norton, D. (1956, July 6). The place of geriatric nursing in training. *Nursing Times*.

Penn State News. (1987). University Park, PA: Department of Public Information.

Phillips, L. R. (1997). Memories of Mary Opal Wolanin: Geriatric nurse, mentor, friend. *Geriatric Nursing, 18*(5), 233.

Quinn, M. J. (2005, February 20). Personal correspondence.

Quinn, M. J. (2005). Guardianships of adults: Achieving justice, autonomy, and safety. *Springer series on ethics, law and aging*. New York: Springer Publishing.

Quinn, M. J. (1986, 1997). *Elder abuse and neglect: Causes, diagnoses, and intervention strategies*. New York: Springer Publishing.

Rader, J. (2005, March 20). Personal correspondence.

Rader, J. (1998). In Gamroth, L. Marilyn Schwab: A vision shared. *Geriatric Nursing, 18*(3), 160–162.

Reiter, F. (1964, April 5). Choosing the better part. *American Journal of Nursing, 64*, 65–68.

Remsburg, R. E. (2005, April 5). Personal correspondence.

Remsburg, R. E., & Crogan, N. L. (2005). NGNA news. *Geriatric Nursing, 26*(2), 88–90.

Resnick, B. (2005, January 3). Personal correspondence.

Resnick, B. in Ebersole, P. R. (2002b). Researchers who have made a difference: Beverly Baldwin, PhD, RN, FAAN, FGSA, and Barbara Resnick, PhD, CRNP, FAAN, FAANP. *Geriatric Nursing, 23*(2), 99–101.

Resnick, S. (1977). Gestalt therapy, the hot seat of personal responsibility. In B. A. Backer, P. M. Dubbert, & E. J. P. Eisenman (Eds.), *Psychiatric mental health nursing: Contemporary readings* (pp. 463–474). New York: D. Van Nostrand.

Robinson, L. (1981). Gerontological nursing research. In I. Burnside (Ed.), *Nursing and the aged*. New York: McGraw-Hill.

Robinson, T. M., & Perry, P. M. (2001). *Cadet nurse stories: The call for and response of women during World War II*. Indianapolis, IN: Sigma Theta Tau International Honor Society of Nursing.

Robinson, V. (1996). The origin of nursing. In M. P. Donahue (Ed.), *Nursing the Finest Art* (2nd ed.). St Louis: C. V. Mosby.

Rondorf-Klym, L. M., & Colling, J. (2003). Quality of life after radical prostatectomy. *Oncology Nursing Forum, 30*(2), E24–32.

Ross, Sr. H. R. (date unknown). *Leprosarium, Carville, Louisiana. 1894–1958*. Material compiled by Sister Hilary Ross on the Louisiana Leper Home 1894–1921, U.S. Public Health Service. (National Leprosarium 1921–1958).

Rosseter, R. (February 28, 2005). ELNEC press release regarding strengthening nursing care. <www.aacn.nche.edu>

Rosseter, R. (2005, February 20). AACN Funds Scholarships. <www.aacn.nche.edu>

Safier, G. (1977). *Contemporary American leaders in nursing: An oral history.* New York: McGraw-Hill.

San Francisco VA Medical Center Nursing Research Committee. (2005, May 20). *The 10th Annual Nursing Research Day: Improving Practice Through Research.* San Francisco VA Medical Center, Unpublished document.

Santo-Novak, D. A., Grissom, K. R., & Powers, R. E. (2004). Mary Starke Harper (Spotlight). *Journal of Gerontological Nursing, 27*(2), 12–14.

Savage, H. (1992). *Notes for Dorothy V. Moses obituary.* San Diego, CA.

Saxon, W. (1999, August 28). Doris R. Schwartz, 84, a nurse who advanced geriatric care. New York: *New York Times.*

Schell, E. (1993). The origins of geriatric nursing. *Nursing History Review, I,* 203–216.

Schorr, T. M. (2005). Meet our members. *The Newsletter of Nurses Educational Funds, Inc., 24*(1), 4.

Schwab, Sr. M. (1986). *A gift freely given: The personal journal of Sister Marilyn Schwab, OSB.* Benedictine Sisters, Mt. Angel, OR.

Schwab, M. (1973). Caring for the aged. *American Journal of Nursing, 731,* 2049.

Schwartz, D. (1996, March 18). *Dear fellow residents of Foulkeways.* Letter to Foulkeways Residents.

Schwartz, D. (1995). *Give us to go blithley: My fifty years in nursing.* New York: Springer Publishing.

Schwartz, D. (1990a, November 15). *Taped interview.* Foulkeways Quaker Retirement Center, Gwynedd, PA.

Schwartz, D. (1990b). Personal reflections. In P. R. Ebersole & P. A. Hess (Eds.), Perspectives of gerontic nurse pioneers. In *Toward healthy aging; Human needs and nursing response* (3rd ed.). St Louis: C. V. Mosby.

Schwartz, D. (1982). *The elderly ambulatory patient: Nursing and psychosocial needs.* New York: Arco.

Schwartz, D. (1969). Aging and the field of nursing. In M. Riley et al. (Eds.), *Aging and society, volume 2, aging and the professions.* New York: Russell Sage Foundation.

Schwartz, D. (1960). Nursing needs of the chronically ill ambulatory patients. *Nursing Research, 9*(4), 185–187.

Shields, A. B. (1990, October 21). Videotaped interview. Vermillion, OH.

Shields-Kyle, E. (2005, March 23). Personal correspondence.

Shields-Kyle, E. (1990, October 21). Videotaped interview. Vermillion, OH.

Smith, J. (1998). In L. Gamroth (1998). Marilyn Schwab: A vision shared. *Geriatric Nursing, 18*(3), 160–162.

Smith, M., Gerdner, L. K., Hall, G. R., & Buckwalter, K. C. (2004). History, development and future of the progressively lowered stress threshold: A conceptual model for dementia care. *Journal of the American Geriatrics Society, 52*(10), 1755–1760.

Smolensky, M. C. (2005). Playing the credentials game. Nursing Spectrum, on line. (Masthead date July 1, 2002).

Springate, J. (2005, March 14). Personal correspondence.

Springate, J. M. (2004). *Curriculum vitae.*

Springer, U. (2005, March 5). Personal correspondence.

Springer, U. (2005, February 24). Personal correspondence.

Steffl, B. (2005, January 30). Personal communication.

Steffl, B. (2004, December 10). Personal correspondence.

Steffl, B. (2003). In Ebersole, P. R. Irene Mortenson Burnside: Her light shines on. *Geriatric Nursing, 24*(4), 232–233.

Steffl, B. (1997). Memories of Mary Opal Wolanin: Geriatric nurse, mentor, friend. *Geriatric Nursing, 18*(5), 233–234.

Steffl, B. (1992, October 22). Taped interview. Phoenix, AZ.

Stilwell, E. (2005, February 20). Personal correspondence.

Stone, V. (1992). Videotaped interview. Durham, NC, November 15, 1990.

Stone, V. (1990). Personal reflections. In P. R. Ebersole & P. A. Hess (Eds.), Perspectives of gerontic nurse pioneers. In *Toward healthy aging: Human needs and nursing response* (3rd ed.). St Louis: C. V. Mosby.

Stone, V. (1986). *Curriculum vitae.*

Stone, V. (1969). Nursing of older people. In E. Busse & E. Pfeiffer (Eds.), *Behavior and adaptation in late life.* Boston: Little Brown and Co.

Stotts, N., & Deitrich, C. (2004). The challenge to come: The care of older adults. *American Journal of Nursing, 104*(8), 40–47.

Strumpf, N. E. (2005, March 20). Personal communication.

Strumpf, N. E. (2003a). *Curriculum Vitae, Neville E. Strumpf, PhD, RN, C, FAAN.*

Strumpf N. E. (2003b). The dynamic partnership of Lois K. Evans and Neville E. Strumpf. In P. R. Ebersole, GN Leaders. *Geriatric Nursing, 24*(2), 110–112.

Strumpf, N. E. (1994). Innovative gerontological practices as models for health care delivery.

Strumpf, N. E. (1982). The relationship of life satisfaction and self-concept to time experience in older women. *Dissertations Abstracts International, 43*(12), 3924–B, 1983. Order #AAC 830 7700.

Strumpf, N. E., & Evans, L. K. (1988). Physical restraint of the hospitalized elderly: Perceptions of patients and nurses. *Nursing Research, 37,* 132–137.

Strumpf, N. E., Evans, L. K., Wagner, J., & Patterson, J. (1992). Reducing physical restraints: Developing an educational program. *Journal of Gerontological Nursing, 18*(11), 21–27.

Sullivan-Marx, E., Strumpf, N., Evans, L., Capezuti, E., & Maislin, G. (2003). The effect of an advanced practice nurse (APN) intervention with hospitalized nursing home residents. *Gerontologist, 43*(1), 358–360.

Tanti, A. (2003). Ode to Books, unpublished poem, school assignment, Capuchino High School Millbrae, California.

Touhy, T. (2003). In P. R. Ebersole, Irene Mortenson Burnside: Her light shines on. *Geriatric Nursing, 24*(4), 232–233.

Travis, S. S. (2005, April 25). Personal correspondence.

Udod, S. A., & Care, W. D. (2004). Setting the climate for evidence-based nursing practice: What is the leader's role? *Canadian Journal of Nursing Leadership, 17*(4), 64–75.

U.S. Department of Defense, Uniformed Services University of the Health Sciences. (2003, December). *Biography: Faye G. Abdellah, RN, EdD, ScD, FAAN, founding Dean, Graduate School of Nursing, Professor Emeritas.* Bethesda, MD.

U.S. Department of Health, Education and Welfare, Public Health Service. Office of Nursing Home Affairs. (1975, July). *Long-term care facility improvement study: Interim report.*

U.S. Department of Health, Education and Welfare. (1971). *Extending the scope of nursing practice: A report of the Secretary's Committee to study extended roles for nurses.* Washington, DC: U.S. Government Printing Office.

U.S. Department Department of Health and Human Services, Agency for Healthcare Research and Quality. (2005, February 22). *AHRQ Press release: Second national reports on quality and disparities find improvements in health care quality, although disparities remain.* <KMigdail@AHRQ.GOV>

U.S. Department Department of Health and Human Services. (1999). *Mental health: A report of the Surgeon General.* Rockville, MD: U.S. Government Printing Office.

U.S. Federal Security Agency. (1950). The U.S. cadet nurse corps 1943–1948. *PHS Publication No. 38*, p. 97. Washington, DC: U.S. Government Printing Office.

Verwoerdt, A. (1981). *Glinical geropsychiatry* (2nd ed.). Baltimore: William & Wilkens.

Vladeck, B. (1980). *Unloving care: The nursing home tragedy.* New York: Basic Books.

Warden-Saunders, G. (2005, March 14). Eliopoulos Joins NADONA/LTC Organization. Email announcement <gary@NADONA.org>.

Warden-Saunders, J. (2001). In P. R. Ebersole, GN Leaders: Joan Warden-Saunders. *Geriatric Nursing, 22*(3), 156–157.

Wells, T. J. (1994). Nursing research on urinary incontinence. *Urologic Nursing, 14*, 109–112.

Wells, T. J. (1990, November 17). Videotaped interview. Boston.

Wells, T. J. (1979). Nursing committed to the elderly. In A. Reinhardt & M. Quinn (Eds.), *Current practice in gerontological nursing.* St. Louis: C. V. Mosby.

Wendt. A. (2003). Mapping gerontological nursing competencies to the 2001 NCLEX-RN test plan. *Nursing Outlook, 51*(4), 152–157.

Whall, A. L. (2005). "Lest we forget": An issue concerning the doctorate in nursing practice (DNP). *Nursing Outlook, 53*(1), 1.

Whall, A. L. (2004). Looking past and looking forward to the preferred gerontological nursing future. *Journal of Gerontological Nursing, 30*(4), 4–6.

Whall, A. (1996). Gerontological nursing in the 21st century: Is there a future? In E. Swanson & T. Reimer (Eds.), *Advances in gerontological nursing* (vol. 2). New York: Springer Publishing.

Williams, C. L., Hyer, K., Kelly, A., Leger-Krall, S., & Tappen, R. (2005). Development of nurse competencies to improve dementia care. *Geriatric Nursing, 26*(2), 1001–1007.

Wilson, R. (1994). Tribute to Virginia Stone (In Memorium). *Geriatric Nursing,* *15*(4),180–181.

Wolanin, M. O. (1990, August 22). Videotaped interview. San Antonio, TX, Air Force Village II.

Wolanin, M. O. (1989). Mary Opal Wolanin biography. Personal communication.

Wolanin, M.O. (1987, June 20). Interview. Airforce Village II, San Antonio, TX.

Wolanin, M.O. (1983). Clinical geriatric research. In H. Werley & J. Fitzpatrick (Eds.), *Annual review of nursing research.* New York: Springer Publishing.

Wolanin, M. O., & Phillips, L. R. (1981). *Confusion: Prevention and care.* St Louis: C. V. Mosby.

Wunderlich E. et al. (1996). *Nursing staff in hospitals and nursing homes.* Washington, DC: National Academy Press.

Wykle, M. L. (2004, summer/fall). Dean's message. *FPB Nursing: A publication of the Frances Payne Bolton School of Nursing.*

Wykle, M. L. (2003). Inside the society. Honor society of nursing, Sigma Theta Tau International. From the president. *Reflections on Nursing Leadership,* *35*(4), 45.

Wykle, M. L. (1999). May L. Wykle, Phd, RN, FAAN. In P. R. Ebersole, Leaders in Geriatric Nursing. *Geriatric Nursing, 20*(1), 50–51.

Wykle, M. L., & McDonald, P. (1997). The past, present and future of gerontological nursing. In Dimond et al. (Eds.), *A National agenda for geriatric education.* New York: Springer Publishing.

Zahorsky, A. C. (1989). *My twenty years in the air force.* Unpublished document.

Index

SPRINGER PUBLISHING COMPANY

End-of-Life Stories
Crossing Disciplinary Boundaries
Donald E. Gelfand, PhD, Richard Raspa, PhD
Sherylyn H. Briller, PhD
Stephanie Myers Schim, PhD, RN, APRN, CNAA, BC, Editors

This book provides a variety of narratives about end-of-life experiences contributed by members of the Wayne State University End-of-Life Interdisciplinary Project. Each of the narratives is then analyzed from three different disciplinary perspectives. These analyses broaden how specific end-of-life narratives can be viewed from different dimensions and help students, researchers, and practitioners see the important and varied meanings that end-of-life experiences have at the level of the individual, the family, and the community. In addition, the narratives include end-of-life experiences of individuals from a variety of ethnic and racial backgrounds.

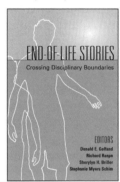

Partial Contents:

2005   218pp   0-8261-2675-8   hardcover

11 West 42nd Street, New York, NY 10036-8002 • Fax: 212-941-7842
Order Toll-Free: 877-687-7476 • Order On-line: www.springerpub.com

SPRINGER PUBLISHING COMPANY

Improving Hospital Care for Persons with Dementia

Nina M. Silverstein, PhD
Katie Maslow, MSW, Editors
With Foreword by Eric Tangalos, MD

"Hospital care of older adults with dementia has received surprisingly little attention among health care professionals. This text represents a new frontier in geriatric care and is an invaluable resource in helping to assure exemplary care for older adults in hospitals nationwide."

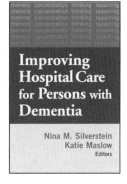

—**Mathy Mezey,** EdD, RN, FAAN, Independence Foundation Professor of Nursing Education Director, The John A. Hartford Foundation Institute for Geriatric Nursing New York University College of Nursing

Broken up into four parts, the book covers the background and issues surrounding hospital care for patients with dementia. In part two, four unique perspectives are shared, including professionals, the assisted living manager, geriatric social worker, emergency department doctor, and that of the person with dementia who lives alone in the community. Part four highlights strategies for different stakeholders in the quest to provide good care for dementia patients in the hospital setting.

Partial Contents:

How Many People with Dementia are Hospitalized? • In Search of Dementia-Friendly Hospitals • Acute Care for Nursing Home Residents with Alzheimer's Disease • Four Perspectives on the Hospital Experience for Persons with Dementia • The In-Patient Experience from the Perspective of the Isolated Adult with Alzheimer's Disease • Promising Approaches Toward Improving Care for Hospitalized Elders with Dementia • Changing Dementia Care in a Hospital System • A NICHE Delirium Prevention Project for Hospitalized Elders • Strategies for Making a Difference • Try This: Best Practices in Nursing Care for Hospitalized Older Adults with Dementia

2005 · 320pp · 0-8261-3915-9 · soft

11 West 42nd Street, New York, NY 10036-8002 • Fax: 212-941-7842
Order Toll-Free: 877-687-7476 • Order On-line: www.springerpub.com

Palliative Care Nursing

2nd Edition
Quality Care to the End of Life

Marianne LaPorte Matzo, PhD, RN, GNP, CS
Deborah Witt Sherman, PhD, RN, ANP, CS
Editors

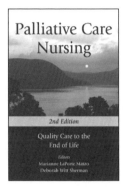

"Palliative Care Nursing is a comprehensive, well-written text that is as appropriate for practicing nurses as it is for undergraduate and graduate nursing students...The editors have paid particular attention to aspects of caring for the dying that have been neglected in nursing education: holistic integrative therapies, communication, caring for families, and peri-death nursing care."
—**Oncology Nursing Forum**

About the new edition:
"These authors and the pages of this text...create the blueprint that will build the kind of care system we all wish for our loved ones."
—From the Foreword by **Betty Rolling Ferrell,** RN, PhD, FAAN

Partial Contents:

Section I: Looking at the Whole Person in Palliative Care • Spirituality and Culture as Domains of Quality Palliative Care • Holistic Integrative Therapies in Palliative Care

Section II: Palliative Care, Society, and the Health Profession • Death and Society • Professional Organizations and Certification in Hospice and Palliative Care Nursing • The Nurse's Role as a Member of the Interdisciplinary Palliative Care Team • Ethical Aspects of Palliative Care • Legal Aspects of End-of-Life Care

Section III: Psychological Aspects of Death and Dying • Communication with Seriously Ill and Dying Patients, Their Families, and Their Health Care Providers

Section IV: Physical Aspects of Dying • Symptom Management in Palliative Care • Pain Assessment and Pharmacologic Interventions

2005   400pp   0-8261-5794-7   hard

11 West 42nd Street, New York, NY 10036-8002 • **Fax: 212-941-7842**
Order Toll-Free: 877-687-7476 • **Order On-line: www.springerpub.com**

SPRINGER / PUBLISHING COMPANY

Safe Patient Handling and Movement

A Practical Guide for Health Care Professionals

Audrey Nelson, PhD, RN, FAAN, Editor

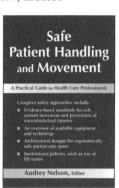

This resource guide presents best practices in safe patient handling and movement, and includes the following approaches to caregiver safety:

- Evidence-based standards for safe patient movement and preventing musculoskeletal injuries
- An overview of available equipment and technology for safe patient handling
- Specific architectural designs for ergonomically safe patient care space
- Institutional policies (such as the use of lift teams) that can be easily implemented in your hospital or health care institution

Partial Contents:

Part I: Introduction

- Scope of the Problem, *J.W. Collins* and *N.N. Menzel* • Myths and Facts about Back Injuries in Nursing, *A.L. Nelson* • Variations in High-Risk Patient Handling Tasks by Practice Setting, *A.L. Nelson*

Part II: Best Practices

- Evidence-Based Standards for Patient Assessment, Care Planning, and Caregiving Practices in Safe Patient Handling and Movement, *A.L. Nelson* • After Action Reviews, *M. Matz* • Unit-Based Peer Safety Leaders to Promote Safe Patient Handling, *M. Matz* • No Lift Policies, *J.W. Collins*

Part III: Special Challenges in Patient Handling

- Preventing Injuries When Taking Care of Special Needs Patients, *H.P. de Ruiter* and *M.A.B. de Ruiter* • Ergonomic Workplace Assessments of Patient Handling Environments, *G. Fragala* and *A.L. Nelson*

Part IV: Future Directions

- Being a Change Agent and Advocate for Safe Patient Handling, *L.G. Doloresco*

December 2005 · 272pp · 0-8261-6363-7 · soft

11 West 42nd Street, New York, NY 10036-8002 • Fax: 212-941-7842
Order Toll-Free: 877-687-7476 • Order On-line: www.springerpub.com

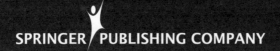
Prostate Cancer

Nursing Assessment, Management, and Care

Meredith Wallace, PhD, RN, CS-ANP
Lorrie L. Powel, PhD, RN, Editors

"The information contained in this text is of vital importance as more men face screening, assessment, diagnosis, and treatment of prostate cancer."

—from the Foreword by
Mary H. Palmer, PhD, RNC, FAAN

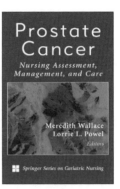

Readers will gain a thorough understanding of symptoms, diagnostic methods, treatment options, and psychosocial effects of this disease. A major focus of the book is on quality of life and the nurses' role in improving this through teaching patients and their families how to manage common symptoms and side effects. Competent nursing care will allow the large numbers of men diagnosed and living with the disease to live the highest possible quality of life.

Partial Contents:

* Prostate Cancer: The Nature of the Problem
* Prostate Cancer: Risk Factors and Prevention
* Assessment, Screening and Diagnosis of Prostate Cancer
* Treatment Choices and the Decision-Making Process
* Quality of Life with Prostate Cancer
* Nursing Care for Radical Prostatectomy
* Nursing Care for Radiation Treatment
* Hormone Therapy
* Watchful Waiting—Managing of Prostate Cancer as a Chronic Disease
* Prevalent Issues in Patient Education
* End of Life Care

Geriatric Nursing Series
2002   232pp   0-8261-8745-5   hard